YOGA

The Indian tradition of yoga, first codified in the *Yoga Sūtra* of Patañjali in the third or fourth century CE, constitutes one of the world's earliest and most influential traditions of spiritual practice. It is a tradition that, by the time of Patañjali, already had an extensive (if obscure) prehistory and one that was to have, after Patañjali, an extraordinarily rich and diverse future. As a tradition, yoga has been far from monolithic. It has embraced a variety of practices and orientations, borrowing from and influencing a vast array of Indic religious traditions down through the centuries.

Recent years have witnessed an increased production in scholarly works on the yoga tradition, which have helped to chart this complex and multifaceted evolution and to demonstrate the important role that it has played in the development of India's religious and philosophical traditions. And yet the popular perception of yoga in the West remains for the most part that of a physical fitness program, largely divorced from its historical and spiritual roots.

The essays collected here provide a sense of the historical emergence of the classical system presented by Patañjali, a careful examination of the key elements, overall character and contemporary relevance of that system, as found in the *Yoga Sūtra*, and a glimpse of some of the tradition's many important ramifications in later Indian religious history.

Ian Whicher is an Associate Professor in the Department of Religion at the University of Manitoba, Canada. His areas of specialization are Hinduism, the Philosophies of India, and yoga theory and practice. He is the author of *The Integrity of the Yoga Darśana: A Reconsideration of Classical Yoga* (1998). His current research interests include an exploration of Indic notions of spiritual liberation and their ethical implications, and the relationship between yoga and Buddhism.

Since completing graduate studies in Theology and the History of Religions at the University of Chicago, **David Carpenter** has taught at St Joseph's University in Philadelphia, where he is currently Associate Professor of the History of Religions. He is the author of *Revelation, History, and the Dialogue of Religions: A Study of Bhartṛhari and Bonaventure* (1995). His research interests include the history of ancient and medieval Indian religions and the comparative study of spiritual practice.

YOGA

The Indian tradition

Edited by Ian Whicher and David Carpenter

Routledge
Taylor & Francis Group
LONDON AND NEW YORK

First published 2003
by Routledge
2 Park Square, Milton Park, Abingdon, Oxon, OX14 4RN

Simultaneously published in the USA and Canada
by Routledge
270 Madison Ave, New York NY 10016

Routledge is an imprint of the Taylor & Francis Group

Transferred to Digital Printing 2010

Typeset in Sabon by
Florence Production Ltd, Stoodleigh, Devon

British Library Cataloguing in Publication Data
A catalogue record for this book is available
from the British Library

Library of Congress Cataloging-in-Publication Data
Yoga: the Indian tradition edited by
Ian Whicher and David Carpenter.
p. cm.
Includes bibliographical references and index.
1. Yoga. 2. Spiritual life – Hinduism. I. Whicher, Ian.
II. Carpenter, David, 1949–
BL1238.52.Y59 2003
181′.45–dc21
2002036708

ISBN10: 0–7007–1288–7 (hbk)
ISBN10: 0–415–60020–0 (pbk)

ISBN13: 978–0–7007–1288–5 (hbk)
ISBN13: 978–0–415–60020–0 (pbk)

CONTENTS

CONTRIBUTORS

John Brockington is Professor of Sanskrit at the University of Edinburgh. Besides numerous articles for various journals (some collected in *Epic Threads*, OUP, Delhi, 2000), he has already published *The Sacred Thread* (1981), *Righteous Rama* (1984), *Hinduism and Christianity* (1992) and *The Sanskrit Epics* (1998). He is also Secretary General of the International Association of Sanskrit Studies.

David Carpenter is Associate Professor of the History of Religions at St Joseph's University in Philadelphia. He is the author of *Revelation, History, and the Dialogue of Religions: A Study of Bhartṛhari and Bonaventure* (1995).

Christopher Key Chapple is Professor of Theological Studies and Director of Asian and Pacific Studies at Loyola Marymount University in Los Angeles. He has published ten books, including *Karma and Creativity* (1986), a co-translation of the *Yoga Sūtra of Patañjali* (1990), *Nonviolence to Animals, Earth, and Self in Asian Traditions* (1993), *Hinduism and Ecology* (2000) and *Reconciling Yogas* (2003). In 2002, he helped establish the yoga Philosophy Program to help yoga teachers and practitioners deepen their understanding of yoga.

Glen Alexander Hayes is Professor of Religion at Bloomfield College in Bloomfield, NJ, USA. Author of numerous essays on the Vaisnava Sahajiya traditions of Bengal, he has also published translations of Bengali Tantric yogic texts in *Religions of India in Practice* (1995) and *Tantra in Practice* (2000). Contributor to *The HarperCollins Dictionary of Religion* (1995) and *The Encyclopedia of Women and World Religions* (1999), he is currently coediting and writing a chapter for *In the Flesh: Eros, Secrecy and Power in the Tantric Traditions of India* (with Hugh B. Urban, forthcoming). In addition to his specialization in medieval Bengali yoga and Tantra, his research interests include contemporary metaphor theory and cognitive linguistics.

Lloyd W. Pflueger is Associate Professor of Philosophy and Religion at Truman State University. He specializes in South Asian Religion, Classical Yoga Philosophy, Indian Philosophy and Classical Sanskrit. He has twenty-seven articles on Hindu and Buddhist topics in the *Oxford Dictionary of World Religions* (1997). He also has an essay, "Discriminating the Innate Capacity: Salvation Mysticism in Classical Sāṃkhya-Yoga" in *The Innate Capacity* (1998) also from Oxford. Dr Pfleger is currently finishing *God and Yoga in Ancient India* for SUNY Press and is working on a manuscript on the *Thousand Names of Vishnu.*

Olle Qvarnström is Associate Professor of the History of Religions at Lund University, Sweden. Recent publications include "Haribhadra and the Beginnings of Doxography in India" in *Approaches to Jaina Studies: Philosophy, Logic, Rituals and Symbols*, N. K. Wagle and O. Qvarnström (eds) (2000); *The Yogaśāstra of Hemacandra: A Twelfth Century Handbook on Jainism* (2002); "Early Vedānta Philosophy Preserved by the Jain Tradition" in *Jainism and Early Buddhism: Essays in Honour of Padmanabh S. Jaini* (2002).

Vidyasankar Sundaresan is currently a research associate in molecular biology at the Scripps Research Institute. He has a wide interest in Indological subjects, particularly in Advaita Vedānta, yoga and the history of Indian monastic traditions. His publications in this area include a study of the prose chapters of Upadeśasāhasrī (*The Adyar Library Bulletin*, 1998), a review of the authorship problem with respect to texts attributed to Śaṅkara (*Philosophy East and West*, 2002) and a comparative study of the major Śaṅkara hagiographies (*International Journal of Hindu Studies*).

Ian Whicher is currently a Professor in the Department of Religion at the University of Manitoba, Canada. His area of specialization is in Hinduism, the Philosophies of India and yoga theory and practice. He is the author of *The Integrity of the Yoga Darśana* (1998, State University of New York Press).

David Gordon White is Professor of Religious Studies at the University of California, Santa Barbara. He is the author of *Myths of the Dog-Man* (1991); *The Alchemical Body: Siddha Traditions in Medieval India* (1996) and *Kiss of the Yoginī: "Tantric Sex" in its South Asian Contexts* (February 2003). He is also the editor of *Tantra in Practice* (2000).

ACKNOWLEDGMENTS

The essays collected together in this volume grew out of a number of conferences over the past several years, and the editors would like to acknowledge the contributions of all those involved. These conferences included an international seminar on the yoga tradition at Loyola Marymount University, Los Angeles, in March 1997, an international workshop on the yoga tradition at the Dharam Hinduja Institute of Indic Research, Faculty of Divinity, University of Cambridge, in October 1998, and an international seminar on the yoga tradition: Inter-Religious Perspectives at the University of California, Los Angeles, in October 2000. Finally, the four essays on Patañjali were originally written for a panel entitled "Revisioning Patañjali's Dualism," given at the annual meeting of the American Academy of Religion in November 2000. Their authors are indebted to T. S. Rukmani, who responded on that occasion.

The editors wish to thank Robert O'Kell, Dean of Arts at the University of Manitoba, and Brice Wachterhauser, Dean of Arts and Sciences at St Joseph's University, for their support in assisting with the costs of production of the index.

ABBREVIATIONS

ĀDS	*Āpastamba Dharma Sūtra*
AP	*Agni Purāṇa*
BDS	*Baudhyāna Dharma Sūtra*
BGBh	*Bhagavadgītā Bhāṣya* of Śaṅkara
BhagP	*Bhāgavata Purāṇa*
BhG	*Bhagavadgītā*
BS	*Brahmasūtra*
BSBh	*Brahmasūtra Bhāṣya*
BU	*Bṛhadāraṇyaka Upaniṣad*
BUBh	*Bṛhadāraṇyaka Upaniṣad Bhāṣya* of Śaṇkara
BUBhV	*Bṛhadāraṇyaka Upaniṣad Bhāṣya Vārttika* of Sureśvara
CU	*Chāndogya Upaniṣad*
CUBh	*Chāndogya Upaniṣad Bhāṣya* of Śaṇkara
GDS	*Gautama Dharma Sūtra*
JAOS	*Journal of the American Oriental Society*
KJñN	*Kaulajñānanirṇaya*
KM	*Kubjikāmata*
Manu	*Manu Smṛti*
MBh	*Mahābhārata*
MU	*Muṇḍaka Upaniṣad*
NI	*The Necklace of Immortality* or *Amṛtaratnāvalī*
NS	*Naiṣkarmyasiddhi* of Sureśvara
RM	*Rāja-Mārtaṇḍa* of Bhoja Rāja
RV	*Ṛg Veda*
RYT	*Rudrayāmala Tantra*
SB	*Svopajña Bhāṣya*
SK	*Sāṃkhya Kārikā* of Īśvara Kṛṣṇa
SV	*Sāma Veda*
TĀ	*Taittirīya Āraṇyaka*
TAS	*Tattvārthasūtra* of Umāsvāti
TU	*Taittirīya Upaniṣad*
TUBh	*Taittirīya Upaniṣad Bhāṣya* of Śaṅkara

TV	*Tattva Vaiśāradī* of Vācaspati Miśra
US	*Upadeśasāhasrī* of Śaṅkara
VaDS	*Vasiṣṭha Dharma Sūtra*
WZKM	*Wiener Zeitschrift für die Kunde des Morganlandes*
WZKSO	*Wiener Zeitschrift für die Kunde Südasiens und Archiv für indische Philosophie*
YS	*Yoga Sūtra* of Patañjali
YSBh	*Yoga Sūtra Bhāṣya*
YSS	*Yoga Sāra Saṃgraha* of Vijñāna Bhikṣu
YV	*Yoga Vārttika* of Vijñāna Bhikṣu

INTRODUCTION

The Indian tradition of yoga, first codified in the *Yoga Sūtra* of Patañjali in perhaps the third or fourth century CE, constitutes one of the world's earliest and most influential traditions of spiritual practice. It is a tradition that, by the time of Patañjali, already had an extensive (if obscure) prehistory and one that was to have, after Patañjali, an extraordinarily rich and diverse future. As a tradition yoga has been far from monolithic. It has embraced a variety of practices and orientations, borrowing from and influencing a vast array of Indic religious traditions down through the centuries.

Recent years have witnessed an increased production of scholarly works on the yoga tradition that have helped to chart this complex and multifaceted evolution and to demonstrate the important role that it has played in the development of India's religious and philosophical traditions. And yet the popular perception of yoga in the West, determined in large part by the commodification of yoga techniques, remains for the most part that of a program of physical fitness, largely divorced from its historical and spiritual roots.

The essays collected here, while not constituting a systematic survey of the yoga tradition, provide a sense of the historical emergence of the classical system presented by Patañjali, a careful examination of the key elements, overall character and contemporary relevance of that system, as found in the *Yoga Sūtra*, and a glimpse of some of the tradition's many important ramifications in later Indian religious history. It is hoped that these essays will contribute not only to the ongoing scholarly study of yoga within its broader Indian context, but will also contribute to a deeper understanding of Pātañjala yoga and its offshoots on the part of the increasing number of its Western practitioners.

The essays

John Brockington's essay on yoga in the *Mahābhārata* introduces Part I, Classical Foundations, and provides a valuable orientation to the historical development of the yoga tradition prior to its initial systematization by

Patañjali. Whether we can speak meaningfully of a "tradition" at this point is of course an important question. In the epic, Brockington argues, the term yoga, as well as the term *sāṃkhya* with which it is often associated, do not refer to the carefully thought out philosophical positions such as we will find later in Patañjali, Īśvarakṛṣṇa and their commentators, but often have the much more general meanings of "practice" and "theory" respectively. Yoga in particular refers to widely diffused spiritual methodologies which on the one hand can be linked with such thoroughly Brahmanical practices as *tapas* or "ascetic heating" and yet, on the other hand, seem clearly to have originated, at least in part, in non-Brahmanical circles and to be widely practiced without regard to specific ideological allegiances. The tension between traditional Brahmanical spiritual practices and widely available yogic alternatives is perhaps what underlies Bhīṣma's promotion, in the *Jāpakopākhyāna* (12.189–193), of the practice of *japa* as an independent discipline and way of life belonging to the Vedic sacrificial tradition and differing from the practice of yoga, even though his actual description of the practices of the *jāpaka* is clearly indebted to yoga.

There is no unanimity concerning which practices properly constitute the practice of yoga in the *Mahābhārata*, but rather a wide variety of configurations, with greater or lesser resemblance to the later classical system. Thus one can find reference to an "eightfold" yoga, but also to the "twelve yogas" and the "seven *dhāraṇas*." Still, according to Brockington, yoga practice as presented in the epic tends to have four main aspects: general preparations through such things as moral conduct; diet, posture and surroundings; the practice of breath-control (*prāṇāyāma*); the withdrawal of the senses (*pratyāhāra*); and concentration and meditation. Thus it seems clear that we find reflected in the epic, especially in the *Mokṣadharmaparvan*, a variety of practices that are in one way or another the precursors of the classical system.

We also find evidence in the epic of yoga's proclivity for theism, in contrast to the non-theistic orientation of Sāṃkhya, whether in the form of a recognition of Īśvara, parallel to what we will find in Patañjali, or in the much more elaborate form of the Bhagavadgītā, with its focus on Kṛṣṇa.

Another theme that makes its appearance in the epic and which continues to be of importance to the later tradition is an ambivalence in regard to the status of the spiritual powers (*aiśvarya*, *siddhi*) that accompany yogic practice. We find clear warnings as to the dangers of such powers for the spiritual aspirant, while at the same time such powers are recognized as an inevitable result of yogic practice and are frequently approved or even made the primary goal of such practice. This is an issue with clear importance for the later tradition, which becomes especially prominent with the emergence of tantra.

The remaining four essays in Part I all focus on the classical formulation of the yoga tradition as presented in Patañjali's *Yoga Sūtra*. The essays are united by a common concern for understanding Pātañjala yoga as a form of practice, as a spiritual path, and for understanding how the metaphysical dualism of *puruṣa* and *prakṛti* that informs Patañjali's worldview, and its association with traditions of world renunciation, affect the character of yoga as a practice, and its place in the world.

Following upon Brockington's examination of yoga in the epic, David Carpenter considers the place of Patañjali's yoga in the context of early classical Brahmanical society. Focusing on the concept of yoga as practice (*abhyāsa*) and in particular on what Patañjali calls *kriyāyoga*, or the "yoga of action," he details the rootedness of these practices in the broader Brahmanical tradition. Carpenter finds a degree of continuity between the traditional formative practices of Brahmanical society and the spiritually formative practices of Patañjali's yoga, and argues that in Patañjali's historical context the renunciatory goals of yoga did not necessarily exclude a real concern for the ritual forms of Brahmanical orthopraxy. A key instance of this assimilation is Patañjali's incorporation of the traditional Brahmanical practice of *svādhyāya* into the practice of *kriyāyoga*. This is in keeping with a general trend of Patañjali's time, namely the appropriation of renouncer values by the Brahmanical mainstream, and recalls Bhīṣma's promotion, noted by Brockington, of the practice of *japa* (which also figures prominently in the *Yoga Sūtra*) as a kind of "Vedic" alternative to the yoga of the renouncers. Thus Patañjali's *kriyāyoga* was a practice that could be appropriate both to the Brahmin "householder," who embodied the values of Brahmanical society, as well as to the "renouncer" who sought to abandon that society.

The final three essays of Part I, while focusing on the *Yoga Sūtra* of Patañjali as a historical document, do so with an eye to questions of its contemporary relevance. Ian Whicher's essay presents a forceful argument that, contrary to some common scholarly representations of it, Patañjali yoga was not as an otherworldly pursuit of spiritual isolation but rather was "a responsible engagement of spirit and matter." Rather than approach Patañjali's thought from the perspective of a set of dualistic metaphysical assumptions derived from Sāṃkhya, Whicher pursues a reading of the *sūtras* that privileges the *experience* of yoga over metaphysical abstraction. While Whicher recognizes that aspects of yoga practice, specifically that attainment of *asaṃprajñāta-samādhi,* entail an actual cessation of all mental activity (*vṛtti*), he argues that it would be a serious misreading of Pātañjala yoga to assume that such cessation is permanent, cutting the yogin off from meaningful engagement with the world. Such an outcome, he notes, would have quickly brought the tradition to an end! Rather, such cessation of mental activity is episodic, and the true goal is not cessation of mental activity *per se*, but the cessation of the *misidentification* with thought. It is not thought itself, or the dynamism of *prakṛti* as a whole, that is the source of suffering (*duḥkha*), but rather one's attachment to it. Through a process of spiritual practice aimed at the progressive purification of the *citta*, a process which Whicher refers to as the "sattvification" of consciousness, it is the mistaken identifications born of ignorance (*avidyā*) that are dissolved, not *prakṛti* itself, which is on the contrary purified and illuminated. The ultimate state of *kaivalya*, "aloneness," at which yoga practice ultimately aims, is not then so much a state of spiritual isolation, as it is frequently interpreted, as it is a state of unattached seeing not only of the transcendence of *puruṣa* but also of the play of *prakṛti*. As Whicher nicely puts it, "Yoga is not simply '*purusa*-realization;' it equally implies 'getting it right with *prakrti*.'" Thus the *yogin* achieves a spiritual freedom that is not only a freedom *from* the world but also a freedom *for* the world, through a balance of theory and practice, metaphysical discrimination of *puruṣa* and ethical engagment with the products of *prakṛti*. For Whicher, Patañjali's *yogin* is what the later tradition will know as a *jīvanmukti*, one liberated in this life, free from the sufferings of *saṃsāra* and yet still active within it.

Lloyd Pflueger's essay offers a counter-point to Whicher's advocacy of what one might call an "engaged yoga." Whereas Whicher sets out to demonstrate the relevance of Pātañjala yoga for contemporary concerns for spiritual renewal, Pflueger cautions that such revisionist projects, while legitimate as part of a living spiritual tradition, nevertheless run the risk, for the scholar, of misrepresenting the significance of Patañjali in his own historical context, a context in which the metaphysical dualism of Sāṃkhya was taken quite seriously. And whereas Whicher begins with the experiential or "epistemological" aspect of yoga, and de-emphasizes this dualist metaphysics, Pflueger accepts as a given that Patañjali's yoga must be properly understood as Sāṃkhya-Yoga, embraces the ontological perspective eschewed by Whicher, and argues that the "mind-boggling, mad, paradoxical dualism" of Sāṃkhya-Yoga is one of its finest achievements. Pflueger argues that while it might be the case that metaphysical dualism is a view with little resonance for contemporary Western practitioners of yoga, nevertheless Patañjali fully accepted the Sāṃkhyan dualism of *puruṣa* and *prakṛti* as the essential theoretical context in which the practice of yoga was to make sense. Key to a retrieval of the significance of Pātañjala yoga today then is a retrieval of the resonance that such a paradoxical dualism had for Patañjali.

What is paradoxical about this dualism is that it is interactive. In addition to the binary opposition between *puruṣa* and *prakṛti* there is also what Pflueger calls a "binary function," in which these two opposite principles "are made to function mysteriously together as a virtual system," a system in which each principle is meaningless without the other. Together, through the mystery of their interaction (*saṃyoga*), they produce the *līlā*, the "play," of phenomenal existence. Furthermore, for Pflueger the real climax of this mysterious play of cosmic opposites is not to be found in the return of each principle to a state of isolation (*kaivalya*), which brings *saṃyoga* to an end, but in the moment just before, which is a "climax of recognition" in which "matter is still manifest but in perfect association, perfect balance with consciousness. They are equally pure."

Pflueger, unlike Whicher, takes the state of *kaivalya* to be a state of otherworldly perfection in quite a strong sense. And yet, for Pflueger, it is not this state that seems most to hold the interest of Īśvarakṛṣṇa and Patañjali. For the former it is the "glory of the complex permutations of matter," for the latter the "glory of the complex meditative states and their dazzling supernormal fruits" that occupy the attention. Thus both Sāṃkhya and Yoga "glorify the path itself," such that the real goal of spiritual practice becomes indistinguishable from the path itself. In the end for Pflueger the paradoxical dualism of Sāṃkhya-Yoga preserves "a sublime and uncompromising spiritual vision" of a "non-dual transcendence" which "enriches the meaning of life."

Ironically, though their approaches to Patañjali differ widely, each being critical of the approach taken by the other, the interpretations offered by Whicher and Pflueger ultimately converge in a common emphasis on yoga as a path, as a spiritual practice which involves an ongoing interaction with the world while leading ultimately beyond it.

Chris Chapple's essay also addresses this issue of yoga's engagement with the world, and like Whicher he is concerned to demonstrate that an ongoing relationship with the world is compatible with ultimate goals of *nirodha* and *kaivalya*. Chapple's approach to this issue is to examine the metaphors of light, lightness and clarity which Patañjali uses to express the actual experience of the "shining forth" of *puruṣa*. Chapple argues that there are numerous passages in the *Yoga Sūtra* where Patañjali describes the pure, clarified witness consciousness of *puruṣa* "with-out insisting that the world itself dissolve." It is this experience of luminosity, somewhat akin perhaps to Pflueger's "climax of recognition," that for Chapple sets Pātañjala yoga apart from Sāṃkhya, for which such dissolution of the world is required. A key passage in this regard is YS 1.41, where Patañjali describes the mind of "diminished fluctuations" (*kṣīṇa-vṛtti*) experiencing a state of unity (*samāpatti*) among the "grasper, grasping, and grasped," in other words, the subject, the act of perception, and the object perceived. The cessation (*nirodha*) of mental fluctuations leads here not to the dissolution of the world as such, but to a non-dual experience of it.

The experience of *samādhi* is also described using metaphors of light, as a "shining forth" of things as they truly are, through the "splendor of wisdom." Such a description, for Chapple, "clearly allows for a world engaged through the aegis of wisdom." The same is true of the "cloud of *dharma samādhi*" with which the *Yoga Sūtra* culminates, and the attendant "power of higher awareness" (*citi-śakti*). As Chapple puts it, "the *Yoga Sūtra* does not conclude with a negation of materiality but with a celebration of the ongoing process of dispassionate yet celebratory consciousness." Such a conclusion casts a new light on the standard image of Pātañjala yoga and Hinduism generally as world denying, and Chapple ends his essay by drawing a parallel between the "dispassionate yet celebratory consciousness" of the liberated yogin and the environmental consciousness of the modern Chipko movement.

In Part II, The Expanding Tradition, the focus shifts away from Patañjali and toward the later deveopment of the yoga tradition in India. As Pflueger noted, no clear Pātañjala teaching lineage or *paramparā* has survived in India, but the historical influence of the *Yoga Sūtra* is beyond doubt. Beyond the extensive commentarial literature on the *Yoga Sūtras* themselves, the classical form that Patañjali gave to the tradition of yoga has had an important influence on other Hindu schools of thought. This is amply illustrated by Vidyasankar Sundaresan's study of the place of yoga in the Advaita Vedānta of Śaṅkara. Sundaresan argues persuasively that the common view that Śaṅkara simply rejected yoga is in need of revision. True, for Śaṅkara liberation comes through self-knowledge, mediated through the *Upaniṣads.* But as Sundaresan demonstrates at length, this does not exclude a significant role for the traditional yogic practices described by Patañjali. In fact, as he notes, "the daily life of the typical *saṃnyāsin* in the Śaṅkaran tradition incorporates a substantial amount of meditation and yoga practice, while the term *aṣṭāṅgayoga-anuṣṭhāna-niṣṭha* is a time-honored title of the Śaṅkaracāryas of Śṛṅgeri . . ." As for Śaṅkara himself, while he clearly rejects the dualism of *puruṣa* and *prakṛti*, he just as clearly endorses many aspects of yoga practice.

Focusing in particular on Śaṅkara's commentary of the Bhagavadgītā and on his Bṛhadāraṇyaka *Upaniṣad* Bhāṣya, as well as on Sureśvara's commentary on the latter, Sundaresan examines Śaṅkara's treatment of the concept of *cittavṛttinirodha,* which Patañjali uses to define yoga at *Yoga Sūtra* 1.2. While it is clearly Śaṅkara's position that *cittavṛttinirodha* is not enjoined in Vedānta, to take this position as a wholesale rejection of yoga would be a serious, if rather common, mistake. Sundaresan shows that what is at stake in this apparent rejection of yoga is actually an opposition to the position of Pūrva Mīmāṃsā concerning the injunctive status of the scriptures generally. Self-knowledge cannot be enjoined. Without the Upaniṣadic teaching of the unity of Ātman and Brahman *cittavṛttinirodha* will reveal nothing. But Śaṅkara doesn't intend to oppose the two. On the contrary, the steady recollection of self-knowledge leads naturally to *cittavṛttinirodha*, and such steady recollection is quite important, given the *saṃnyāsin's* karmic tendency toward action even after the dawn of liberating knowledge.

In his subsequent examination of Śaṅkara's references to the traditional eight limbs of Pātañjala yoga, Sundaresan is able to show that each one of them plays a role in Advaita Vedānta as well. In fact, Śaṅkara's discussion of them at times exhibits a close verbal dependance on the *Yoga Sūtra* and its commentarial tradition, as when he uses the technical terms *pūraka*, *recaka* and *kumbhaka* in commenting on Bhagavadgītā 4.29, even though this passage makes no use of these terms. Śaṅkara was clearly not averse to incorporating elements of yoga practice into his own understanding of the spiritual path. As Sundaresan notes, Śaṅkara's attitude here is best reflected in his disciple Sureśvara, who explicitly recommends the practice of yoga, *yogābhyāsa*, for one who has renounced *karma*. Yoga practice, if not its metaphysical underpinnings, thus occupied a significant place in the life of the Advaitin.

Beyond the influence that it has exerted on Hindu schools such as Advaita Vedānta, Pātañjala yoga has also had made itself felt beyond the Hindu tradition itself. This is made particularly clear by Olle Qvarnström who, in discussing the concept of yoga in Śvetāmbara Jainism, speaks of the influence of the classical tradition of yoga associated with Patañjali in creating the "pan-Indian debate" on yoga in which the Jains took part. Qvarnström examines the terminology used by a series of Jain teachers in discussing the path to liberation (*mokṣamārga*). As described in the *Tattvārthasūtra* of Umāsvāti, a rough contemporary of Patañjali, this path, like that described in the *Yoga Sūtras*, involved the repeated practice of meditation (*dhyāna*) in order gradually to bring about the cessation of the activity of the mind, *cittanirodha*. And yet quite unlike Patañjali's definition of yoga as precisely this cessation of mental activity (YS 1.2: *yogaś cittavṛtiinirodhaḥ*), in the *Tattvārthasūtra* Umāsvāti uses the term yoga to refer to activity itself, rather than to the process of its reduction. By the time of Haribhadra in the eighth century, however, the term yoga has come to refer to the entire Jaina soteriological path and we find an appropriation of Patañjali's "eight limbs" (*aṣṭāṅga*) in an explicit attempt to assimilate the yoga system of Patañjali into that of the Jains. Indeed, according to Qvarnström, Hemacandra was himself familiar with the *Yoga Sūtra* and the doctrine of yoga presented in the twelfth chapter of his major work, the *Yogaśāstra*, while still differing somewhat is terminology and detail, is consistent with a pan-Indian yogic doctrine that was systematized by Patañjali.

It is noteworthy, given the issue raised by Whicher and Pflueger concerning the *yogin*'s relationship to the world of everyday activity, that the Jains explicitly recognize the possibility of an enlightened sage who remains active in the world. Such a person is called a *sayogin* or a *sayogakevalin*, one who possesses enlightenment while in a state of activity (yoga). At the same time, the Jains also recognize a state beyond this, the state of the *ayogin* or *ayogakevalin*, for whom all activity, mental, verbal and physical, has come to an end.

While the *Yogaśāstra* of Hemacandra provides clear evidence of the lasting influence of the *Yoga Sūtra* in the Indian tradition of yoga as a whole, it has also apparently been influenced by a further permutation of that tradition, namely the development of haṭhayogic practices of the Kānphaṭa or Nāth Siddha tradition said to have originated with Matsyendranātha, and associated particularly with the name of Gorakhnātha. Qvarnström argues that some of the key terminology used by Hemachandra in the twelfth chapter of his *Yogaśāstra* derived from sources that came to be part of the Nāth Sampradāya, another example of the cross-fertilization of yogic traditions in India, even across traditional religious boundaries. Terms for the state of complete mental cessation such as *amanaskatā* and *unmānībhāva* are unknown to the earlier Jain tradition and are yet present both in the *Yogaśāstra* and in key Nāth texts such as the *Amanaskayoga* attributed to Gorakhnātha. And as yet another indication of the complex interweavings of India's yogic traditions, Qvarnström notes that some of this terminology, while new to Jain texts, can be traced back as far as the *Upaniṣads*.

Qvarnström's reference to the Nāth Siddhas provides a helpful connection to the next two essays in the volume, which shift away from the classical forms of yoga influenced by Pātañjala tradition. Starting perhaps as early as the sixth century CE a strikingly original form of yoga, which came to be known as *haṭha* yoga, appeared in India. *Haṭha* yoga seems to have only tenuous ties to the practice described by Patañjali. These tantric forms of practice gave new prominence to the role of the body, not only through greatly expanded interest in the physical postures or *āsanas* that Patañjali mentions only briefly, but in particular to the notion of a "subtle" body, the system of energy centers or *cakras* that make up its structure, the feminine energy that flows through these centers, and the powers (*siddhis*) which result from its mastery.

David White begins his essay on yoga in early Hindu tantra by discussing the status of powers or *siddhis* in yoga practice. As we have seen, this is an issue that dates back at least to the *Mahābhārata*, if not before. The ambivalent attitude toward such powers in the epic has been noted, and the same ambivalence can be found in the *Yoga Sūtra*. Whereas Patañjali, at YS 3.37, warns that *siddhis* can distract the yogin from the pure practice of *samādhi*, he nevertheless devotes a substantial portion of his work to the description of such powers and the means of their attainment, without a hint of disapproval. These powers, long recognized by the tradition as a result of yogic practice, take on a new prominence within the *haṭha* yoga tradition associated with Hindu tantra.

The main focus of White's essay is not the *siddhis*, however, but the historical emergence of the notion of the subtle body and its structure in a variety of Hindu and Buddhist texts dating from the eighth to the twelfth centuries. Contrary to the impression created by Arthur Avalon's widely read work, *The Serpent Power*, the system of the *cakras* presented there as if normative is actually the result of a complex historical evolution and expresses but one of many possible configurations. In the earliest discussions of the *cakras*, dating from the eighth century, we find reference to only four. Some early sources speak of five. Nor are they necessarily called *cakras*. This term is first applied to them in the ninth- to tenth-century *Kaulajñānanirṇaya* of Matsyendranātha, which enumerates seven *cakras* as well as an expanded list of eleven. This system of eleven cakras was subsequently appropriated by Abhinavagupta.

Of particular interest is the description of a ritual of self-sacrifice revealed by Bhairava in the tenth-century *Kubjikāmata* wherein the practitioner lays out a *maṇḍala* traced in his own blood and proceeds to offer a series of fearsome goddesses parts of his own body, including semen and blood, parts which correlate with the seven *dhātus* of the Hindu medical tradition. In exchange the goddesses confer supernatural knowledge upon the practitioner. This ritual is presented in the text as a special form of "bolt practice" that "impels the crooked one upward." White argues that we can see in this ritual a rudimentary form of *haṭha* yoga, noting that elsewhere in the text one finds goddesses correlated with locations within the subtle body of the practitioner, as well as references to a "feminine energy" (*śakti*) in the form of a sleeping serpent, a possible reference to *kuṇḍalinī*. A closer examination of early tantric material leads White to conclude that what we have in the classic *haṭha* yoga practices involving the "flying up" of *kuṇḍalinī* through the *cakras* to unite with Śiva is, when viewed historically, an internalization of what was originally a system of ritual transactions of actual sexual fluids. Furthermore, these transactions seem to have been grounded historically in the cremation-ground offerings to Yoginīs and Ḍākinīs such as those described in the *Kubjikāmata*.

White notes that, unlike the phonematic metaphors that one finds in the Trika Kaula system of Abhinavagupta, in the classical haṭhayogic texts attributed to Gorakhnātha one finds transactions and transfers involving *kuṇḍalinī* conveyed through fluid metaphors. Glen Hayes notes that the same is true of the Vaiṣṇava Sahajiyā tradition of medieval Bengal, where one finds a preference for metaphors of fluids and substances rather than metaphors of energy, sound, power and light. In what is methodologically the most self-conscious essay in the volume, Hayes argues for the importance of attention to metaphor for our understanding of tantric texts. Drawing upon the work of George Lakoff and especially upon Mark Johnson's notions of "image schemata" and "metaphorical projections" Hayes examines the metaphorical structure of the cosmophysiology (*dehatattva*) and the psychophysical ritual practices (*sādhana*) of the Sahajiyās, focusing on the *Amṛtaratnāvalī* or *Necklace of Immortality* attributed to the seventeenth-century Sahajiyā author Mukunda-dāsa. Like White, Hayes is primarily interested in the representation of the subtle body, or what he refers to as the "spiritual" or "yogic" body that is both "within" and "above" the physical body.

In the *Amṛtaratnavali* the journey to final liberation requires the transformation of the physical body into a subtle, interior "divine body" (*devadeha*). As a "container" this divine body is generated by means of initiation into a *sādhana,* which is received like a second birth from one's guru as father and from the secret mystical community of Sahajiyā adepts as one's mother. The "substance" of the divine body, however, is generated through the ritual exchange of sexual fluids. These fluids are made to "flow upwards against the current" along the "crooked river" toward the four "inner lotus ponds" and the Sahajiyā heavens. This propensity for fluid metaphors is exemplified in the use of the term *rasa*, literally "juice" or "essence," but which is used to refer both to aesthetic experience and sexual substance, both of which can "flow" like a river. Thus unlike the more familiar system of *nāḍīs* and *cakras*, one finds in the Sahajiyā tradition a system of "rivers" and "ponds," and a journey through the subtle inner world that reflects in many ways the natural topography of Bengal. Tantric *sādhana* can be understood as the enactment of such metaphoric structures through the medium of the human body.

Part I

CLASSICAL FOUNDATIONS

1
YOGA IN THE *MAHĀBHĀRATA*

John Brockington

In this essay I survey not only the main passages on yoga in the *Mahābhārata* (*Mokṣadharma*, *Bhagavadgītā* and *Sanatsujātīya*) but also references to yoga more generally and I seek to place these in the context of the emergence of the Sāṃkhya and Yoga systems.[1] Besides the more obviously philosophical passages, there are many more which incorporate elements which we can identify as Yoga or Sāṃkhya; even the *Bhīṣmastavarāja* (12.47), comprising Bhīṣma's *dhyāna* on Kṛṣṇa, for example, is introduced by a question about which yoga he adopted. Various individuals are associated with such expositions of yoga; indeed, Vyāsa himself is the main teacher of yoga, as well as being once termed *vyāso vogavidāṃ varaḥ* (12.26.4b) in a standardly formed epithet (cf., for example, *vyāso vedavidāṃ varaḥ* at 15.38.19b). Yoga and *yogins* in fact occur quite widely in the *Mahābhārata* in contexts which suggest a wider and to some extent different understanding of the terms than that found in classical yoga, while the older practice of *tapas* and that of yoga are often linked; I shall explore the reasons for and possible explanations of this feature, along with the actual terminology employed in the epic. It is, however, worth emphasizing at the start the prevalence in the *Mahābhārata* of various other views, such as those which elevate *kāla*, *daiva*, *svabhāva* or the like to the status of supreme principle.

There has been, of course, a long-running debate over the origins of Sāṃkhya and Yoga, in which two main positions have been adopted. One regards them as ancient, non-Brahmanical systems which predate the rise of Buddhism, while the opposite view is that Sāṃkhya and Yoga as philosophical systems can hardly be attested before the *Sāṃkhya Kārikā* of Īśvarakṛṣṇa and the *Yoga Sūtra* of Patañjali, and so, far from belonging to the beginnings of Indian philosophy, they are late, derivative systems influenced by the *Upaniṣads*, early Buddhism, the *Mokṣadharma* and the *Bhagavadgītā*. To state my own position on this controversy at the outset, Sāṃkhya and Yoga probably were ancient trends of thought that owed much to groups outside Vedic orthodoxy and for which texts such as the *Upaniṣads* and the *Mokṣadharma* are valuable sources of information, but they cannot be regarded as fully-fledged systems before the time of Īśvarakṛṣṇa and Patañjali.

When, from the 1920s on, Frauwallner examined in detail the texts of the *Mokṣadharma*, he divided them into the two categories of Sāṃkhya and non-Sāṃkhya, including in the latter the yoga passages.[2] However, the exact meaning of the terms is crucial: there are several contexts in which *sāṃkhya* and *yoga* seem to mean little more than theory and practice respectively. Edgerton has rightly insisted that to assume the existence of the systems whenever the terms occur in the *Mokṣadharma*, *Bhagavadgītā* and other early texts is to commit a fundamental error in historical judgement.[3] In all of these texts the terms refer not so much to philosophical positions as to spiritual methodologies; for example, Vasiṣṭha in his dialogue with Karāla Janaka (12.291–296, to which I shall return later) defines yoga in terms of *ekāgratā* and *prāṇāyāma* (12.294.8) while affirming that the basis of Sāṃkhya is discrimination and enumeration (12.294.41).

Since both the meditative discipline of yoga and the cosmological theories of Sāṃkhya or its precursors were frequently utilized by other authors and schools, many texts with a different orientation incorporate these ideas, of which the best known instance is the *Bhagavadgītā*. There are also various pointers to suggest that both Sāṃkhya and Yoga originated, at least in part, in the same milieu as the unorthodox systems. In both, the goal of *mokṣa* is significantly termed *kaivalya*, which has traditionally been interpreted as "aloneness, isolation" of the selves both from *prakṛti* and from each other, as self-contained monads. While in the classical schools there is a fairly clear distinction between Sāṃkhya and Yoga, this is not necessarily true in the epic or other popular presentations. Indeed, the *Śāntiparvan* contains not infrequent assertions of their essential identity (as expounding the twenty-five *tattvas* at 12.228.28, 295.42 and 304.3, as emphasizing purity of conduct and observance of vows at 289.9, and so on).

For example, at 12.187 (repeated with some significant variations at 12.239–241), in the varying usage of the terms *bhāva* and *guṇa,* there are traces of a synthesis between ancient cosmological speculations and yogic theories of evolution. This is the passage on which Frauwallner bases his interpretation of the earliest Sāṃkhya, seeing it as "der epischen Grundtext des Sāṃkhya."[4] In addition, as Frauwallner has indicated, beside the apparent archaism of its ideas, the fact that this text-group is textually so corrupt is another indication of an early date. Within this passage the goal of yoga as the direct vision of the *ātman* is presented when it is declared that to one who controls his mind through yoga, the *ātman* shines forth like a lamp blazing forth from a pot (187.44, cf. 240.15 and, more generally, 232.18). The next chapter is the *Dhyānayoga* passage on the fourfold yoga of meditation (12.188, to be discussed below). There then follows, however, the *Jāpakopākhyāna* (12.189–193), which deals with the importance of *japa* and the *jāpaka* and in which Bhīṣma declares that *japa* constitutes an independent discipline and way of life belonging to the Vedic sacrificial tradition and different from Sāṃkhya and Yoga (or Sāṃkhyayoga, i.e. the Sāṃkhya type of yoga), while propounding as its observances much of the yoga practice; Bhīṣma stresses to Yudhiṣṭhira that a *jāpaka* practising *japa* is equal to a *yogin* in terms of achievements. This is just one of several indications that yoga techniques were widely diffused already throughout the period of the epics and were not limited to a specific school, another indicator being the frequency of occurrence of yoga or *yogin* even in the core battle books of the epic.[5]

A significant difference between Yoga and Sāṃkhya as found in the *Mahābhārata* is that Sāṃkhya is typically *anīśvara,* though not denying the existence of the Vedic gods. Evidence for this can be found in 12.289 (the *Yogakathana*); here *sāṃkhyayoga* is clearly differentiated from other kinds of yoga and it is stated that Sāṃkhya is non-theistic, emphasizes knowledge as the only means of salvation, and relies mainly on accepted teaching as a means of knowledge; Yoga, on the other hand, is theistic, emphasizes the power and strength of bodily discipline, and relies primarily on immediate perception as a means of knowledge; the passage also declares at verse 9 that the "views" (*darśana*) are not the same in the two systems, although it is not made clear just what this means. However, some of the passages which assert a twenty-sixth principle do not imply the later yoga notion of a lord as a kind of super-soul, but rather mean the *puruṣa* or *kṣetrajña* in its enlightened state (e.g. 12.296.11), and in several passages a non-theistic doctrine seems clearly implied: for example, in 12.241.1 the *kṣetrajña* is equated with the *īśvara.* Nevertheless, in the *Bhagavadgītā* the tendency is to relate the highest principle which is beyond the twenty-five to Kṛṣṇa. In one *Mokṣadharma* passage Yājñavalkya explains in detail the distinction between *kṣetra* and *kṣetrajña* and distinguishes this perceiving self from the twenty-four categories of *prakṛti* constituting the sphere of empirical knowledge (12.306.27–55; cf. 12.187.37–39, 240.19–21, 296.22–26 and 303.13–18). This perceiving self is not the real doer and enjoyer but simply the pure witness-consciousness that forms the background of our empirical existence. But both it and *prakṛti,* though independent of each other, are dependent on a further principle, *puruṣottama,* which is the final abode of the whole creation. While there are various differences from classical Sāṃkhya and Yoga, this passage definitely says that all sufferings are due to false identification of *prakṛti* and *kṣetrajña* and that final liberation will be effected by recognition of the distinction between spirit and matter.

The *Vārṣṇeyādhyātma* (12.203–210), though incorporating elements of an early form of Sāṃkhya, does not use that term but refers rather to yoga and operates in a basically theistic framework. To his pupil's initial question about where they both had come from, its anonymous teacher replies that Vāsudeva is everything and that he causes the emanation and dissolution of the universe, being the unmanifest, eternal Brahman (203.7–9). After indicating the usefulness of yoga techniques, the dialogue then emphasizes the role of intuition in being freed from the mortal world and becoming Brahman, which is going to the blessed, unborn, divine Viṣṇu, who is called the unmanifest (210.28–30).

The clearest theistic emphasis is found in the *Bhagavadgītā*.[6] Its earlier chapters are mainly concerned with yogic techniques of isolating the self. In the second chapter *sāṃkhyayoga* is defined as a kind of yoga which stands apart from *karmayoga*, *dhyānayoga*, and so on, and Kṛṣṇa declares that it is possible to recognize the eternal *ātman* through the practice of yoga, by learning to detach oneself completely from the results of actions; by abandoning desires such a person reaches peace and the stillness of Brahman (2.71–72). This specialized understanding of detachment accounts for the fact that *saṃnyāsa* and *karmayoga* are contrasted at 5.1–2 but identified at 6.2. Mislav Ježić regards the extant *Bhagavadgītā* as built up on an original epic poem (ending at 2.37) and has identified a first yogic layer extending this in 2.39–4.42, with certain exceptions, before an overall *bhakti* outlook synthesizes the successive layers.[7] The start of the fourth chapter declares that this yoga was first revealed to Vivasvat and now after its disappearance is being revealed again to Arjuna by Kṛṣṇa (4.1–3); yoga as revelation is certainly rather different from the classical view (but paralleled elsewhere, as when Yājñavalkya affirms that the eightfold yoga is found in the Vedas, 12.304.7). The transition from yoga to *bhakti* is presented as a generalization of yoga (e.g. 4.9–11, 6.30–31 and 46–47).

The fifth chapter, which is similar in its ideas to the second, reverts to the theme of Brahman, with even more emphatic exaltation of Brahman as both the goal of yoga and as an external agency. The self-discipline of yoga is reached by intense concentration of one's attention on a single point and those integrated in this way realize that the *ātman* is never the author of any action (5.14 and 27–28, cf. 6.13 and 8.10). In the seventh chapter a clearly theistic account of *sāṃkhyayoga* is presented: the eightfold *prakṛti* is called Kṛṣṇa's "lower nature" (7.4) and described as his *māyā*. The eighth chapter again presents the method of meditation in yoga as the way to release from a more clearly theistic perspective, while in the thirteenth chapter yet another account appears, which seems considerably later and close to the classical scheme. However, neither Yoga nor Sāṃkhya had assumed their later distinctive shape even by the end of the epic period, where in fact the nearest approach to the classical systems is found (at 14.40–42) within the very late *Anugītā*, the supposed recapitulation of his teachings by Kṛṣṇa after the battle (14.16–50), which also refers to the unequalled science of yoga (*ataḥ paraṃ pravakṣyāmi yogaśāstram anuttamam*, 14.19.14ab) in a passage directed towards seeing the self in the self, using also the term *ekāntaśīla* "devoted to one purpose" (at 14.19.18c + 30c, cf. *ekāntaśīlin* at 1.110.33a and also 12.304.12b, but *adhyātmaśīlin* at the parallel 12.232.3b) as perhaps a later equivalent for *ekāgramanas.*

As indicated in the opening paragraph, yoga and *yogins* occur quite widely in the *Mahābhārata* – indeed, the terms occur well over 300 times in the *Śāntiparvan* and not far short of 900 times in the *Mahābhārata* as a whole – and do so in contexts which often suggest a broader and rather different understanding of the terms from that found in classical yoga; indeed, relatively specific references, such as that to the rules of yoga (*vidhiṃ ca yogasya,* 9.49.53c), occur in passages which are clearly late.[8] Also, I have noted elsewhere that the older practice of *tapas* and the discipline of yoga are often linked.[9] For example, in the *Āraṇyakaparvan* Śaunaka urges Yudhiṣṭhira to pursue success by *tapas* and by yoga (*tapasā siddhim anviccha yogasiddhiṃ ca bhārata,* 3.2.77cd – c is repeated at 78c and its purpose given as support of the twice-born), holding out the example of the gods who attained their sovereignty because they possessed the power of yoga (*yogaiśvaryeṇa saṃyuktāḥ,* 3.2.76c); similarly, in the next *adhyāya,* in the late context of the 108 names of the sun, Yudhiṣṭhira, duly resorting to austerity (*tapa āsthāya dharmeṇa,* 3.3.12c) to support the twice-born, undertook the supreme austerity (*tapa ātiṣṭhad uttamam,* 13d) and, after resorting to yoga (*yogam āsthāya,* 14c), practised breath control (*prāṇāyāmena tasthivān,* 14f). However, by the late *Nārāyaṇīya* (12.321–339), *tapas* and yoga are both alike subordinated to *bhakti,* with Nārāyaṇa identifying himself as the goal of yoga proclaimed in yoga texts (326.65cd, cf. 335.74c), while the juxtaposition of Sāṃkhya and Yoga has become a commonplace and so, for example, at 327.64–66 the seven mind-born sons of Brahmā – Sana, Sanatsujāta, Sanaka, Sanandana, Sanatkumāra, Kapila and Sanātana – are collectively described as the foremost knowers of Yoga and knowers of the Sāṃkhya *dharma.*

Elsewhere specific practices are linked, for example breath control and plucking out the hair (3.81.51cd, where the variant *svalomāni* seems better than the *śvalomāni* of the text). Indeed, *tapas* and other yoga practices are often simply efficacious methods to achieve mundane ends, since they produce power which can be manipulated and used to force one's will on others, and this is a feature which persists even into the *Mokṣadharmaparvan*; examples include the magical power, *prabhāva,* of flying through the air mentioned at 12.312.8cd (where Vyāsa cautions his son Śuka not to be tempted to use it), a long list of such powers at 12.228.21–37, and even simply *aṣṭaguṇam aiśvaryam* at 12.326.51c (cf. 3.388*7).[10] The same term *aiśvarya* is used when Bhīṣma declares that a *jāpaka* who is intent on powers (*athaiśvaryapravṛttaḥ saj jāpakaḥ,* 12.190.7ab) goes to hell for ever; here, then, the attitude to these magical powers is condemnatory, in accordance with the outlook of Pātañjala yoga, rather than neutral or even commendatory.

One of the most striking instances occurs in 12.278, the episode of Kāvya Uśanas – described as *yogasiddho mahāmuniḥ* (9b) – who uses his yogic power to deprive Kubera of his wealth and then to evade Śiva's trident and enter his mouth (13–20), for he is finally granted a boon by Śiva and adopted by Pārvatī as her son, indicating that "the god of yoga" is content to overlook this misuse of yogic powers. Elsewhere, more positively since on behalf of the gods, king Kuvalāśva, as a *yogin* by his yoga (*yogī yogena*, 3.197.27c), quenches the fieriness of the Asura Dhundhu. Again, in the *Anuśāsanaparvan*, in a somewhat similar incident (13.40–43) to that of Kāvya Uśanas, Vipula guards the chastity of Ruci, the wife of his guru Devaśarman, against Indra's attempts at seducing her by taking yogic possession of Ruci (*yogenānupraviśyeha gurupatnyāḥ kalevaram*, 40.50ab) and so preventing her from responding to Indra's advances; this exercise of his powers is clearly seen as praiseworthy in the context of the episode as a whole. Elsewhere in that book, after Bharadvāja enters him by yoga, Pratardana immediately he is born grows into a thirteen-year-old (13.31.29–30) and goes out to defeat the descendants of Vītihavya.

Even the term *ekāgramanas* is used not only of yogic discipline proper but also more or less as a general term of commendation. For example, the Kurus as they march out against the Pāṇḍavas are Veda-knowing heroes, all having performed their vows well and all having concentrated minds (5.197.3–4, cf. 6.53.3). In some very late passages this is taken to the extent of directly comparing the disciplined *yogin* and the warrior slain in battle, in that both are able to pierce the orbit of the sun (for example, at 5.178*). Even among the occurrences of *ekāgramanas* in the *Śāntiparvan* (12.20.2d, 35.9d, 56.28d, 322.29a, 323.32e and 325.3a) half are in a Pāñcarātrin context, in the *Nārāyaṇīya*, as is exclusively the case with the similar term *ekāntin* (13 occurrences between 12.323 and 336).

Perhaps the two most striking features in the religious aspects of yoga are the concern with techniques of dying and the link with ideas of light and radiance. One example is the *Sanatsujātīya* (5.42–45) which begins by declaring that there is no killing or being killed and has as a refrain in its final chapter, directed towards the *puruṣa*, "the yogins behold him, the eternal blessed one" (*yoginas taṃ prapaśyanti bhagavantaṃ sanātanam*, 5.45.1ef etc.); analogies are obvious with the message of the *Bhagavadgītā*, the yoga elements of which have been discussed already. Another example comes in the *Brāhmaṇavyādhasaṃvāda*, the dialogue of the brāhman and the butcher (3.198–206), where, after an exposition of the Sāṃkhya categories and the role of the *prāṇas*, the butcher declares that if one disciplines the mind during the night, eats little and is pure of soul, one sees the self within oneself and that, as though with a lighted lamp, ones sees with the lamp of the mind that the self is separate and is then released (3.203.37–38). At the humblest level, this light image is widespread in the simile of the steady lamp applied to the *yogin* (e.g. BhG 6.19a, Mbh 3.203.36c, 12.187.44d, 238.11c, 240.15d, 294.18ab, 304.19ab).

The most striking example, however, is found in the description of Droṇa's death.[11] This states that – as Droṇa resolves to die, abandons his weapons and applies himself to yoga (*yogayuktavān*) – he who possesses great austerities assents to it, resorts to yoga (*yogam āsthāya*, a standard phrase), becoming a light, and ascends to heaven; as he goes it seems to those below that there are two suns and that the atmosphere is entirely filled with lights (7.165.35–40). Although the degree of duplication within the whole account of Droṇa's death points to the existence of more than one layer in its narration, this particular passage shows that it hasbeen homologated with accounts of yogic experience in terms of incomparable radiance. There are pronounced similarities to this in the account of Kṛṣṇa's death (16.5), as Peter Schreiner demonstrates, while the term *jyotirbhūta* used within this description is used elsewhere of Kṛṣṇa as the supreme deity (13.143.35a), as well as of mythical figures or those achieving liberation (6.9.11d, 7.159.46b, 12.224.37b, 262.22d and 335.12c), and seems almost a synonym of *brahmabhūta*. It is also worth noting that there is quite a close parallel to the themes apparent in Droṇa's death in that of Bhūriśravas, also described as *yogayukta*, earlier in the *Droṇaparvan* (7.118.16–18), while in the *Karṇaparvan* the dying Droṇa is called *yuktayoga* (8.5.61); in the later stages of the epic, the dying Vidura, resorting to the power of yoga and as it were blazing with splendour, enters the body of Yudhiṣṭhira who feels himself strengthened (15.33.26–28).

Descriptions of yoga are quite frequent in the *Mokṣadharmaparvan* and a common feature of them is a strong emphasis on discipline and meditation. As already noted, Vasiṣṭha in his dialogue with Karāla Janaka (12.291–296) defines yoga in terms of *ekāgratā* and *prāṇāyāma* (12.294.7–8, cf. *prāṇāyāma* being recommended at BhG 4.29d),[12] while he also declares that by ten or twelve *codanās*, presumably restraints of breath, one should urge the self to what is beyond the twenty-fourth (12.294.10cd, repeated in a modified context by the *Anugītā* at 14.48.4cd, cf. also 12.304.11, cited on p. 22).[13] In this dialogue there is a strong tendency to identify Sāṃkhya and Yoga with each other but in *adhyāya* 294 Vaṣiṣṭha is particularly concerned with the nature of yoga, while the last chapter of the dialogue introduces a twenty-sixth principle, the *puruṣa* or *kṣetrajña* in its enlightened state (12.296.11, noted earlier).

Yoga practice, as presented in the *Mahābhārata*, comprises four main aspects of general preparations through moral conduct; diet, posture and surroundings; breath control; and withdrawal of the senses, concentration and meditation. Moral conduct, besides being indicated positively as in the list "meditation, study, giving, truth, modesty, honesty, patience, purity, cleanliness of food and restraint of the senses" at 12.232.10, is also defined negatively as avoidance of the five faults (*doṣas* – the epic term corresponding to the *kleśas* of the *Yoga Sūtra*) of "lust, anger, greed, fear and sleep" at 12.232.4, or "passion, delusion, affection, lust and anger" at 12.289.11 (cf. also a similar Sāṃkhya listing at 12.290.53–54), or the activities of the five senses (12.304.13). The fruit of the *niyamas* is seen directly according to 13.74.9 but the context is one of *vratas* rather than yoga. The *yogin* should be abstemious (*laghvāhāra*, 12.180.28c and 266.17b), living on coarsely ground grain, vegetables, fruit and roots (12.208.21, 289.43–44) and fasting for an entire month (12.289.46). He should practice yoga during the first and last watches of the night (12.180.28, 232.13, 294.13) or else three times a day (12.232.23), selecting as the site for his practice a mountain-top, a *caitya*, tree-tops, mountain caves, temples or empty houses (12.232.23 + 26).

The *āsanas* are at most indirectly indicated in this last passage but one, the *vīrāsana,* is specifically named at 12.292.8d and also in the *Anuśāsanaparvan*, where Śiva, detailing the various types and practices of extreme asceticism to Umā, lists it as one form (13.130.8–10). Breath control or *prāṇāyāma* is defined as being *saguṇa* in contrast to *dhāraṇa* as *nirguṇa* (12.304.9, cf. 12.294.8); however, these two verses contain the only four occurrences of the term *prāṇāyāma* in the entire *Śāntiparvan*, while even more strikingly the term *āsana* as such occurs only at 12.178.16c and 193.18c. The *Dhyānayoga* passage, already noted, gives one of the fullest descriptions from the standpoint of suppression (*nirodha*), while the main passage for the yoga of heightened consciousness (*jñānadīptiyoga*) is the *Yogakathana* (12.289).

In the *Dhyānayoga* chapter (12.188), Bhīṣma outlines to Yudhiṣṭhira the fourfold yoga of meditation (*dhyānayogaṃ caturvidham*, 1b), where one should collect together all the senses, fix the mind on a single point and sit like a log of wood and, after passing through further stages of meditation (*vitarka*, *vicāra* and *viveka*, 15ab) and finally withdrawing the senses through concentration, one becomes completely tranquil and gains *nirvāṇa* (22cd); this passage is echoed in *Bṛhannāradīya Purāṇa* 44.83–105. In the final chapter of the *Anugītā*, by contrast, *dhyānayoga* is evidently seen as the climax of the path of spiritual ascent, since by it noble ones free from possessiveness and egoism obtain or enter the great further world (14.50.22–24); incidentally, this contrasts with the declaration earlier in the *Anugītā* that yoga has the nature of activity (*pravṛttilakṣaṇo yogaḥ*, 14.43.24c). According to 12.209.20, it is possible through *pratyāhāra* to know the unmanifest Brahman, whereas elsewhere withdrawal of the senses is expressed through various images, such as the reins of the senses being controlled by the *manas* (12.187.44), the senses being calm like water in which a reflection is seen (12.197.2), or when the senses have returned from their pastures and remain in their stalls (12.242.6).[14]

Within the *Śukānupraśna* (12.224–247) – which is in fact a distinctly heterogeneous collection of passages, including, for example, both the *Vedarahasya* (238) and an account of the *yogin*'s direct vision (245) – there is a marked emphasis on *dhāraṇā* in 12.228, which begins by declaring that, after the faults have been cut off one should practice the twelve yogas (not otherwise defined here, but cf. *Manu* 12.120–121), and then launches into an extended metaphor identifying the parts of a warrior's chariot with the requirements of yoga; this leads into a description of seven *dhāraṇās* (12.228.13–15; cf. also 12.289.39–57, which contains the striking image that it is easier to stand on sharpened razor edges than to undertake the *dhāraṇās* of yoga for the uncontrolled, 54),[15] and concludes with the assertion that he who has passed beyond yogic domination (*yogaiśvaryam atikrānto*, 37c) is released. Again, also within the *Śukānupraśna*, Vyāsa's exposition of Sāṃkhya (12.231), which implies that Sāṃkhya and Yoga are alternative ways to attain Brahman, is followed by his presentation of yoga (12.232.2–22), which begins by describing the purpose of this complete *yogakṛtya* (2a) as "unification of *buddhi* and *manas* and of the senses as a whole" (2cd) and by defining its activities at verse 10 (cf. above); it proclaims the goal as being the attainment of the state of Brahman (17) or identity with the imperishable (*gacched akṣarasātmyatām*, 20d) and concludes with an indication of the magical or supernatural powers achieved by its practices but to be disregarded by the true yogin (21–22), while in its terminology it is quite close to the *Yoga Sūtra*. Near the end of the *Śukānupraśna* Vyāsa then provides an account of the *yogin*'s direct vision of the inner subtle self (12.245), quoting Śāṇḍilya's dictum that yoga consists mainly of *samādhi* (245.13cd), with which may be compared Vasiṣṭha's affirmation that the essence of yoga lies in *dhyāna*, which is twofold: concentration of the mind and control of the breath (294.7).

The main passage concerned with the yoga of heightened consciousness (*jñānadīptiyoga*), the *Yogakathana* (12.289, in which the terms *yoga* and *yogin* occur particularly frequently), explicitly contrasts this form of yoga with the lengthy account of Sāṃkhya presented in the following *adhyāya* (*Sāṃkhyakathana*, 12.290, containing no fewer than 110 verses against sixty-two in the *Yogakathana*, and referring to various yogas, *yogāṃś ca vividhān*, 34b); this and other features suggest that it is relatively close to the classical yoga of Patañjali. Nevertheless, among its many analogies for powerful *yogins* is that "a yogin who has become strong, mighty with flaming energy, like the sun at the time of the end of the world, might dry up the whole world" (12.289.21, cf. also 33). Also in a specifically Sāṃkhya or Yoga context, Sulabhā, a female teacher of Sāṃkhya, assumes by means of yoga the form of a beautiful woman as she visits king Janaka of Mithilā, uses her powers to enter his mind and test his claims to detachment, binding him with bonds of yoga (12.308.10–17); she is called a *bhikṣukī*, established in *yogadharma* and wandering the earth alone (308.7). So, too, within the *Śukacarita* (the life-story of Śuka, 12.310–320) Śuka, to whom tradition attributes even greater sanctity as the ideal renouncer than to his father Vyāsa, is intent on gaining *mokṣa* and, when he returns to his father, *yogayukta*, he flies like an arrow, uninterrupted by trees or mountains (314.27) and subsequently by means of yoga, he becomes like the wind and enters the sun (318.53).[16] These various feats are implicitly commended rather than avoided, as Vyāsa advises at 12.232.21–22, and indeed they are at odds with Vyāsa's advice a few chapters earlier in this same episode (312.8cd, on which I commented above), cautioning his son against flying through the air.

Somewhat similarly to the *Yogakathana*, in the *Yājñavalkya-janakasaṃvāda* (12.298–306), Yājñavalkya follows an exposition of Sāṃkhya with one of Yoga (12.304, which has similarities with 12.232, mentioned already), in which he views Sāṃkhya in terms of knowledge and Yoga in terms of power (*nāsti sāṃkhyasamaṃ jñānaṃ nāsti yogasamaṃ balam*, 2ab) and, while regarding them as one, affirms that the eightfold yoga is found in the Vedas (*vedeṣu cāṣṭaguṇitaṃ yogam āhur manīṣiṇaḥ*, 7ab) and, as we have seen, declares yoga's two components to be breath control, which is *saguṇa*, and concentration of the mind, which is *nirguṇa* (8–9). Yājñavalkya then mentions twelve practices of concentration (*codana*), coupled with breath control, to be performed by an aspirant at the beginning and end of the night (11, cf. 12.129.10cd above).[17] Later in this passage there is the graphic picture of the man of concentration as one who could carry a full vessel of oil up a staircase while menaced by men armed with swords without spilling a single drop (22–23, cf. 289.32) and Yājñavalkya declares of the *yogin* who meditates on *īśāna* and Brahman that "like a flame in a windless place, like a mountain peak, he beholds Brahman, which is like a fire in great darkness" (19 + 25cd).

Nevertheless, the identity of Yoga with Sāṃkhya as far as its basic teachings are concerned is repeatedly affirmed, not only at 12.304.3, as mentioned above, but also, for example, at 295.42 and at 228.28, where their common acceptance of twenty-five *tattvas* is noted; on the other hand, such stress on identity quite possibly represents an aspiration rather than a reality. Certainly, statements distinguishing Sāṃkhya from Yoga (or *sāṃkhyayoga* from *karmayoga*, *dhyānayoga* and so on, such as 12.304.2ab and 289.2–5, or the well-known BhG 2.39) may well represent the first stage in their gradual differentiation into separate schools. The distinctiveness of Yoga lies in its techniques for *dhyāna* or meditation, as even more of the passages cited indicate. There is even at times a suggestion that the Sāṃkhya is preliminary to the Yoga, as in the metaphorical likening of yoga to curds or whey (295.44cd). These two paths – they are not yet developed systems, even in the latest passages – are certainly prominent in the *Śāntiparvan*, mainly in the *Mokṣadharma-*

parvan, but it contains much else besides, bringing together as it does so many divergent views. Equally, the extent to which incidental mention of yoga occurs through the whole *Mahābhārata* indicates that some of its ideas already enjoyed wide currency. However, much work is still needed to disentangle the origins of the various strands of thought which we see here at a formative stage.

Notes

1 This essay develops my treatment of epic Sāṃkhya and yoga in *The Sanskrit Epics*, Leiden, E. J. Brill, 1998, pp. 302–312. It also shares some material with my paper at the Conference on Sāṃkhya and Yoga in Lausanne, 6–8 November 1998, and is indebted to Peter Schreiner's paper at the same conference. See John Brockington, "Epic Sāṃkhya: Texts, Teachers, Terminology," *Asiatische Studien/Études Asiatiques*, 1999, vol. 53, pp. 473–490, and Peter Schreiner, "What Comes First (in the *Mahābhārata*): Sāṃkhya or Yoga?" *Asiatische Studien/Études Asiatiques*, 1999, vol. 53, pp. 755–777.

2 Eric Frauwallner, "Untersuchungen zum Mokṣadharma" (3 parts), *JAOS*, 1925, vol. 45, pp. 51–67, *WZKM*, 1925, vol. 32, pp. 179–296 and *WZKM*, vol. 33, pp. 57–68; also his *Geschichte der indischen Philosophie*, Salzburg, Müller, 1953, vol. I, pp. 275–408.

3 Franklin Edgerton, *The Beginnings of Indian Philosophy*, London, Allen & Unwin, 1965, pp. 35–48 and 255–334 (quotation from p. 36 at the end of the next paragraph).

4 Frauwallner, "Untersuchungen zum Mokṣadharma," II, pp. 179–180. In the Bombay edition there are three versions of this passage but its 12.286[5] is lacking in several manuscripts and its readings are given by the Critical Edition in App.II.1 as variants to 12.187; it also recurs at *Bṛhannāradīya Purāṇa*, 44.21–82. It is translated by Edgerton, *The Beginnings of Indian Philosophy*, pp. 256–260, and analysed by J. A. B. van Buitenen, "Studies in Sāṃkhya (I)," *JAOS*, 1956, vol. 76, pp. 153–157; the latest study is by Hans Bakker and Peter Bisschop, "Mokṣadharma 187 and 239–241 reconsidered," in *Asiatische Studien/Études Asiatiques*, 1999, vol. 53. pp. 459–472.

5 The terms occur forty-three, twenty-two and twenty-six times in books 7–9, and 131 times in book 6, of which, however, well over half occur in the *Bhagavadgītā*; there is no book of the *Mahābhārata* from which they are absent. These data come from Peter Schreiner's paper mentioned in note 1.

6 For more on the *Bhagavadgītā* see my "The Bhagavadgītā: Text and Context," in J. Lipner (ed.), *The Fruits of Our Desiring: An Enquiry into the Ethics of the Bhagavadgītā for Our Times*, Calgary, Bayeux, 1997, pp. 28–47.

7 Mislav Ježić, "The first yoga layer in the Bhagavadgītā," in J. P. Sinha (ed.), *Ludwik Sternbach Felicitation Volume*, part 1, Lucknow, Akhila Bharatiya Sanskrit Parishad, 1979, pp. 545–557, continuing his "Textual Layers of the Bhagavadgītā as Traces of Indian Cultural History," in Wolfgang Morgenroth (ed.), *Sanskrit and World Culture: Proceedings of the Fourth World Sanskrit Conference*, Berlin, Akademie Verlag, 1986, pp. 628–638.

8 An early and still useful treatment, despite certain limitations, is that by E. W. Hopkins, "Yoga-technique in the Great Epic," *JAOS*, 1901, vol. 22, pp. 333–379.

9 See my *The Sanskrit Epics*, Leiden, E. J. Brill, 1998, pp. 237–240.

10 The specific terms *aṇimā* and *laghimā* occur at 12.291.15c, apparently equated with the formless self (*amūrtātmā*).

11 On this passage, and more generally on these themes, see my "Mysticism in the Epics," in Peter Connolly (ed.), *Perspectives on Indian Religion: Papers in Honour of Karel Werner*, Delhi, Sri Satguru, 1986, pp. 9–20, and Peter Schreiner, "Yoga – Lebenshilfe oder Sterbetechnik?" *Umwelt & Gesundheit* (Köln), 1988, vol. 3/4, pp. 12–18.

12 However, it should be noted that the term *ekāgratā* occurs only at 198.6c and 294.8a and *prāṇāyāma* only at 294.8bc and 304.9bc in the entire *Śāntiparvan*. In view of the infrequency of technical vocabulary in any of these passages, their occurrence here must raise the suspicion that 12.294 is particularly late in the growth of the *Mokṣadharmaparvan*.

13 V. M. Bedekar, however, understands these *codanās* as successive stages of withdrawal, which "are probably directed to the withdrawal respectively from the 10 objects of senses corresponding to the 5 senses of action and 5 senses of knowledge and of the mind and intellect," in his "Yoga in the Mokṣadharmaparvan of the *Mahābhārata*," *WZKSO*, 1968–1969, vols 12–13, pp. 43–52 (quoting p. 48).

14 In the *Śāntiparvan* the term *pratyāhāra* otherwise only occurs at 224.74a, within a context which enumerates the divisions of time (though not specifically *kālavāda*, a view which is propounded at 12.217, for example), and is opposed to *sarga*, which means that it is operating at the macrocosmic level.

15 The term *dhāraṇā* occurs in the *Śāntiparvan* at 159.32d, 36b, 210.24e, 27d(iic), 228.13a, 289.30b, 37b, 54c, 55a, 56b and 304.9a (also, for example, at 3.200.4b), but not always with its technical meaning; contrast the use of *prāṇadhāraṇa* at 12.139.36d, 55b, 58d, 185.33, 13ad and 330.20b.

16 The *Śukānucarita* has been studied by Cheever Mackenzie Brown, "Modes of Perfected Living in the *Mahābhārata* and the Purāṇas: The Different Faces of Śuka the Renouncer," in Andrew O. Fort and Patricia Y. Mumme (eds), *Living Liberation in Hindu Thought*, Albany, SUNY Press, 1996, pp. 157–183, also by David Dean Shulman, *The Hungry God, Hindu Tales of Filicide and Devotion*, Chicago, University of Chicago Press, 1993, pp. 108–129, and by Alf Hiltebeitel, *Rethinking the Mahābhārata: A Reader's Guide to the Education of the Dharma King*, Chicago, University of Chicago Press, 2001, pp. 279–312.

17 There is a full discussion of this passage on pp. 339–43 of E. W. Hopkins, "Yoga-technique in the Great Epic," *JAOS*, 1901, vol. 22, pp. 333–379.

2

PRACTICE MAKES PERFECT

The role of practice (*abhyāsa*) in Pātañjala yoga[1]

David Carpenter

Introduction

In the *Yoga Sūtra* Patañjali describes the practice of yoga as *abhyāsa*, which literally means repetition. Though we may not often reflect on the fact, the practice of yoga as Patañjali understands it is in an important sense a form of repetitive activity. This is particularly true of what he calls *kriyāyoga* or the yoga of action. Key elements of *kriyāyoga* involve specific forms of repetition, and a strong case can be made for the importance of *kriyāyoga* to Patañjali's understanding of yoga as a whole.[2] Forms of repetitive activity are in fact of central importance for Pātañjala yoga, and thus there would seem to be a clear basis for speaking of the practice of yoga, inasmuch as it involves repetition, as a form of ritual.[3] But in an Indian context this sounds odd. Isn't it Brahmanical ritualism with its concerns for dharma that is opposed by the "renunciatory" traditions such as yoga with their concerns for *mokṣa* or *kaivalya*, an opposition reflected in the aloof *puruṣa* standing apart from the captivating activities of *prakṛti*? Certainly there is much evidence to suggest that such an opposition was indeed operative at different points in India's past, but how appropriate is it when applied to Pātañjala yoga? I think that an examination of Patañjali's understanding of practice in general as *abhyāsa*, and the specific practices involved in what he calls *kriyāyoga*, when combined with a consideration of Patañjali's likely historical context, may shed some helpful light on this question.

In the first part of this essay I will examine each of the three practices constitutive of *kriyāyoga*, which Patañjali defines in the first sūtra of the *Sādhanapāda* as consisting of *tapas* or asceticism, *svādhyāya* or personal recitation, and *Īśvarapraṇidhāna* or fixing one's mind upon the Īśvara.[4] These practices will be considered in the light of Patañjali's notions of practice as *abhyāsa* and the closely connected virtue of *vairāgya* or dispassion. In the *Samādhipāda* Patañjali tells us that the goal of yoga is the attainment of the condition of *nirodha*, or the cessation of the fluctuations of the mind, and that this requires two things: *abhyāsa* or repeated practice, and *vairāgya* or "dispassion." The three specific practices of *kriyāyoga* in fact concretize what is meant by *abhyāsa* and *vairāgya*. *Tapas* is a means for the cultivation of the necessary virtue of dispassion, *vairāgya*. *Svādhyāya* and *Īśvarapraṇidhāna* are specific instances of what Patañjali means by *abhyāsa*, which he defines (at YS 1.13) as effort applied to the maintenance of mental calm or stability (*sthiti*). Thus *abhyāsa* and *vairāgya*, as embodied in the three practices of *kriyāyoga*, are key to understanding yoga's transformative potential. In particular, *abhyāsa* or repetition generally may be seen as productive of the dispositions (*saṃskāras*) that in large part determine the quality of mental life. These *saṃskāras* or dispositions, depending on their type, may be either the source of mental agitation or the key to its removal. Repetition in the strict sense of spiritual practice, as the repeated effort (*yatna*) to achieve and maintain a condition of calm, is productive of the type of dispositions that make this state of calm an enduring quality or virtue of the body–mind. The cultivation of such dispositions through practice in turn makes possible states of *samādhi* or mental unification, and the repeated achievement of such states of *samādhi* leads ultimately to the state of *nirodha* and makes possible the experience of liberation (*kaivalya*) through insight into one's true nature. Repetition and the dispositions that it creates thus seem to lie at the heart of the practice of yoga as Patañjali presents it.

Later in the essay I will ask whether this notion of spiritual practice as repetition aimed at the construction of *saṃskāras* might not provide a link between the concerns of the renunciatory traditions of which yoga was in some way a part, and the traditional concerns of the Brahmanical householder. Specifically I will ask whether the goals of social formation and spiritual formation, while distinct, might not share some common ground, namely the positive valuation of the temporal process of repetition required by the formative process itself, as an essentially ritual process aimed at the construction of *saṃskāras* through repeated practice. The process of formative action, or repetitive actions as formative, is essential to the concept of *saṃskāra*, and might help us relate the *saṃskāras* cultivated by the *yogī* to the well-known *saṃskāras* that structure the life of the householder. In the light of what we know about Patañjali's most likely social and historical context it becomes possible to imagine Patañjali's *yogī* not as someone who simply stands in opposition to the householder, but as someone who himself has much in common with the householder's own religious practice, who understands the participation in the traditional *saṃskāras* of the householder as the foundation for the cultivation of the liberative *saṃskāras* of the *yogī*.

Kriyāyoga

Patañjali introduces his notion of *kriyāyoga*, the yoga of action or the yoga of performance, at the beginning of the second book of his *Yoga Sūtra*, the *Sādhanapāda*, or book on spiritual practice. In explaining the transition from the first book or *Samādhipāda*, in which the yoga of the recollected or concentrated mind (*samāhitacitta*) had been the focus, Vyāsa tells us that the present book will explain how yoga applies to the agitated mind (*vyutthitacitta*).[5] The purpose of yogic *sādhana*, then, is the transformation of the mind that is *vyutthita* into one that is *samāhita*, from a mind that is agitated or excited, scattered or distracted, into one that is calm and collected, concentrated and one-pointed, a mind in which all mental fluctuations (*vṛttis*) have ceased.

The initial means for effecting this transformation are the three practices involved in *kriyāyoga*. Patañjali explains the goal of each of these three practices at 2.43–45. Specifically, the perfection (*siddhi*) of the body and the senses comes from *tapas*, which destroys impurity (*aśuddhi*) (2.43),[6] contact with one's chosen deity comes from *svādhyāya* (2.44),[7] and the attainment of *samādhi* comes from *Īśvarapraṇidhāna* (2.45).[8] Before considering each of these practices separately, it is worth noting that this particular list of practices resembles other such lists found elsewhere in Patañjali and in Vyāsa's commentary. Thus, at 4.1 we find *mantra* (an important content of *svādhyāya*), *tapas* and *samādhi* (the goal of *Īśvarapraṇidhāna*) listed as three of the five sources of spiritual attainments (*siddhis*).[9] This sequence of *mantra*, *tapas* and *samādhi* is repeated by Vyāsa in his commentary on 4.6, as sources of the "created minds" (*nirmāṇacittāni*) of the *yogī*. It appears again in Vyāsa's comment on 4.7, where Patañjali speaks of the *yogī*'s action as being neither black nor white and thus implicitly divides action into four types: black, black and white, white, and neither black-nor-white. "White" actions, says Vyāsa, belong to those who are possessed of *tapas*, *svādhyāya* and *dhyāna*. It is action that is directed to the *manas* alone, is independent of external means, and does not harm others.[10] Here we find *mantra* rather than *svādhyāya*, and *dhyāna* rather than *samādhi*, but in each case the two terms are closely related. Finally, Vyāsa's comment here can be compared to his comment on 2.12, which addresses the ripening of *karma*. Here Vyāsa says that meritorious *karma* can be produced by *mantras*, *tapas* or *samādhi*, as well as by worship of great powers such as Īśvara, *devatās*, and *mahārṣis*.[11]

The practice of *tapas* is common to all of these lists. But the close connections between *mantra* and *svādhyāya*, and between *samādhi* and *Īśvarapraṇidhāna*, are worth noting as well. Thus beyond the explicit formulation of *kriyāyoga* there seems to be a more generalized notion of a threefold approach to spiritual practice, involving asceticism, some methodic use of sacred speech (*mantra*, *svādhyāya*), and the cultivation of meditative states (*dhyāna*, *samādhi*), sometimes through a focus on a divine being. One thing that I will want to emphasize is that this threefold model is not unique to the *Yoga Sūtra*, but is basic to Brahmanical spiritual practice as a whole.[12] This will become more clear as we proceed. At present, it is clear that spiritual practice as understood here involves the purification both of the body and the mind (*citta*), and that such purification is a means of generating merit and cultivating *samādhi*. This dual aim of purification and *samādhi* is made explicit. Directly after introducing his concept of *kriyāyoga*, Patañjali tells us that its purpose is to cultivate *samādhi* and to weaken the *kleśas* or defilements.[13] Let us now look at each of the three practices constitutive of *kriyāyoga* in more detail, beginning with *tapas*.

Tapas

Patañjali's own direct comments on *tapas* are limited to four *sūtras* (2.1, 2.32, 2.43 and 4.1). Three of these classify it among other related practices: as a component of *kriyāyoga*, as one of the five *niyamas*, and as one of the five sources of *siddhis*. Only at 2.43 does he describe its purpose, which is the destruction of impurity and the perfection of the body and the senses. For more detail we must turn to Vyāsa.

Vyāsa expands upon the role of *tapas* in purification. Commenting on 2.1 he says that without *tapas* yoga is not successful. Without *tapas* there is no destruction of impurity, namely the various subliminal impressions (*vāsanās*) that result from *karma* and cognitive and affective defilements (*kleśas*). The purpose (*upādāna*) of *tapas* is thus the destruction of such impurity.[14] By its means an unobstructed (*abādhyamāna*) clarity of thought (*cittaprasādana*) is to be cultivated.[15]

Vyāsa's most expansive description of *tapas* is found in his commentary on the five *niyamas*. *Tapas*, he tells us, is the patient endurance of the pairs of opposites (*dvandvasahanam*), such as hunger and thirst, cold and heat, standing and sitting, absence of all expression and absence of speech.[16] He adds that *tapas* can also involve the performance of vows: "According to the situation there are also vows (*vrata*): painful vows, lunar vows and heating vows."[17] Here Vyāsa is referring to the different vows prescribed for various offenses in the Dharma Sūtras and Dharma Śāstras, primarily forms of fasting.

Vyāsa's comments on 2.43 add little to what Patañjali himself says. *Tapas* purifies the body and the senses by removing the "covering" (*āvaraṇa*) of impurity, thus making possible the perfection of the body and senses, and the attendant powers, such as seeing or hearing at a distance. More significant is his comment on 2.52, where the repeated practice (*abhyāsa*) of the restraint of breath, *prāṇāyama*, is presented as the means for destroying the *karma* that covers over discriminative knowledge.[18] Vyāsa ends his comment by quoting a saying to the effect that there is no *tapas* higher than *prāṇāyāma*, a view found also in the Dharma literature.[19] From it comes purity from defilement (*viśuddhir malānāṃ*) and the light of knowledge (*dīptiś ca jñānasya*).[20]

Finally it is worth noting that Vyāsa also lists *tapas* as one of the means for firmly establishing repeated practice (*abhyāsa*). This recalls Patañjali's own linking of *abhyāsa* with the virtue of *vairāgya* or dispassion. Commenting on 1.14, Vyāsa says that repeated practice is accomplished, given due care and provided with a firm foundation through *tapas*, *brahmacarya* (one of Patañjali's *yamas*), *vidyā* and *śraddhā*.[21] Clearly the repeated practice of *tapas*, as an ascetic restraint of the body, is related here to the cultivation of an attitude of dispassion or detachment (*vairāgya*), without which effective practice for Patañjali is impossible. The two cannot be simply equated, however, since the value of *vairāgya* entails an overall detachment from the world that is not necessarily implied in the practice of *tapas*. I will return to this contrast in meaning below.

As regards their view of *tapas* itself as a means of purification, however, it is clear that Patañjali and Vyāsa are here well rooted in the Brahmanical tradition. As early as the Brāhmaṇas *tapas* was recognized as a vital form of ascetic purification voluntarily undertaken by the *yajamāna* as part of his *dīkṣā* or preparation for the sacrifice.[22] The ascetic life was also prescribed for the entire period of Vedic studentship, a state known of course as *brahmacarya*, one of Patañjali's five *yamas*, and for the life of the forest hermit, or *vānaprastha*, who entered a kind of permanent *dīkṣā* or consecration. It is also worth noting that *tapas* is frequently associated, in the *Mahābhārata*, with both *brahmacarya* and *svādhyāya*. Thus it would appear that Patañjali's notion of asceticism as a component of *kriyāyoga* has much in common with the traditional practice of the young *brahmacārin* and his older counterpart, a kind of permanent student, the *vānaprastha*. This will become increasingly clear as we now turn to Patañjali's discussion of *svādhyāya*.

Svādhyāya

Patañjali mentions *svādhyāya* three times in his *sūtras*, at 2.1, 2.32 and 2.44, and refers to the practice of *japa* once, at 1.28. In his commentary on 2.1, where Patañjali introduces *svādhyāya* as a part of *kriyāyoga*, Vyāsa defines *svādhyāya* as the "chanting (*japa*) of purifying prayers such as the syllable *Oṃ* or the going over (*adhyayana*) of treatises on spiritual liberation,"[23] a definition that he repeats in commenting on 2.32, where Patañjali lists *svādhyāya* as one of the five *niyamas*. The first part of this definition, which defines *svādhyāya* in terms of *japa*, borrows a phrase commonly found in the Dharma Śāstras: *pavitrāṇi japet*, "let him chant purifying texts."[24] Such a purifying chant was a basic part of the Brahman householder's religious obligations. Even "treatises on spiritual liberation," if we can accept the *Upaniṣads* as such, had already been recognized as such purifying texts. The term *adhyayana* used here comes from the verbal root *adhy-i*, noted above in connection with the memorization of the Veda, and means to turn something over in the mind repeatedly, to recite something until it is memorized. Thus it seems clear that, at least on Vyāsa's reading, Patañjali's understanding of *svādhyāya* shares many of the features of the practice as known within the Brahmanical traditions of his time.

Patañjali nowhere describes the actual practice of *svādhyāya* in detail, and Vyāsa's comments are quite brief. Later commentators such as Vācaspati Miśra and Vijñānabhikṣu do not comment on *svādhyāya* at all, saying that its meaning is obvious. It seems clear why. Like *tapas*, *svādhyāya* was an integral part of the religious practice of the typical post-Vedic Brahman householder. Both were a part of the assumed context of any serious spiritual practice. For a better understanding of *svādhyāya*, and the closely associated practice of *japa*, then, we must look to the broader Brahminical tradition.

In its original Vedic context, the practice of *svādhyāya* was the recitation (*adhyāya*) on the part of an individual (*sva*, "own") of a Vedic text. The practice dates back to a very early period and was central to the education of a young Brahman or *brahmacārin*. Literally years were spent "going over" (*adhy-i*, to go over, learn by heart) the version of the Vedic compositions used by the *brahmacārin*'s family until they were known by heart. The practice of *svādhyāya* was thus initially a process of memorization. In this oral tradition, one "became" the Veda by committing it to memory.

As early as the Śathapatha Brāhmaṇa the *svādhyāya* developed into an important religious practice in and of itself, which was to be performed not only by the young Brahman student but also by the adult Brahman householder. Here previously memorized texts were recited daily in a practice that came to be seen as equal to, and in some cases even superior to, the actual performance of the Vedic sacrifices.[25] *Svādhyāya* itself came to be thought of as a form of sacrifice, and was known as *brahmayajña*, the "sacrifice of and to brahman," *brahman* here referring to the sacred and powerful speech of the Veda itself and to its ultimate source, the god Prajāpati, counterpart of the Ṛg Vedic *Puruṣa*. With or without the external performance of the sacrificial ritual one identified one's self (*ātman*) with Prajāpati, through the *incorporation* – first by memorization and then by recitation – of the *language* of the sacrifice, the Veda, which was itself *brahman*. Through the ritual repetition of the *svādhyāya* one became an *ātmayājī*, a sacrificer to the self rather than a sacrificer to the gods (*devayājī*), and acquired a body made of the Vedic hymns themselves, and with this new body one passed to the heavenly world.[26] Significantly, as described in Taittirīya Āraṇyaka 2.11.1–8, the *svādhyāya* was always to begin with the chanting of the syllable *Oṃ*, followed by the three *vyāhṛtis* and the Gāyatrī verse. The sacred syllable *Oṃ* symbolized the totality of the Vedic corpus with which one identified oneself through assimilating its language, the *brahman*, in the *svādhyāya*. Thus in the Baudhāyana Dharma Sūtra we read that the Vedic renouncer, the *saṃnyāsī*, should continue to recite (*japet*) the Vedic *mantras* used in the Agnihotra, and, according to a verse that Baudhāyana cites, remain silent except during the *svādhyāya*. He abides at the root of the tree that is the Veda, itself rooted in the syllable *Oṃ*: "The syllable *Oṃ* is the quintessence of the Veda. Prajāpati has declared: 'Meditating on *Oṃ*, containing *Oṃ* within himself, he becomes fit for becoming Brahman.' "[27] As in the outward performance of the sacrifice one became identified with the god Prajāpati through identification with the sacrifice, one here becomes identified with *brahman* through identification with the language of the Veda.[28] Charles Malamoud has noted that in this unification of the sacrificer with the Veda through the *svādhyāya* we have the model for what will later, in the *Upaniṣads*, be the unity of *ātman* and *brahman*.[29] What is most striking here is that this identification is brought about by a ritual process, the process of memorization and recitation.

Svādhyāya was closely associated with the asceticism (*tapas*) that we have discussed above. The two terms are found in compound (*tapaḥsvādhyāya*, *svādhyāyatapas*) in the *Mahābhārata*,[30] just as we find them associated in Patañjali's description of *kriyāyoga*. In particular the practice of *svādhyāya* came to be associated with "highest tapas" (*paraṃ tapas*), namely the restraint of the breath (*prāṇāyāma*). In a verse found both in a late section of the *Baudhāyana Dharma Sūtra* (4.1.22) and in the *Vasiṣṭha Dharma Sūtra* (25.4) the practice of *svādhyāya* is to be undertaken with controlled breath: "Seated with purificatory grass in hand, he should control his breath and recite the purificatory texts, the *vyāhṛtis*, the syllable *Oṃ*, and the daily portion of the Veda."[31] Indeed in a verse found slightly later in these same two texts (at 4.1.28 and 25.13 respectively) *prāṇāyāma* is *defined* as reciting of *Oṃ*, the *vyāhṛtis* and the Gāyatrī three times "while controlling the breath" (*āyataprāṇa*).[32]

Closely associated with the *svādhyāya* is the practice of *japa*, the chanting of *mantras* or prayers in a low voice. The verb *jap* is quite common in the Brāhmaṇas, referring to the low muttering of the priest in the course of the sacrifice. In the Kalpasūtras, according to Renou, *japa* appears as a technical term for the recitation of *Oṃ* and the *vyāhṛtis*.[33] The term is clearly used this way in the Dharma Sūtras and Śāstras,[34] and this of course brings it into close association with the *svādhyāya*, which always begins in this way, as do the morning and evening devotions (*saṃdhyā*) which were the daily duty of every Brahmin. Thus in describing the proper way to begin Vedic recitation Manu (2.74ff) refers to the chanting of the opening *Oṃ*, *vyāhṛtis* and Gāyatrī as *japa*, meaning that these were to be chanted in a low voice. But *japa* could also extend the recitation of a much broader group of texts, much like the *svādhyāya*. This is made clear in the Dharma Sūtras, when *japa*, along with *tapas*, is presented as a prominent form of penance. In this context, *japa* involves the recitation of purificatory texts (*pāvanāni*). These texts are enumerated in very similar terms in three of the four extant Dharma Sūtras. All three lists have in common the *Upaniṣads*, the conclusions of the Vedas (*vedānta*, however this is to be construed), the hymn collections of all the Vedas (*sarvacchandaḥsu saṃhitā*), the "Honey" verses (RV 1.90.6–8), the Aghamarṣaṇa hymn (RV 10.190), the Atharvaśiras, the Rudra hymn, the Puruṣasūkta (RV 10.90), the Rājana and Rauhiṇi Sāmans (SV 1.318 = RV 7.27.1), the Kūṣmāṇḍa verses (TA 2.3), the Pāvamānī verses, and of course the Sāvitrī.[35] Similarly, in the *Jāpakopākhyāna* or account of the *jāpaka* in the *Mokṣadharma* of the *Mahābhārata* (MBh 12.189–193), Bhiṣma recommends the recitation of a *saṃhitā*, a suitable text, which may or not refer to a Vedic *saṃhitā*, but clearly seems to indicate something more than *Oṃ*, the *vyāhṛtis* and Gāyatrī.[36] It would seem, then, that the practice of *japa*, like the practice of *svādhyāya*, involved a wide variety of texts, including, significantly, the *Upaniṣads*. At the same time, just as *japa* could consist only of chanting *Oṃ*, the *vyāhṛtis* and Gāyatrī, there is evident in the Dharma literature a tendency to abbreviate the *svādhyāya*. At *Baudhāyana Dharma Sūtra* 2.11.6 the Brahmin is told to do the *svādhyāya* every day even if it is just reciting the syllable *Oṃ*, symbolically identical with the entire Veda and thus with *brahman*. Thus the full practice of the *svādhyāya* could be condensed into the recitation of the single syllable *Oṃ*. Whether a single syllable or a more extensive text, *japa* and *svādhyāya* were obviously closely associated and in some contexts probably identical (when recitation was done silently or in a low voice). As we have seen, this close association of the two terms is precisely what we find in the *Yoga Sūtra*, especially as interpreted by Vyāsa.

Just as the *svādhyāya* is described as the "sacrifice to *brahman*" so *japa* is described as a sacrifice, the "sacrifice consisting of *japa*" (*japayajña*),[37] which is elevated in the *Bhagavadgītā* as the best of all sacrifices,[38] reminescent of the status given to *svādhyāya* in the Dharma Sūtras as a "great sacrifice" (*mahāyajña*). The practice of *japa* also reveals the clear process of the interiorization of the sacrifice also at work in the development of the *svādhyāya*. *Japa per se* is performed in a low voice rather than out loud. But, more importantly, the *japayajña* is considered to be ten times better than an outward sacrifice on an animal, just as the *svādhyāya*, as the "sacrifice of *brahman*," is sometimes said to be superior to external sacrifice. When *japa* is done silently, it is said to be one hundred times more valuable than an outward sacrifice, and when it is entirely mental it is a thousand times better.[39] This tendency to attribute higher value to silent or mental recitation is a general characteristic of the Dharma literature generally. It is interesting to note that while the *svādhyāya*, unlike *japa*, was typically done aloud, it too could be done silently, as in the case of the *vānaprastha* who has withdrawn from the life of the village.[40]

Japa, like *svādhyāya*, is a form of *tapas*, involving the control of breath (*prāṇāyāma*), and is an important means of purification.[41] This is particularly clear in the eleventh chapter of Manu, where the practice of *japa* accompanied by *prāṇāyāma* is frequently mentioned as a form of penance. This conjunction of *prāṇāyāma* with recitation as a means of purification is in fact a commonplace in the Dharma literature. Also prominent is the value attributed to repeated recitation of single texts. As a source of purification the Sāvitrī verse in particular is often to be recited as many as one thousand times.[42] Baudhāyana prescribes the recitation of an entire Vedic *saṃhitā* once, twelves times, or multiples of twelve, up to a thousand. "Should he recite the Vedic Collection one thousand times without eating, becoming Brahman and free from stain, he becomes Brahman."[43]

Finally, one more aspect of the practice of both *japa* and *svādhyāya* is particularly important for understanding their role in the *Yoga Sūtra*, and that is that these practices are to be performed in a state of mental concentration. The Brahmin, while performing his ritual duties, is to be in a recollected or concentrated state (*samāhita*).[44] Being in a state of mental concentration is a prerequisite for the practice of *japa*.[45] The householder should be always intent (*nityayukta*) upon the *svādhyāya*,[46] and upon *Oṃ* and the *vyāhṛtis*.[47] In the *Mokṣadharma* we read that the sage should keep his mind one-pointed (*ekāgram*), joined to *svādhyāya* (*svādhyāyasaṃśliṣṭam*).[48] Occasionally, especially in the late portions of the Dharma Sūtras and in Manu, we find explicit references to the practice of yoga (though of course these should not be simply equated with Pātañjala yoga). Thus a passage found in the late sections of both Baudhāyana and Vasiṣṭha, which discusses the practice of recitation, especially of *Oṃ* and the *vyāhṛtis*, we read: "By yoga one obtains knowledge. Yoga is the mark of the Law (*dharma*). All good qualities are rooted in yoga. Therefore, one should constantly practise yogic practice (*yuktaḥ sadā bhavet*)."[49] Āpastamba also recommends yogic practices to the Brahmin, both as a means of self-knowledge and for the eradication of faults.[50] In describing the practice of the ascetic or *yati*, Manu prescribes not only yoga in general as a means for meditating on the supreme soul and destroying defilements, but also the specific practices of *dhāraṇa*, *pratyāhāra* and *dhyāna*, which of course are key practices in Patañjali's system.[51]

The practices of *svādhyāya* and *japa*, then, each understood as a form of *tapas* and as involving the practice of controlling the breath (*prāṇāyāma*) and concentrating the mind, were central religious practices in the

Brahmanical world of the post-Vedic period. It is these well-established practices that Patañjali has incorporated into his system of yoga.

At 2.44 Patañjali describes the *result* of the practice of *svādhyāya* as "communion with one's chosen divinity."[52] Commenting on this *sūtra* Vyāsa says: "one who is accustomed to the practice of *svādhyāya* sees the gods, seers and realized beings."[53] Thus the purification of the mind (*citta*) facilitated by *svādhyāya* and related *niyamas* would appear to facilitate a type of visionary experience. To fully appreciate this aspect of *svādhyāya* in Pātañjala yoga we need to look closely at the discussion of *japa* in the first book of the *Yoga Sūtra*, which also leads us to a discussion of the third component of *kriyāyoga* as well, namely, *Īśvarapraṇidhāna*.

Īśvarapraṇidhāna

At 1.23 Patañjali tells us that *Īśvarapraṇidhāna*, "fixing one's attention upon the Lord (Īśvara)" is one of the means for attaining the state of contemplative calm or *samādhi*, a point he also makes clearly in his sūtra explaining *Īśvarapraṇidhāna* as a component of *kriyāyoga*, at 2.45.[54] This association of *Īśvarapraṇidhāna* and *samādhi* has also been noted above, through the implication of references to *mantra*, *tapas* and *samādhi*. After describing the nature of Īśvara in 1.24–26 Patañjali tells us first, at 1.27, that Īśvara is expressed by the *praṇavaḥ* or syllable *Oṃ*,[55] and consequently (1.28) that through the chanting (*japa*) of that syllable its meaning (Īśvara) becomes manifest.[56] Vyāsa explains that the *yogī* who practices in this way attains a single-pointed mind (*cittam ekāgram*), or in other words attains *samādhi*, and ends his comment on the *sūtra* by citing a verse from *Viṣṇu Purāṇa* 6.6.2: "After *svādhyāya* let him abide in yoga; after yoga, he abides in *svādhyāya*. Through the fulfillment of *svādhyāya* and yoga the supreme *Ātman* shines forth."[57] Patañjali's next *sūtra* provides further information on the results of this practice: "From it comes the attainment of interiority and the absence of obstacles" (1.29).[58] Vyāsa defines interiority here as seeing one's own self (*svarūpadarśanam*), which echoes the verse just quoted. As for the obstacles, these "distractions" or "perplexities" of the mind (*cittavikṣepas*) are listed at 1.30–31, and include sickness, idleness, doubt, negligence, sloth, dissipation, confused vision, non-attainment of a basis in yoga and restlessness,[59] and are accompanied by suffering, despair, unsteadiness of the limbs, and irregular breathing.[60] Finally, as a kind of concluding statement, we are told that repetitive practice (*abhyāsa*) focused on a single reality (*ekatattva*), in this context clearly the repetition of the syllable *Oṃ* as a means of fixing one's mind upon Īśvara, is intended for the prevention of these problems.[61]

The practice of *Īśvarapraṇidhāna* is thus explained in terms of the practice of *svādhyāya*, and more specifically in terms of the practice of *japa*, focused on the syllable *Oṃ*, which, as Lloyd Pflueger has well said, in discussing this practice, "carries the whole Indian tradition on its back."[62] Its purpose is expressly stated to be the cultivation of *samādhi*. Although Vyāsa tends to give *Īśvarapraṇidhāna* a devotional cast, Pflueger has shown that Patañjali's own description of it in the YS focuses more on practice (*abhyāsa*) than on piety.[63] It is perhaps significant that the term *praṇidhāna* itself is most familiar in a Buddhist context, where it refers to a firm resolve or aspiration on the part of a bodhisattva to attain the supreme perfect enlightenment of a Buddha.[64] It is much less common to earlier Brahmanical literature, appearing only three times in the *Mahābhārata*, for instance, and not at all in the Dharma Sūtras or in Manu.[65] As Pflueger has noted, the use of the term in the *Yoga Sūtra* is in fact very close to the Buddhist meaning.[66] Just as the bodhisattva's *praṇidhāna* places him or her on the path to Buddhahood, so the yogī's practice of *Īśvara-praṇidhāna* conduces to the achievement of *samādhi*.

Given the centrality of the crucial concept of *abhyāsa* or repeated spiritual practice both to *svādhyāya* and to *Īśvarapraṇidhāna*, let us now examine it closely, along with the closely associated notion of dispassion (*vairāgya*).

Abhyāsa and *vairāgya*

As we have seen, Patañjali's most general statement on the nature of spiritual practice is that it aims at the cessation of the various disturbances or "turnings" (*vṛttis*) of the mind (*citta*) through repeated practice (*abhyāsa*) and dispassion (*vairāgya*).[67] What is most striking about this formulation, at least in the present context, is that the *cessation of the activity* of the *citta* is said to derive from a form of *activity*. Repeated practice, repetitive activity, leads beyond activity. Thus the key to the cessation of action is action itself, properly carried out. This formulation of the essential nature of spiritual practice is not unique to the *Yoga Sūtra*. It is found, in precisely these terms, in the *Bhagavadgītā* as well, at 6.35, where Kṛṣṇa tells Arjuna that the mind, while unsteady, can be grasped by practice and dispassion (*abhyāsena ... vairāgyeṇa ca gṛhyate*).[68] In Patañjali's formulation what is needed is the gradual reduction of the activities or processes (*vṛttis*) which occur in the mind complex (*citta*) due to the influence of subliminal dispositions (*saṃskāras*) and habit-patterns (*vāsanās*) laid down in that mind-complex by its own earlier activities. Mental life is made up largely of the interplay of mental processes or *vṛttis* (which Patañjali classifies in five types: valid cognition, false knowledge, conceptualization, sleep and memory),[69] which in turn are, to a large extent, manifestations of the accumulated *samskāras* and *vāsanās* which are collectively known as one's "karmic stockpile" (*karmāśaya*). The interactions between conscious thoughts and emotions and subliminal dispositions which are their "seed" (*bija*) constitute a reciprocal process that knows no beginning. The practice of yoga aims at the gradual attenuation of this karmic burden and eventual spiritual release through a different kind of activity and the different type of *saṃskāras* that result from it. Through a process of mind–body purification one aspires to enhance the reflectivity of the "material" components of the mind-complex to such a degree that, by way of its reflection in the mirror of the *buddhi*, free from all distortions introduced by the dispersive activities (*vṛttis*) of the senses, emotions and thoughts, the Spirit might recognize itself as Spirit. It is repeated practice (*abhyāsa*) and ascetic detachment (*vairāgya*) that help bring this about. But how?

In order to answer this question we need to look more carefully at Patañjali's understanding of *abhyāsa* and *vairāgya*. Vyāsa's commentary on 1.12 employs the image of the two steams of the mind, flowing in opposite directions. One stream flows towards the good and one towards evil; one tends towards the state of spiritual liberation (*kaivalya*) and the other towards *saṃsāra*.[70] Using this image, then, *vairāgya* "dries up" the stream flowing out into the world of *saṃsāra* while *abhyāsa* opens up the stream flowing towards liberation. Both are necessary.[71] Let us look first at *vairāgya*.

Vairāgya

Patañjali defines *vairāgya* as referring to the mastery over the thirst for objects that are seen and heard (1.15), and adds that beyond this there is the state of complete absence of thirst for the *guṇas* themselves, i.e. from material nature or *prakṛti* as a whole, that results from the discriminative knowledge of *Puruṣa* or Spirit (1.16). This higher state of *vairāgya* is virtually equivalent to *kaivalya*, the ultimate goal of yoga practice, the state of spiritual liberation. As for the "lower" *vairāgya*, it of course literally refers to the absence of *rāga* or passion, hence the quite literal translation "dispassion," or what the Stoics called *apatheia*. Vyāsa gives a rather long-winded definition of *vairāgya* which runs as follows.

Dispassion is a technical term[72] for the mastery which is empty of what is to be rejected and what is to be acquired, has the essential character of impassibility (*anābhoga*), and comes from the power of meditation to the mind which is free of thirst for visible things, such as women, food and drink, and power, which is free of thirst for things that have been reported, such as the attainment of heaven, a disembodied state or absorption in *prakṛti*, and which, even when in contact with divine and worldly things, sees their faults.[73]

The affinity between *vairāgya* so defined and the practice of *tapas* is clear. We have seen that *tapas* involves precisely detachment from women (*brahmacarya*) and food (the various *vratas*). It also involves detachment from the pairs of opposites, such as here, what is to be rejected and what is to be acquired. But whereas *tapas* is a term closely associated with Vedic ritual and the values of early Brahmanical society, the term *vairāgya* is of a different provenance.[74] It is not found in the early Vedic literature, and only appears once in the classical *Upaniṣads* (at Maitri Upaniṣad 1.2). Nor does it appear in the Dharma Sūtras and Dharma Śāstras. And while it appears ten times in the *Mahābhārata*, in each instance this is in sections that are recognized as quite late.[75] Unlike the term *tapas*, then, the Vedic pedigree of which is beyond doubt, the term *vairāgya* seems to derive originally from the non-Vedic context of the renouncers. The term *vitṛṣṇa*, which Patañjali uses to define it, recalls the Buddhist use of the term *tṛṣṇa* or thirst (not to mention the term *rāga*) in a very similar context, i.e. as being the cause of suffering. And just as the Buddhist seeks liberation from *saṃsāra* through the cessation (*nirodha*) of *tṛṣṇa* or *rāga*, which is *nirvāṇa*, so the *yogī* seeks liberation from *prakṛtic* existence through the same means, the complete absence of *tṛṣṇa* or *rāga* in the higher *vairāgya* which is *kaivalya*.

A non-Vedic context also seems to be indicated by Vyāsa's use of the term *anābhoga* in his comment on 1.12. I have translated this term as "impassibility," following Sylvain Lévi. [76] The term does not seem to appear in classical Sanskrit, but it is frequent in the *Mahāyānasūtrālaṃkāra*, a Yogācāra Buddhist text. Lévi translates it in that text as "impassibility" and notes that at *Mahāyānasūtrālaṃkāra* 20.16 it is used to gloss *upekṣaka*, "apathy."[77] This recalls Patañjali's use of the term *upekṣa* in 1.33 and (implicitly) at 3.23, where he is clearly being inspired by Buddhist sources. Woods takes the use of the term *anābhoga* here as further evidence of the close connection between Patañjali (or at least Vyāsa) and the Mahāyāna.[78]

Thus while there is certainly an affinity between the concepts of *tapas* and *vairāgya*, they originally belonged to different worlds. *Tapas*, as ascetic practice aimed at generating innner heat, is central to Vedic ritualism, whereas *vairāgya* as a dispassionate attitude toward the world as a whole, is central to renunciatory traditions and their associated spiritual practices. The fact that Patañjali brings them together is, I believe, highly significant. More will be said about this in due course.

For Patañjali, just as *tapas* goes hand in hand with *svādhyāya* and *Īśvarapraṇidhāna*, so *vairāgya* itself goes hand in hand with *abhyāsa*. It is now time to look more closely at this concept of *abhyāsa*, and its relations with components of *kriyāyoga*.

Abhyāsa

As noted, the Sanskrit term *abhyāsa* means repetition, and Monier-Williams gives the meanings of repeated or permanent exercise, discipline, use, habit, and custom. In the Dharma Sūtras, as one might expect, the term typically refers to repeated actions generally, the term *karmābhyāsa* being common.[79] Interestingly in Manu, however, the term refers almost exclusively to Vedic recitation, in other words, to *svādhyāya*,[80] and is closely linked with *tapas*.[81] In the *Mahābhārata* its uses are of course many. It can be used to describe Arjuna's practice with the bow under Droṇa's guidance, when he discovers the power of practice to develop lasting skill.[82] It can refer to any learned behavior, cultivated through practice, whether its object is sublime[83] or mundane.[84] It can also refer explicitly to the practice of yoga, *yogābhyāsa*.[85] Especially in the *Bhagavadgītā abhyāsa* takes on a meaning close to what we find in Patañjali. We have already noted the reference to *abhyāsa* and *vairāgya* as the essential means of restraining the mind at 6.35. The meaning of *abhyāsa* as spiritual practice is predominant throughout the *Gītā*, however, as for instance in the compound *abhyāsayoga*.[86] In the twelfth book in particular *abhyāsayoga* or the "discipline of practice" seems to describe a spiritual practice intermediate between external actions and inward contemplation or knowledge, similar perhaps to Vyāsa's notion of "white" action.[87] In the *Gītā abhyāsa* can also refer to the karmic influence of previous actions.[88] Instances of *abhyāsa* referring specifically to spiritual practice are also to be found in the *Mokṣadharma*.[89]

Thus just as the term *vairāgya* begins to appear in the late epic and especially in the *Gītā*, so too does *abhyāsa* in the specific meaning of spiritual practice. This would suggest a degree of similarity in viewpoint between the redactors of the didactic portions of the *Mahābhārata* and the author of the *Yoga Sūtra*, a point to which we will return.

In the *Yoga Sūtra abhyāsa* has a meaning very close to that of the Gītā, but it is now presented with a psychological sophistication lacking in the latter text. As we saw at the outset, Patañjali defines *abhyāsa* as effort (*yatna*) expended on behalf of stability or calm (*sthiti*) (1.13). He then adds that practice is firmly grounded when one devotes one's full attention (*satkāra*) to it uninterruptably over a long period of time (1.14). *Abhyāsa* is thus the repeated effort to maintain a state of mental stability which Vyāsa describes, not as a state of stasis, but as a "calm flowing" (*praśāntavāhitā*) of the mind which is without fluctuations (*vṛttis*). Vyāsa further characterizes *abhyāsa* as the performance of the means for the realization of this stability.[90] The performance (*anuṣṭhāna*) of the "means" (*sādhana*) here is clearly a reference to the full practice of yoga as laid out in the second book, the *Sādhanapāda*, and especially the practice of the eight "limbs" of Patañjali's yoga, as is clear from 2.28 as well as Vyāsa's comment on it. The performance of yoga (*yogānuṣṭhāna*), says Patañjali, leads to the destruction of impurity, and Vyāsa elaborates that the more the means (*sādhanāni*) are performed (*anuṣṭhīyante*), the more one weakens impurity,[91] explicitly identifying the means with the eight limbs. As regards practice becoming "firmly grounded," employing a formula found also in the Praśna Upaniṣad,[92] Vyāsa comments that this is accomplished by means of *tapas*, *brahmacarya*, knowledge (*vidyā*) and faith (*śraddhā*), thereby making successful practice dependent upon *tapas* generally and *brahmacarya* specifically.[93] When practice is thus well rooted its object is not easily overcome by "dispersive dispositions" (*vyutthānasaṃskāras*), in other words, one with a firm practice is not easily distracted by old dispersive habit patterns.[94]

An examination of the occurrences of the term *abhyāsa* in the *Yoga Sūtra* and *bhāṣya* reveals a series of increasingly interior practices. On the most external level, *abhyasa* can refer to the cultivation of the pleasures of the senses themselves (*bhogābhyāsa*), something that is not practice at all in the yogic sense and merely reinforces attachment to sense objects and cannot lead to dispassion.[95] More basic is *abhyāsa* as purification. Thus Vyāsa refers to *abhyāsa*, along with *vairāgya*, as a means for the elimination of spiritual obstacles (*vikṣepas*) which obstruct *samādhi*.[96] The term *abhyāsa* is used to refer to the repeated practice of *prāṇāyāma*, which removes the "covering" (*āvaraṇa*) that obscures true knowledge, and is thus described as the highest form of *tapas*.[97] Nevertheless, once a certain level of mastery is reached, the *yogī* is no longer dependent upon this form of purificatory practice.[98] *Abhyāsa* then moves to a higher level.

At this level we find the repeated practice of *dhyāna* (*dhyānābhyāsa*, 1.48 *bhāṣya*), practice which has some objective support (*sālambana abhyāsa*, 1.18 *bhāṣya*), repeated practice directed to a single entity (*ekatattvābhyāsa*, 1.32). Here there is a clear correlation with the practice of *svādhyāya* and *Īśvarapraṇidhāna*, and with what Vyāsa calls "white" or virtuous action that is largely inward. Finally, at the highest level we find the "repeated practice of the dispositions tending toward cessation" (*nirodhasaṃskārābhyāsa*, 3.10 *bhāṣya*), the "repeated practice of the stopping of thought" (*virāmapratyayābhyāsa*, 1.18), and the "repeated practice of the vision of Puruṣa" (*puruṣadarśanābhyāsa*, 1.16 *bhāṣya*).

Thus just as *kriyāyoga* has as its purpose both the purification of the *citta* from its defilements (*kleśas*) and the cultivation of *samādhi*, so too *vairāgya* and *abhyāsa* begin as a means of purification, as a removal of "obstructions" (*vikṣepas*) and the cultivation of *samadhi*. What for Patañjali is the "lower dispassion" of 1.15 constitutes an initial stage of ascetic detachment and purification that correlates well with the practice of *tapas* as a component of *kriyāyoga*. And the initial stages of *abhyāsa*, what one might call the "lower practice," correlate well, as we have just seen, with the practices of *svādhyāya* and *Īśvarapraṇidhāna*. But the range of *abhyāsa* extends beyond such "lower practice," just as *vairāgya* extends beyond the lower dispassion and *tapas*. At its highest stages *abhyāsa* aims at *nirodha* and the vision of Puruṣa. Ultimately one must learn detachment from *abhyāsa* itself, along with the objects that support it, in order to realize the higher dispassion which is equated with the discernment of

Puruṣa, a state that finally goes beyond practice and constitutes spiritual liberation (*kaivalya*). Thus the spiritual path that Patañjali sets out leads from a lower to a higher dispassion by way of increasingly internalized and unifying forms of practice. Viewed in terms of the components of *kriyāyoga* we might say that the practice of *tapas* lays the foundation for the practice of *svādhyāya*, with which it is frequently associated, and that *svādhyāya* reaches its fulfillment in the specific form of *Īśvarapraṇidhāna* or the continual repetition of the syllable *Oṃ*, which in turn sustains the "cognitive *samādhis*" (*saṃprajñātasamādhis*) that finally make possible the "higher dispassion" that is spiritual liberation itself. We find here, then, in a detailed analysis of Patañjali's uses of the terms *vairāgya* and *abhyāsa*, the same threefold approach to spiritual practice mentioned earlier, namely one that progresses from asceticism, through the methodical and repetitive use of sacred speech, to the cultivation of the meditative state of *samādhi*. At the same time, however, it becomes clear that the range of *abhyāsa* and *vairāgya*, while inclusive of the traditional practices included within *kriyāyoga*, extends beyond them, leading finally to the liberative knowledge of Puruṣa and the state of *kaivalya*.

Saṃskāra

The *Yoga Sūtra* provides a sophisticated picture of the process of gradual purification and unification of the *citta* through sustained practice. The key to this process, in all its stages, is the systematic transformation, through repetition, of the *saṃskāras* or dispositions that determine the quality of mental life. Repeated practice is important, indeed necessary, because it is through such practice that *saṃskāras* can be deliberately modified, making possible a deliberate transformation of the mind. This deliberate construction of *saṃskāras* through repetitive practice (*abhyāsa*) is described as a process of cultivation (*bhāvana*). And it is this deliberate cultivation of the *saṃskāras* that counteracts the afflictive states and prepares the mind for the state of contemplative calm or *samādhi*. Patañjali's understanding of the *saṃskāras* takes us into the heart of his spiritual psychology.

In its early stages the purpose of practice is to restrain the type of mental activities known as "afflicted" (*kliṣṭa*) processes. These processes arise primarily from ignorance (*avidyā*), as well as from the closely associated "vices" of egoism (*āsmitā*), desire (*rāga*), hatred (*dveṣa*) and attachment to life (*abhiniveśa*), the five *kleśas* or "afflictions."[99] Each of these afflicted states of mind produce *saṃskāras* or subliminal dispositions which tend to perpetuate them. The purpose of practice (*abhyāsa*) and ascetic detachment (*vairāgya*) is to modify these dispositions and thus break this self-perpetuating cycle. Through the practice of *kriyāyoga* one purifies the disruptive dispositions latent in the mind, thereby freeing the mind from the influence of the *kleśas* and from the afflictive states that arises from them. Of equal importance, however, are the new dispositions that are cultivated and which prepare the mind for the complete cessation of mental activity (*samādhi*) that will lead to spiritual liberation. This twofold role of the *saṃskāras* in Patañjali is a key to understanding his positive valuation of spiritual practice as requiring repetitive activity.

Vyāsa tells us that the *kleśas* are attenuated through a process known as *pratipakṣabhāvana*, or cultivation of their opposites.[100] Patañjali discusses this process in some detail at 2.33–34, in the context of a discussion of the *yamas* and *niyamas*, of which *kriyāyoga* is a part:

> Negative thoughts are blocked by the cultivation of their opposites. The cultivation of opposites is the realization that negative thoughts such as those of violence, whether done, caused to be done or [merely] approved, whether preceded by desire, anger or delusion and whether slight, moderate or excessive, bear the fruit of endless ignorance and suffering.[101]

The practice of *svādhyāya* in particular would appear to contribute to the attenuation of *kleśas* by planting the mind with the seeds (i.e. *saṃskāras* as specific memory traces) in the form of virtuous ideas found in a variety of traditional religious texts, including undoubtedly in the present context, the *Yoga Sūtra* itself. This internalization of texts and the resultant transformation on the memory is made possible through the repetitive character of the practice as a form of *bhāvana*, which Vācaspati Miśra defines as repeated absorption in the mind.[102] Through such conscious cultivation "afflicted" contents of the mind (the *kleśas*) are countered by the deliberate creation of positive *saṃskāras*, which we might refer to as virtues, and at the same time the dispersive activities of the mind (its *vṛttis*) are restricted by the very process of repetition. Thus *svādhyāya* becomes a means not only for the attenuation of the *kleśas* but also for the cultivation of *samādhi*. Continual repetition leads to one-pointedness of mind.

With the cultivation of calmness through repetition of a particular mental content, whether a memorized text, the single syllable *Oṃ*, or virtually any other object, wisdom arises and with it a special type of *saṃskāra* which Vyāsa refers to as a *prajñākṛtasaṃskāra*, a *saṃskāra* that is produced by wisdom (*prajñā*). Wisdom here is the direct insight into a thing's nature which results from the complete calmness of the mind. Once all conscious mental activity and subconscious coloring of experience has been brought temporarily to a halt the objects of experience appear in the clear, undisturbed mirror of the *buddhi* or intellect as they truly are. This is the state that Patañjali calls *samprajñatasamādhi* or *samādhi* with a specific content. Unlike the dispersive dispositions (*vyutthānasaṃskāras*) produced by normal mental activity, the dispositions produced by the wisdom arising from meditative calm predispose the mind to further states of calm in a process that culminates in the experience of cessation itself, *nirodha*, a state of *samādhi* without object, or *asamprajñatasamādhi*. This state in turn produces a *nirodhasaṃskāra*, a kind of self-annuling disposition that leaves the mind totally without dispositional residue and thereby frees it from all involvement in the activities of *prakṛti*. At this point the culminating insight into the otherness of *prakṛti* and *puruṣa* becomes possible and with it the state of final spiritual liberation (*kaivalya*) which is the ultimate goal of yoga practice.

This twofold status of the *saṃskāras* as both factors of bondage and factors of liberation, which Lakshmi Kapani has called their "ambivalence,"[103] is crucial for appreciating the role of practice in Patañjali's yoga. There is a need for intermediary states of the *citta* between pure distraction and *nirodha*. Before there can be action that is "neither black nor white" there must be the "white" action of those possessed of *tapas*, *svādhyāya* and *dhyāna*,[104] or in other words, of those who practice *kriyāyoga*. There must be *akliṣṭa vṛttis*, i.e. virtuous acts, which give rise to *akliṣṭasaṃkāras*,[105] i.e. pure, sattvic, *saṃskāras* that predispose the mind to the calm of *samādhi* and ultimately *nirodha*. In other words, there must be a level of spiritual culture or practice (*abhyāsa* in the sense of *bhāvana*) that mediates between the realm of suffering and the realm of pure spiritual freedom represented by *kaivalya*, between the realms respectively of Prakṛti and Puruṣa. But the word "culture" can have two meanings. It can refer to the type of cultivation that we have just been discussing. But it can also refer to the broader context in which such practice takes place, to Indian culture, or more specifically to Brahmanical culture. The word *saṃskāra*, referring most basically, as an agent noun, to a process of cultivation or formative action, can function on both of these levels. In particular, this term points us in the direction of some tentative conclusions concerning the possible social location of the practice of Pātañjala yoga in the context of early classical India.

From social formation to spiritual formation and back

The term *saṃskāra* is of course well known outside the context of the tradition of yoga. It is especially prominent in two quite different contexts, namely, Brahmanical ritual and Buddhist psychology.

Although the term *saṃskāra* as such does not appear in the Vedic corpus, its prominence in Brahmanical ritual contexts stems from the prominence of the verb *saṃskṛ* in Vedic literature, and especially in the Brāhmaṇas, where it refers to the process of ritual construction, and has the sense not merely of construction, but of making perfect, and of ritual purification. In the Dharma literature, where we do find the term *saṃskāra*, it refers specifically to the *śarīrasaṃskāras*, or the rites intended to purify or perfect the human body, the so-called Hindu "sacraments," the two most prominent of which are initiation and marriage. Initiation or *upanayana* in particular introduces the male Brahmin child to a period of studentship or *brahmacarya*, which involves many of the same practices and ascetic restrictions that Patañjali prescribes for the practice of *kriyāyoga*: *brahmacarya* in the sense of chastity, *tapas* generally, and the specific practice of *svādhyāya*. As we have seen, there is a deep affinity between the practice of *kriyāyoga* and this aspect of traditional Brahmanical life.

In the context of Buddhism, on the other hand, the connotations of the term *saṃskāra* are quite different. The Pali *saṃkhāra* refers to composite or constructed things, which are equated with the realm of *dukkha* or suffering.[106] The most prominent use of the term is of course in the context of the well-known five aggregates or *skandhas* which include all conditioned existence or *saṃsāra*. The fourth of the aggregates is *saṃskāra*, disposition or "karmic formation," with "formation" being taken in both an active and passive sense, as both the result of action and as the ground out of which future action arises. This understanding of *saṃskāra* as disposition, which played an essential role in the elaboration of Buddhist psychology, is virtually identical to that found in Patañjali. For the Buddhist as for Patañjali, the *saṃskāras* may be sources of distraction and continued suffering, or they may be virtuous dispositions that aid in the ending of suffering.

Thus the term *saṃskāra* can refer both to ritual action and to a psychological disposition. Admittedly Patañjali doesn't use the term in the former sense, but his interpretation of the *kriyāyoga*, comprised for the most part of traditional Brahmanical practices, in terms of *abhyāsa* and *vairāgya*, with their meanings of spiritual practice and renunciation, provides a bridge between the traditional Brahmanical understanding of *saṃskāra* as ritual purification and the understanding of *saṃskāra* as an inner disposition. Indeed, this bridge had already been at least partially built. As we saw, there is a development in the use of the term *abhyāsa* from the Dharma Sūtras to the Dharma Śāstras, from referrring to overt actions in the former to focusing almost exclusively on recitation or *svādhyāya* in the latter. And there is a tendency for the *svādhyāya* itself, and the closely connected practice of *japa*, to be increasingly internalized and associated with states of mental concentration. This development needs to be understood in the context of an important change in Brahmanical culture in the centuries that preceded Patañjali. As I have argued elsewhere,[107] in the course of the transformation of the old Brahmanical ritual system in the late Vedic period *svādhyāya*, as the ritual practice of the learned Brahmin or *śiṣṭa*, took on a new centrality. The memorization and recitation of the Veda and of other sacred texts, in short the pratice of study, came to have an importance for the *smārta* Brahmin analogous to what the *śrauta* system had had for his ancestors. The rituals of the sacrificer were transformed into the rituals of the scholar. The ritual of study was an essential aspect of the Brahmin's fulfillment of dharma, and was sustained by a belief in the dharmic character of correct or *saṃskṛta* speech. Just as the overt actions of the learned Brahmin or *śiṣṭa* were considered authoritative, as *śiṣṭācāra*, so their linguistic practice was also a manifestation of correct form. What we find in Patañjali, in his incorporation of the practice of *svādhyāya,* and *kriyāyoga* generally, into his system of yogic practice, is the further transformation of the rituals and linguistic practices of the scholar into the rituals of the *yogī*.

What Patañjali provided to the new *smārta* ritual of the scholar was an adequate spiritual psychology, one that neither the Brahmanical tradition nor the Sāṃkhya system had provided.[108] Such a psychology would provide a way to link the traditional understanding of the *saṃskāras* as means of purification through conformity to the norms of dharma (through such rites as the *upanayana* or initiation of the Vedic student or *brahmacārin*, and through the correct linguistic practice of the *śiṣṭa* in the *svādhyāya*), with the *saṃskāras* of the inner life, the dispositions of what Patañjali, most probably infuenced by Buddhist usage, calls the *citta*.[109] In doing so it would also create a kind of synthesis between traditional Brahmanical values and those of the renouncers, or between the values and practices involved in social formation and those involved with the spiritual formation of the individual. In doing this he would have been very much the child of his time, as the many parallels between Patañjali and such texts as the late sections of the Dharma Sūtras, the Dharma Śāstras, the epic, and particularly the *Bhagavadgītā*, make plain.

Pātañjala yoga's debt to Buddhist psychology is widely recognized. Indeed, it is precisely the crucial psychological notions of *saṃskāra*, *vāsanā*, *citta*, and *kleśa* that make their appearance first in Buddhist sources and appear to have been appropriated by Patañjali, whether directly or indirectly.[110] By providing the practices of *kriyāyoga*, among them *svādhyāya*, with a psychological rationale Patañjali is able to clarify and accentuate the transformative potential of traditional Brahmanical practices while at the same time placing these practices into a new context of spiritual practice (*abhyāsa*) and renunciation (*vairāgya*). The repetition of the formal norms of Brahmanical society could thus be interpreted as a process of purification that is continuous with rather than opposed to the spiritual practice of the *yogī*. What joins them is the positive value of repeated formative action, gradually internalized, which first socializes and then transforms the agent.

It is well known that the renunciatory tradition of Buddhism became increasingly integrated into the social status quo in such places as South East Asia, Tibet and Japan. The same can be said for the renunciatory traditions within what came to be known as Hinduism. One manifestation of this tendency is the Gītā's presentation of *karmayoga* as a solution to the conflict between renunciation and the demands of the *varṇāśramadharma*. Another, I think, is Patañjali's concept of *kriyāyoga*, which consists of practices that, as we have seen, are in continuity with mainstream post-Vedic Brahmanical practice but also aim at the spiritual goals of *samādhi* and *kaivalya*, to the spiritual realization of the renouncers. *Kriyāyoga*, with its ritual overtones, is not marginal to Patañjali's conception of yoga but central to it. Here I would have to take issue with Georg Feuerstein, who seems to want to distance yoga from any association with ritual. While he rightly rejects the position that *kriyāyoga* is a ritual preliminary to eight-limbed yoga, which would marginalize the practice of *kriyāyoga* in a way that is inconsistent with what Patañjali actually says, he goes further to insist that *tapas*, *svādhyāya* and *Īśvarapraṇidhāna* are not rituals, even though he admits that they were understood in this way (i.e. as rituals) in the preclassical traditions and in later Puranic traditions: "This leads one to conclude that only in the strictly philosophical *yogadarśana* did *tapas*, *svādhyāya* and *Īśvarapraṇidhāna* acquire a non-ritualistic meaning."[111] This opposition of ritual to the "strictly philosophical" is unwarranted. What sense does it make to refer to Patañjali's system of yoga as "strictly philosophical"?[112] Why oppose yoga and ritual in this way? Only due to a modern, and largely Western prejudice against ritual, I suspect. But clearly the purpose of repeated practice in yoga is to create *saṃskāras*, just as the purpose of repeated ritual action is to produce *saṃskāras*. Even though the ultimate goal of yoga is the realization of a reality that transcends the operation of the *saṃskāras*, their systematic cultivation through practice is a necessary means to that end. The *yogī*, by Patañjali's account, is not merely an exception to Brahmanical society but in some ways an exemplification of many of its ideals, though ideals which themselves had been transformed through the influence of the traditions of renunciation. We do not have opposition here, but accommodation, made possible by the common theme of the positive formative role of repeated action.

Notes

1 This essay was first presented as a paper at the annual meeting of the American Academy of Religion in November 2000. I would like to thank Fred Smith who carefully read and commented upon the original draft. I would also like to acknowledge my debt to Peter Schreiner who made available to me his electronic edition of the YS and YB.

2 Indeed, Georg Feuerstein has argued that *kriyāyoga* is the original and most important contribution of Patañjali, and that eight-limbed yoga is an independent tradition that he grafted onto his own *kriyāyoga* when composing the *Yoga Sūtra*. See his *The Yoga-Sūtra of Patañjali: An Exercise in the Methodology of Textual Analysis*, New Delhi, Arnold-Heinemann, 1979, pp. 90–104. Whatever one may make of Feuerstein's argument, it will become

clear as we proceed that *kriyāyoga* is an integral part of the practice of yoga as presented in the *Yoga Sūtra.*

3 The underlying issue here is the relationship between what we call "spiritual practice" and what we call ritual. We tend to use the terms in very different contexts, and describing one in terms of the other can seem odd. This is due in part, I think, to a deficient understanding of the nature of spiritual practice, which precisely as a practice, necessarily shares some common ground with ritual. For an interesting example of this connection, see the discussion of the practice of Zen as a form of ritual by Ronald L.Grimes, "Modes of Zen Ritual," in his *Beginnings in Ritual Studies*, Columbia, SC, University of South Carolina Press, 1995, pp. 104–117.

4 YS 2.1: *tapaḥ-svādhyāyeśvarapraṇidhānāni kriyā-yogaḥ*

5 YB 2.1: *uddiṣṭaḥ samāhita-cittasya yogaḥ / katham vyutthita-citto api yoga-yuktaḥ syād ity etad ārabhyate /.*

6 YS 2.43: *kāyendriyasiddhir aśuddhikṣayāt tapasaḥ.*

7 YS 2.44: *svādhyāyād iṣṭa-devatā-saṃprayogaḥ.*

8 YS 2.44: *samādhi-siddhir īśvara-praṇidhānāt.*

9 YS 4.1: *janmauṣadhimantratapaḥsamādhijāḥ siddhayaḥ.* The other two are previous births and herbs.

10 YB 4.7: *śuklā tapaḥsvādhyāyadhyānavatām / sā hi kevale manasy āyatatvād bahiḥ sādhana-an-adhīnā parān pīḍayitvā bhavati /.*

11 YB 2.12: *tatra tīvrasaṃvegena mantratapaḥsamādhibhir nirvartita īśvarade-vatāmahā-ṛṣi-mahānubhāvānām ārādhanād vā yaḥ pariniṣpannaḥ sa sadyaḥ paripacyate puṇyakarmāśaya iti /.*

12 It might even be worth comparing this sequence with the well-known Christian sequence of purgation, illumination and union.

13 YS 2.2: *samādhibhāvanārthaḥ kleśatanūkaraṇārthaś ca.*

14 YB 2.1: *anādikarmakleśavāsanācitrā pratyupasthitaviṣayajālā cāśuddhir nāntareṇa tapaḥ saṃbhedam āpadyatae iti tapasa upādānam /.*

15 YB 2.1: *tac ca cittaprasādanam abādhyamānam anenāsevyam iti manyate /.*

16 YB 2.32: *tapo dvandvasahanam / dvandvaś ca jighatsāpipāse śītoṣṇe sthānāsane kāṣṭhamaunākāra-maune ca /.*

17 YB 2.32: *vratāni caiṣāṃ yathā-yogaṃ kṛcchra-cāndrāyaṇa-sāṃtapana-ādīni /.*

18 YB 2.52: *prāṇāyāmān abhyasyato asya yoginaḥ kṣīyate vivekajñāna-āvaraṇīyaṃ karma /.*

19 See, for instance, BDS 4.1.23, VaDS 25.5 and Manu 2.83.

20 YB 2 52: *tathā cauktam / tapo na paraṃ prāṇāyāmāt tato viśuddhir malānāṃ dīptiś ca jñānasyaiti.*

21 YB 1.14: *tapasā brahmacaryeṇa vidyayā śraddhayā ca saṃpāditaḥ satkāravān dṛḍhabhūmir bhavati.*

22 For an extensive discussion of the Brahmanical understanding of *tapas*, see Walter O. Kaelber, *Tapta Mārga: Asceticism and Initiation in Vedic India*, Albany, State University of New York Press, 1989.

23 YS 2.1: *bhāṣya: praṇavādipavitrāṇāṃ japo mokṣaśāstrādhyayanaṃ vā.*

24 See, for instance, Viṣṇusmṛti 46.25 and 64.36; Yājñavalkya Smṛti 3.325 and Parāśara Smṛti 8.41.

25 See in particular Charles Malamoud's study, *Le Svādhyāya: Recitation Personnelle du Veda* (*Taittirīya Āraṇyaka Livre II*), Paris, Institut de Civilisation Indienne, 1977.

26 Śatapatha Brāhmaṇa 11.2.6.13: *sa ṛṇmayo yajurmayaḥ sāmamaya āhutimayaḥ svargaṃ lokamabhisambhavati.*

27 BDS 2.18.25–26: *vedo vṛkṣaḥ/tasya mūlaṃ praṇavaḥ/praṇavātmako vedaḥ // praṇavaṃ dhyāyan sapraṇavo brahmabhūyāya kalpata iti hovāca prajāpatiḥ //.*

Translated by Patrick Olivelle, *The Dharmasūtras: The Law Codes of Ancient India*, Oxford, Oxford University Press, 1999, p. 209.

28 TA 2.11.4: *dakṣiṇottarau pāṇī pādau kṛtvā sapavitrāv om iti prati padyata etad vai yajus trayīṃ vidyāṃ praty eṣā vāg etat paramam akṣaram.*

29 Malamoud, *Le Svādhyāya*, p. 11.

30 See MBh 3.180.5, 3.287.5, 12.19.11, 12.37.34, 12.192.79 and 99.

31 *prāṇāyāmān pavitrāṇi vyāhṛtīḥ praṇavaṃ tathā / pavitrapāṇir āsīno brahma naityakam abhyaset //*. Translated (slightly modified) by Olivelle, *The Dharmasūtras*, pp. 229 and p. 315–316.

32 BDS 4.1.28: *savyāhṛtikāṃ sapraṇavāṃ gāyatrīṃ śirasā saha / triḥ paṭhed āyataprāṇaḥ prāṇāyāmaḥ sa ucyate //*.

33 Louis Renou, *Vocabulaire du rituel Védique*, Paris, Klincksieck, 1954, p. 68, cited by André Padoux, "Contributions à l'étude de *Mantraśāstra*. III: Le *japa*," *Bulletin de l'École Française d'Extrême-Orient*, 1987, vol. 76, p. 118.

34 See, for instance, Baudhāyana Dharma Sūtra 4.2.7 and Yājñavalkya Smṛti 1.23.

35 See BDS 3.10.9–10; GDS 19.11–12, and VaDS 22.8–9.

36 On the practice of *japa* as described in the *Mahābhārata*, see V. M. Bekedar, "The Place of *Japa* in the Mokṣadharmaparvan (MBh. XII 189–193) and the *Yoga-Sūtras*: A Comparative Study," *Annals of the Bhandarkar Oriental Research Institute*, 1963, vol. 44, 63–74.

37 Vasiṣṭha Dharma Sūtra 26.10.

38 BhG 10.25.

39 See Vasiṣṭha Dharma Sūtra 26.9 and Manu 2.85.

40 See Āpastambha Dharma Sūtra 2.22.19.

41 See, for instance, Āpastamba Dharma Sūtra 1.26.14.

42 See ĀDS 1.26.14–27.1; BDS 2.7.5; 2.8.10; 2.17.41.

43 BDS 3.9.15: *anaśnan saṃhitā sahasram adhīyīta/brahma. bhūto virajo brahma bhavati //*. Translated by Olivelle, *Dharmasūtras*, p. 225.

44 See ĀDS 1.13.19, 1.20.8; BDS 4.4.1, 4.5.18; Manu 2.104, 2.222, 11.262.

45 Manu 2.222, 4.93, 11.194.

46 Manu 3.75, 4.35, 6.8.

47 BDS 4.1.27; VaDS 25.9.

48 MBh 12.188.5.

49 BDS 4.1.25 and VaDS 25.8. Translated by Olivelle, *Dharmasūtras*, p. 230.

50 See ĀDS 1.22.1, 1.23.3ff.

51 See Manu 6.69ff, esp. 6.72.

52 YS 2.44: *svādhyāyād iṣṭadevatāsamprayogaḥ.*

53 YS 2.44: *bhāṣya: devā ṛṣayaḥ siddhāś ca svādhyāyaśīlasya darśanaṃ gacchanti.*

54 YS 2.45: *samādhi-siddhir īśvara-praṇidhānāt.*

55 YS 1.27: *bhāṣya: tasya vācakaḥ praṇavaḥ.*

56 YS 1.28: *tajjapas tadarthabhāvanam.*

57 YS 1.28 *bhāṣya: svādhyāyād yogam āsīta, yogāt svādhyāyam āsate //. svādhyāyayogasampattyā paramātmā prakāśate //.*

58 YS 1.29: *tataḥ pratyakcetanādhigamo 'py antarāyābhāvaś ca.*

59 YS 1.30: *vyādhistyānasaṃśayapramādālasyāviratibhrāntidarśanālabdhabhūmikatvānavasthitatvāni cittavikṣepās. te 'ntarāyāḥ.*

60 YS 1.31: *duḥkhadaurmanasyāṅgamejayatvaśvāsapraśvāsā vikṣepasahabhuvaḥ.*

61 YS 1.32: *tatpratiṣedhārtham ekatattvābhyāsaḥ.*

62 Lloyd Pflueger, "Discriminating the Innate Capacity: Salvation Mysticism of Classical Sāṃkhya-Yoga," in Robert K. C. Forman (ed.) *The Innate Capacity: Mysticism, Philosophy, and Philosophy*, New York, Oxford University Press, 1998, p. 66.

63 Pflueger, "Discriminating Innate Capacity," p. 59.
64 For a discussion of its Buddhist meaning see Har Dayal, *The Bodhisattva Doctrine in Buddhist Sanskrit Literature*, London, Trubner, 1932, pp. 64–67.
65 See MBh 3.387.19, 5.47.11 and 5.101.21.
66 Lloyd William Pflueger, "God, Consciousness, and Meditation: The Concept of Īśvara in the Yogasūtra," PhD dissertation, University of California, Santa Barbara, 1990, p. 269.
67 YS 1.12: *abhyāsavairāgyābhyāṃ tannirodhaḥ*.
68 BhG 6.35: *asaṃśayaṃ mahābāho mano durnigrahaṃ calam abhyāsena tu kaunteya vairāgyeṇa ca gṛhyate*.
69 YS 1.6: *pramāṇa-viparyaya-vikalpa-nidrā-smṛtayaḥ*.
70 YS 1.12: *bhāṣya: citta-nadī nāma ubhayato-vāhinī vahati kalyāṇāya vahati. pāpāya ca / yā tu kaivalya-prāg-bhārā viveka-viṣaya-nimnā sā kalyāṇa-vahā / saṃsāra-prāg-bhārā a-viveka-viṣaya-nimnā pāpa-vahā /.*
71 *tatra vairāgyeṇa viṣaya-srotaḥ khilī-kriyate, viveka-darśana-abhyāsena viveka-srota udghāṭyata ity ubhaya-adhīnaś citta-vṛtti-nirodhaḥ.*
72 Here I follow Lloyd Pflueger in translating *saṃjñā* as "technical term." See Pflueger, "God, Consciousness, and Meditation," p. 425, n. 15. Hariharānanda Āraṇya, *Yoga Philosophy of Patañjali*, Albany, State University of New York, 1983, p. 38, also takes vaśīkārasaṃjñā as a proper name, following Vācaspati Miśra who distinguishes four levels of *vairāgya: yatamāna-saṃjñā*, consciousness of endeavor; *vyatireka-saṃjñā*, consciousness of discrimination; *ekendriya-saṃjñā*, consciousness of a single sense; and *vaśīkāra-saṃjñā*, consciousness of mastery.
73 YS 1.15: *bhāṣya: striyo anna-pānam aiśvaryam iti dṛṣṭaviṣaye vitṛṣṇasya svarga-vaidehya-prakṛtilayatva-prāptāv ānuśravikaviṣaye vitṛṣṇasya divya-adivya-viṣaya-saṃprayoge api cittasya viṣaya-doṣa-darśinaḥ prasaṃkhyānabalād, anābhoga-ātmikā heya-upādeya-śūnyā vaśī-kāra-saṃjñā vairāgyam /.*
74 *Tapas* was originally aimed primarily at the acquisition of power, and not necessarily connected with ideas of renunciation and salvation. In the didactic portions of the Epic one seems to find a spiritualizing and ethicizing of *tapas* that is analogous to what we find in Patañjali. See Brockington, *The Sanskrit Epics* Leiden: Brill, 1998, pp. 238–289, who cites Minoru Hara, *Koten Indo no kugyō [Tapas in the Mahābhārata]*, Tokyo: Shunjūsha, 1979, and Monika Shee, *Tapas und Tapasvin in den erzählenden Partien des Mahābhārata*, Reinbek: Dr I. Wezler Verlag, 1986.
75 MBh 1.2.30, 3.203.9, 6.28.35, 6.35.8, 6.40.52, 12.210.21, 12.308.29, 12.308.144, 13.16.63, and 14.19.9. On the relative lateness of these passages see Brockington, *Sanskrit Epics*, pp. 130–155.
76 See *Mahāyānasūtrālaṃkāra: Exposé de la Doctrine du Grand Véhicule selon le Systême Yogācāra*, Sylvain Lévi (ed. and trans.), Paris, Libraire Honor, Champion, 1911, p. 8.
77 Ibid.
78 James Woods, *The Yoga-System of Patañjali*, Cambridge, MA, Harvard University Press, 1914, p. 36.
79 See, for instance, Āpastamba Dharmasūtra 1.9.26.7 and 1.10.29.18, Baudhāyana Dharmasūtra 2.1.1.17 and Gautama Dharmasūtra 21.1.
80 The one exception is Manu 12.74, where it refers, as in the Dharmasūtras, to repeated action in general.
81 See Manu 2.166, where *abhyāsa* is *tapaḥ param*.
82 See MBh 1.123.4.
83 Thus at MBh 3.192.24 it refers to the habit of devotion to God.
84 Thus at Mbh 3.201.3 it refers to devotion to the senses.

85 At MBh 5.27.8.
86 See BhG 8.8 and 12.9.
87 qSee BhG 12.9–12.
88 See BhG 6.44.
89 See, for instance, MBh 12.226.7 and 12.284.25.
90 YS 1.13: *bhāṣya: tatsādhanānuṣṭhānam abhyāsaḥ.*
91 YS 2.28: *bhāṣya: yathā yathā ca sādhanāny anuṣṭhīyante tathā tathā tanutvam a-śuddhir āpadyate /.*
92 Praśna Upaniṣad 1.10: "Those who seek the self by means of austerity, chastity, faith, and knowledge, on the other hand, proceed by the northern course and win the sun." (*athottareṇa tapasā brahmacaryeṇa śraddhayā vidyayātmānam anviṣyādityam abhijayante*) (Olivelle's trans.).
93 YS 1.14: *bhāṣya: tapasā brahmacaryeṇa vidyayā śraddhayā ca saṃpāditaḥ sat-kāravān dṛḍha-bhūmir bhavati.*
94 YS 1.14: *bhāṣya: vyutthāna-saṃskāreṇa drāg ity evānabhibhūta-viṣaya ity arthaḥ.*
95 YS 2.15: *bhāṣya: na caindriyāṇāṃ bhogābhyāsena vaitṛṣṇyaṃ kartuṃ śakyam / kasmāt ? / yato bhogābhyāsam anu vivardhante rāgāḥ kauśalāni caindriyāṇām iti /.*
96 YS 1.31: *bhāṣya: ete vikṣepāḥ samādhipratipakṣās tābhyām evābhyāsavairāgyābhyāṃ niroddhavyāḥ.*
97 YS 2.52: *bhāṣya: prāṇāyāmān abhyasyato asya yoginaḥ kṣīyate vivekajñānāvaraṇīyaṃ karma* [. . .] *tad asya prakāśāvaraṇaṃ karma saṃskāranibandhanaṃ prāṇāyāmābhyāsād durbalaṃ bhavati pratikṣaṇaṃ ca kṣīyate / tathā coktam / tapo na paraṃ prāṇāyāmāt tato viśuddhir malānāṃ dīptiś ca jñānasyaiti.*
98 YS 1.40: *bhāṣya: tadvaśīkārāt paripūrṇaṃ yoginaś cittaṃ na punar abhyāsakṛtaṃ parikarmāpekṣata.*
99 YS 2.3: *avidyāsmitārāgadveṣābhiniveśāḥ kleśāḥ.*
100 YS 2.4: *bhāsya: pratipakṣabhāvanopahatāḥ kleśās tanavo bhavanti.*
101 YS 2.33–34: *vitarkabādhane pratipakṣabhāvanam / vitarkā hiṃsādayaḥ kṛtakāritānumoditā lobhakrodha-mohapūrvakā mṛdumadhyādhimātrā duḥkhājñānānantaphalā iti pratipakṣabhāvanam.*
102 Vācaspati Miśra on YS 1.28: *punaḥ punaś citte niveśanam.*
103 See Lakshmi Kapani, *La Notion de Saṃskāra dans L'Inde Brahmanique et Bouddhique*, Paris, Éditions-Diffusion de Boccard, 1993, pp. 475–503.
104 YB on 4.7, discussed above, p. 4.
105 See TV 1.5: *akliṣṭābhir vṛttibhir akliṣṭāḥ saṃskārā ity arthaḥ*, and Kapani, *Notion de Saṃskāra*, p. 486.
106 So the Dhammapāda 203: *saṃkhārā paramā dukkhā.*
107 See David Carpenter, "Language, Ritual and Society: Reflections on the Authority of the Veda in India," *Journal of the American Academy of Religion* 1992, vol. 60, pp. 57–77. More recently Timothy Lubin has traced a parallel development, by which a group of rites which he calls "consecrations" (especially the *vrata*-s, the *dikṣā*, *upanayana* and *brahmacarya*) became increasingly central to Brahmanical domestic practice, and shifted the focus away from the sacrificial cult to the spiritual condition of the individual. Lubin notes that it was these very Brahmanical consecrations which "became models for explicitly antisacrificial or at least antidomestic forms of religious life." See Timothy Lubin, "Consecration and Ascetical Regimen: A History of Hindu Vrata, Dikṣā, Upanayana and Brahmacarya," unpublished PhD dissertation, Columbia University, 1994, p. 200.

108 On the lack of sophistication of the Sāṃkhya system on this score, see Gerald James Larson, "An Old Problem Revisited: The Relation between Sāṃkhya, yoga and Buddhism," *Studien zur Indologie und Iranistik*, 1989, vol. 15, pp. 129–46, and more recently, "Classical Yoga as Neo-Sāṃkhya: A Chapter in the History of Indian Philosophy," *Asiatische Studien,* 1999, vol. 53, pp. 723–732.

109 See Larson, "Classical Yoga as Neo-Sāṃkya," p. 728: "The term 'citta,' of course, appears variously in the ancient literature, both Brahmanical and Buddhist, but it is hard to avoid the parallel with discussions of 'citta' in Sautrāntika and Vijñānavāda Buddhist contexts in particular."

110 See the study of Louis de la Valleee Poussin, "Le Bouddhisme et le Yoga de Patañjali," *Mélanges Chinois et Bouddhiques,* 1936–1937, vol. 5, pp. 223–242, recently reviewed and extended by Gerald Larson in the article "An Old Problem Revisited" just noted above.

111 Feuerstein, *The Yoga-Sūtra of Patañjali: An Exercise in the Methodology of Textual Analysis*, New Delhi, Arnold-Heinemann, 1979, p. 104.

112 T. S. Rukmani has pointed out some of the difficulties involved in considering the *Yoga Sūtra* as a strictly philosophical system. She concludes that "it is best to accept it [yoga] as a discipline to be followed rather than to be understood intellectually." See T. S. Rukmani, "Tension between Vyutthāna and Nirodha in the Yoga-Sūtras," *Journal of Indian Philosophy*, 25, 1997, 623.

3

THE INTEGRATION OF SPIRIT (*PURUṢA*) AND MATTER (*PRAKṚTI*) IN THE *YOGA SŪTRA*

Ian Whicher

Introduction

This essay centers on the thought of Patañjali (*c.* second to third century CE), the great exponent of the authoritative classical Yoga school (*darśana*) of Hinduism and the reputed author of the *Yoga Sūtra*. I will argue that Patañjali's philosophical perspective has, far too often, been looked upon as excessively "spiritual" or isolationistic to the point of being a world-denying philosophy, indifferent to moral endeavor, neglecting the world of nature and culture, and overlooking the highest potentials for human reality, vitality, and creativity. Contrary to the arguments presented by many scholars, which associate Patañjali's yoga exclusively with extreme asceticism, mortification, denial, and the renunciation and abandonment of "material existence" (*prakṛti*) in favor of an elevated and isolated "spiritual state" (*puruṣa*) or disembodied state of spiritual liberation, I suggest that Patañjali's yoga can be seen as a responsible engagement, in various ways, of "spirit" (*puruṣa* = intrinsic identity as Self, pure consciousness) and "matter" (*prakṛti* = the source of psychophysical being, which includes mind, body, nature) resulting in a highly developed, transformed, and participatory human nature and identity, an integrated and embodied state of liberated selfhood (*jīvanmukti*).

The interpretation of Patañjali's Yoga Darśana presented in this essay – which walks the line between a historical and hermeneutic-praxis (some might say theological or "systematic") orientation – counters the radically dualistic, isolationistic, and ontologically oriented interpretations of yoga[1] presented by many scholars and suggests an open-ended, epistemologically oriented hermeneutic which, I maintain, is more appropriate for arriving at a genuine assessment of Patañjali's system.

It is often said that, like classical Sāṃkhya, Patañjali's yoga is a dualistic system, understood in terms of *puruṣa* and *prakṛti*. Yet, I submit, yoga scholarship has not clarified what "dualistic" means or why yoga had to be "dualistic." Even in avowedly non-dualistic systems of thought such as Advaita Vedānta we can find numerous examples of basically dualistic modes of description and explanation.[2]

Elsewhere[3] I have suggested the possibility of Patañjali having asserted a provisional, descriptive, and "practical" metaphysics, i.e. in the *Yoga Sūtra* the metaphysical schematic is abstracted from yogic experience, whereas in classical Sāṃkhya, as set out in Īśvara Kṛṣṇa's *Sāṃkhya Kārikā*, "experiences" are fitted into a metaphysical structure. This approach would allow the *Yoga Sūtra* to be interpreted along more open-ended, epistemologically oriented lines without being held captive by the radical, dualistic metaphysics of Sāṃkhya. Despite intentions to render the experiential dimension of yoga, purged as far as possible from abstract metaphysical knowledge, many scholars have fallen prey to reading the *Yoga Sūtra* from the most abstract level of the dualism of *puruṣa* and *prakṛti* down to an understanding of the practices advocated. Then they proceed to impute an experiential foundation to the whole scheme informed not from mystical insight or yogic experience, but from the effort to form a consistent (dualistic) world view, a view that culminates in a radical dualistic finality[4] or closure.

Patañjali's philosophy is not based upon mere theoretical or speculative knowledge. It elicits a practical, pragmatic, experiential/perceptual (not merely inferential/theoretical) approach that Patañjali deems essential in order to deal effectively with our total human situation and provide real freedom, not just a theory of liberation or a metaphysical explanation of life. Yoga is not content with knowledge (*jñāna*) perceived as a state that abstracts away from the world removing us from our human embodiment and activity in the world. Rather, yoga emphasizes knowledge in the integrity of being and action and as serving the integration of the "person" as a "whole." Edgerton concluded in a study dedicated to the meaning of yoga that: "yoga is not a 'system' of belief or of metaphysics. It is always a way, a method of getting something, usually salvation."[5] But this does not say enough, does not fully take into account what might be called the integrity of Patañjali's yoga. Yoga derives its real strength and value through an integration of theory and practice.[6]

Cessation (*nirodha*) and the "return to the source" (*pratiprasava*): transformation or elimination/negation of the mind?

In Patañjali's central definition of yoga, yoga is defined as "the cessation (*nirodha*) of [the misidentification with] the modifications (*vṛtti*) of the mind (*citta*)."[7] What kind of "cessation" we must ask is Patañjali actually referring to in his classical definition of yoga? What does the process of cessation actually entail for the yogin ethically, epistemologically, ontologically, psychologically, and so on? I have elsewhere suggested[8] that *nirodha* denotes an epistemological emphasis and refers to the transformation of self-understanding brought about through the purification and illumination of consciousness; *nirodha* is not (for the yogin) the ontological cessation of *prakṛti* (i.e. the mind and *vṛttis*). Seen here, *nirodha* thus is not, as is often explained, an inward movement that annihilates or suppresses *vṛttis*, thoughts, intentions, or ideas (*pratyaya*), nor is it the non-existence or absence of *vṛtti*; rather, *nirodha* involves a progressive unfoldment of perception (*yogi-pratyakṣa*) that eventually reveals our true identity as *puruṣa*. It is the state of affliction (*kleśa*) evidenced in the mind and not the mind itself that is at issue. *Cittavṛtti* does not stand for all modifications or mental processes (cognitive, affective, emotive), but is the very seed (*bīja*) mechanism of the misidentification with *prakṛti* from which all other *vṛttis* and thoughts arise and are (mis)appropriated or self-referenced in the state of ignorance (*avidyā*), that is, the unenlightened state of mind. Spiritual ignorance gives rise to a malfunctioning or misalignment of *vṛtti* within consciousness that in yoga can be corrected thereby allowing for a proper alignment or "right" functioning of *vṛtti*.[9] It is the *cittavṛtti* as our confused and mistaken identity, not our *vṛttis*, thoughts, and experiences in total that must be brought to a state of definitive cessation. To be sure, there is a temporary suspension of all the mental processes as well as any identification with an object (i.e. in *asaṃprajñāta-samādhi*, this being for the final purification of the mind[10]), but it would be misleading to conclude that higher *samādhi* results in a permanent or definitive cessation of the *vṛttis* in total, thereby predisposing the yogin who has attained purity of mind to exist in an incapacitated, isolated, or mindless state and therefore to be incapable of living a balanced, useful, and productive life in various ways.

From the perspective of the discerning yogin (*vivekin*) human identity *contained* within the domain of the three *guṇas* of *prakṛti* (i.e. *sattva*, *rajas*, and *tamas*) amounts to nothing more than sorrow and dissatisfaction (*duḥkha*).[11] The declared goal of classical Yoga, as with Sāṃkhya and Buddhism, is to overcome all dissatisfaction (*duḥkha*, YS II.16) by bringing about an inverse movement or counter-flow (*pratiprasava*)[12] understood as a "return to the source"[13] or "process-of-involution"[14] of the *guṇas*, a kind of reabsorption into the transcendent purity of being itself. What does this "process-of-involution" – variously referred to as "return to the origin," "dissolution into the source,"[15] or "withdrawal from manifestation" – actually mean? Is it a definitive ending to the perceived world of the yogin comprised of change and transformation, forms and phenomena? Ontologically conceived, *prasava* signifies the "flowing forth" of the primary constituents or qualities of *prakṛti* into the multiple forms of the universe in all its dimensions, i.e. all the processes of manifestation and actualization or "creation" (*sarga*, *prasarga*). *Pratiprasava* on the other hand denotes the process of "dissolution into the source" or "withdrawal from manifestation" of those forms relative to the personal, microcosmic level of the yogin who is about to attain freedom (*apavarga*).

Does a "return to the origin" culminate in a state of freedom in which one is stripped of all human identity and void of any association with the world including one's practical livelihood? The ontological emphasis usually given to the meaning of *pratiprasava* – implying for the yogin a literal dissolution of *prakṛti's* manifestation – would seem to support a view, one which is prominent in yoga scholarship, of spiritual liberation denoting an existence wholly transcendent (and therefore stripped or deprived) of all manifestation including the human relational sphere. Is this the kind of spiritually emancipated state that Patañjali had in mind (pun included)? In YS II.3–17 (which set the stage for the remainder of the chapter on yogic means or *sādhana*), Patañjali describes *prakṛti*, the "seeable" (including our personhood), in the context of the various afflictions (*kleśas*) that give rise to an afflicted and mistaken identity of self. Afflicted identity is constructed out of and held captive by the root affliction of ignorance (*avidyā*) and its various forms of karmic bondage. Yet, despite the clear association of *prakṛti* with the bondage of ignorance (*avidyā*), there are no real grounds for purporting that *prakṛti* herself is to be equated with or subsumed under the afflictions. In yoga, the world is clearly affirmed; *prakṛti* is deemed to be real (YS IV.13–14), all forms of *prakṛti* being comprised of the three *guṇas*: *sattva*, *rajas*, and *tamas*. To equate *prakṛti* with affliction itself implies that as a product of spiritual ignorance, *prakṛti*, along with the afflictions, is conceived as a reality that the yogin should ultimately abandon, condemn, avoid, or discard completely. Patañjali leaves much room for understanding "dissolution" or "return to the source" with an epistemological emphasis thereby allowing the whole system of the Yoga Darśana to be interpreted along more open-ended lines. In other words, what actually "dissolves" or is ended in yoga is the yogin's misidentification with *prakṛti*, a mistaken identity of self that – contrary to authentic identity, namely, *puruṣa* – can be nothing more than a product of the three *guṇas* under the influence of spiritual ignorance. Understood as such, *pratiprasava* need not denote the definitive ontological dissolution of manifest *prakṛti* for the yogin, but rather refers to the process of "subtilization" or sattvification of consciousness so necessary for the uprooting of misidentification – the incorrect worldview born of *avidyā* – or incapacity of the yogin to "see" from the yogic perspective of the seer (*draṣṭṛ*), our authentic identity as *puruṣa*.

The discerning yogin sees (YS II.15) that this guṇic world or cycle of saṃsāric identity is in itself dissatisfaction (*duḥkha*). But we must ask, what exactly is the problem being addressed in yoga? What is at issue in Yoga philosophy? Is our ontological status as a human being involved in day-to-day existence forever in doubt, in fact in need of being negated, dissolved in order for authentic identity (*puruṣa*), immortal consciousness, finally to dawn? Having overcome all ignorance, is it then possible for a human being to live in the world and no longer be in conflict with oneself and the world? Can the *guṇas* cease to function in a state of ignorance and conflict in the mind? Must the guṇic constitution of the human mind and the whole of prakṛtic existence disappear, dissolve for the yogin? Can the ways of spiritual ignorance be replaced by an aware, conscious, non-afflicted identity and activity that transcend the conflict and confusion of ordinary, saṃsāric life? Can we live, according to Patañjali's yoga, an embodied state of freedom?

"Aloneness" (*kaivalya*): implications for an embodied freedom

In the classical traditions of Sāṃkhya and Yoga, *kaivalya*, meaning "aloneness,"[16] is generally understood to be the state of the unconditional existence of *puruṣa*. In the *Yoga Sūtra*, *kaivalya* can refer more precisely to the "aloneness of seeing" (*dṛśeḥ kaivalyam*) which, as Patañjali states, follows from the disappearance of ignorance (*avidyā*) and its creation of *saṃyoga*[17] – the conjunction of the seer (*puruṣa*) and the seeable (i.e. *citta*, *guṇas*) – explained by Vyāsa as a mental superimposition (*adhyāropa*, YB II.18). "Aloneness" thus can be construed as *puruṣa's* innate capacity for pure, unbroken, non-attached seeing/perceiving, observing, or "knowing" of the content of the mind (*citta*).[18] In an alternative definition, Patañjali explains *kaivalya* as the "return to the origin" (*pratiprasava*) of the *guṇas*, which have lost all soteriological purpose for the *puruṣa* that has, as it were, recovered its transcendent autonomy.[19] This *sūtra* (YS IV.34) also classifies *kaivalya* as the establishment in "own form/nature" (*svarūpa*), and the power of higher awareness (*citiśakti*).[20] Although the seer's (*draṣṭṛ/puruṣa*) capacity for "seeing" is an unchanging yet dynamic power of consciousness that should not be truncated in any way, nevertheless our karmically distorted or skewed perceptions vitiate against the natural fullness of "seeing." (Patañjali defines spiritual ignorance (*avidyā*), the root affliction, as: "seeing the non-eternal as eternal, the impure as pure, dissatisfaction as happiness, and the non-self as self" (YS II.5)). Having removed the "failure-to-see" (*adarśana*), the soteriological purpose of the *guṇas* in the saṃsāric condition of the mind is fulfilled; the mind is relieved of its former role of being a vehicle for *avidyā*, the locus of egoity and misidentification, and the realization of pure seeing – the nature of the seer alone – takes place.

According to yet another *sūtra* (YS III.55), we are told that *kaivalya* is established when the *sattva* of consciousness has reached a state of purity analogous to that of the *puruṣa*.[21] Through the process of subtilization or "return to the origin" (*pratiprasava*) in the *sattva*, the transformation (*pariṇāma*) of the mind (*citta*) takes place at the deepest level bringing about a radical change in perspective: the former impure, fabricated states constituting a fractured identity of self are dissolved resulting in the complete purification of mind. Through knowledge (in *saṃprajñāta-samādhi*) and its transcendence (in *asaṃprajñāta-samādhi*) self-identity overcomes its lack of intrinsic grounding, a lack sustained and exacerbated by the web of afflictions in the form of attachment (*rāga*), aversion (*dveṣa*), and the compulsive clinging to life based on the fear of extinction (*abhiniveśa*). The yogin is no longer dependent on liberating knowledge (mind-*sattva*),[22] is no longer attached to *vṛtti* as a basis for self-identity. Cessation, it must be emphasized, does not mark a definitive disappearance of the *guṇas* from *puruṣa's* view.[23] For the liberated yogin, the *guṇas* cease to exist in the form of *avidyā* and its *saṃskāras*, *vṛttis*, and false or fixed ideas (*pratyaya*) of selfhood that formerly veiled true identity. The changing guṇic modes cannot alter the yogin's now purified and firmly established consciousness. The mind has been liberated from the egocentric world of attachment to things prakṛtic. Now the yogin's identity (as *puruṣa*), disassociated from ignorance, is untouched, unaffected by qualities of mind,[24] uninfluenced by the *vṛttis* constituted of the three *guṇas*. The mind and *puruṣa* attain to a sameness of purity (YS III.55), of harmony, balance, evenness, and a workability together: the mind appearing in the nature of *puruṣa*.[25]

Kaivalya, I suggest, in no way destroys or negates the personality of the yogin, but is an unconditional state in which all the obstacles or distractions preventing an immanent and purified relationship or engagement of person with nature and spirit (*puruṣa*) have been removed. The mind, which previously functioned under the sway of ignorance coloring and blocking our perception of authentic identity, has now become purified and no longer operates as a locus of misidentification, confusion, and dissatisfaction (*duḥkha*). *Sattva*, the finest quality (*guṇa*) of the mind, has the capacity to be perfectly lucid/transparent, like a dust-free mirror in which the light of *puruṣa* is clearly reflected and the discriminative discernment (*vivekakhyāti*)[26] between *puruṣa* and the *sattva* of the mind (as the finest nature of the seeable) can take place.[27]

The crucial (ontological) point to be made here is that in the "aloneness" of *kaivalya prakṛti* ceases to perform an obstructing role. In effect, *prakṛti* herself has become purified, illuminated, and liberated[28] from *avidyā's* grip including the misconceptions, misappropriations, and misguided relations implicit within a world of afflicted identity. The mind has been transformed, liberated from the egocentric world of attachment, its former afflicted nature abolished; and self-identity left alone in its "own form" or true nature as *puruṣa* is never again confused with all the relational acts, intentions, and volitions of empirical existence. There being no power of misidentification remaining in *nirbīja-samādhi*,[29] the mind ceases to operate within the context of the afflictions, karmic accumulations, and consequent cycles of *saṃsāra* implying a mistaken identity of selfhood subject to birth and death.

The *Yoga Sūtra* has often been regarded as calling for the severance of *puruṣa* from *prakṛti*; concepts such as liberation, cessation, detachment/dispassion, and so forth have been interpreted in an explicitly negative light. Max Müller, citing Bhoja Rāja's commentary[30] (eleventh century CE), refers to yoga as "separation" (*viyoga*).[31] More recently, numerous other scholars[32] have endorsed this interpretation, that is, the absolute separateness of *puruṣa* and *prakṛti*. In asserting the absolute separation of *puruṣa* and *prakṛti*, scholars and non-scholars alike have tended to disregard the possibility for other (fresh) hermeneutical options, and this radical, dualistic metaphysical closure of sorts surrounding the nature and meaning of Patañjali's yoga has proved detrimental to a fuller understanding of the Yoga Darśana by continuing a tradition based on an isolationistic, one-sided reading (or perhaps misreading) of the *Yoga Sūtra* and Vyāsa's commentary. Accordingly, the absolute separation of *puruṣa* and *prakṛti* can only be interpreted as a disembodied state implying death to the physical body. To dislodge the sage from bodily existence is to undermine the integrity of the pedagogical context that lends so much credibility or "weight" to the yoga system. I am not here implying a simple idealization of yoga pedagogy thereby overlooking the need to incorporate a healthy critical approach to the guru–disciple dynamic. Rather, I am suggesting that it need not be assumed that, in yoga, liberation coincides with physical death.[33] This would only allow for a soteriological end state of "disembodied liberation" (*videhamukti*). What is involved in yoga is the death of the atomistic, egoic identity, the dissolution of the karmic web of *saṃsāra* that generates notions of one being a subject trapped in the prakṛtic constitution of a particular body–mind.

Not being content with mere theoretical knowledge, yoga is committed to a practical way of life. To this end, Patañjali included in his presentation of yoga an outline of the "eight-limbed" path (*aṣṭāṅga-yoga*)[34] dealing with the physical, moral, psychological, and spiritual dimensions of the yogin, an integral path that emphasizes organic continuity, balance, and integration in contrast to the discontinuity, imbalance, and disintegration inherent in *saṃyoga*. The idea of cosmic balance and of the mutual support and upholding of the various parts of nature and society is not foreign to yoga thought. Vyāsa deals with the theory of "nine causes" (*nava kāraṇāni*) or types of causation according to tradition.[35] The ninth type of cause is termed *dhṛti* – meaning "support" or "sustenance." Based on Vyāsa's explanation of *dhṛti* we can see how mutuality and sustenance are understood as essential conditions for the maintenance of the natural and social world. There is an organic interdependence of all living entities wherein all (i.e. the elements, animals, humans, and divine bodies) work together for the "good" of the whole and for each other.

Far from being exclusively a subjectively oriented and introverted path of withdrawal from life, classical yoga acknowledges the intrinsic value of "support" and "sustenance" and the interdependence of all living (embodied) entities, thus upholding organic continuity, balance, and integration within the natural and social world. Having achieved that level of insight (*prajñā*) that is "truth-bearing" (*ṛtaṃbharā*),[36] the yogin perceives the natural order (*ṛta*) of cosmic existence, "unites" with, and embodies that order. To fail to see clearly (*adarśana*) is to fall into disorder, disharmony, and conflict with oneself and the world. In effect, to be ensconced in ignorance implies a disunion with the natural order of life and inextricably results in a failure to embody that order. Through yoga one gains proper access to the world and is therefore established in the right relationship to the world. Far from being denied or renounced, the world, for the yogin, has become transformed, properly engaged.

We need not read Patañjali as saying that the culmination of all yogic endeavor – *kaivalya* – is a static finality or inactive, isolated, solipsistic state of being. *Kaivalya* can be seen to incorporate an integrated, psychological consciousness along with the autonomy of pure consciousness, yet pure consciousness to which the realm of the *guṇas* (e.g. psychophysical being) is completely attuned and integrated. On the level of individuality, the yogin has found his (her) place in the world at large, "fitting into the whole."[37]

In the last chapter of the *Yoga Sūtra* (*Kaivalya-Pāda*), "aloneness" (*kaivalya*) is said to ensue upon the attainment of *dharmamegha-samādhi*, the "cloud of *dharma*" *samādhi*. At this level of practice, the yogin has abandoned any search for (or attachment to) reward or "profit" from his or her meditational practice; a non-acquisitive attitude (*akusīda*) must take place at the highest level of yogic discipline.[38] Vyāsa emphasizes that the identity of *puruṣa* is not something to be acquired (*upādeya*) or discarded (*heya*).[39] The perspective referred to as "Pātañjala Yoga Darśana" culminates in a permanent state of clear "seeing" brought about through the discipline of yoga. Yoga thus incorporates both an end state or "goal" and a process.[40]

Dharmamegha-samādhi presupposes that the yogin has cultivated higher dispassion (*para-vairāgya*) – the means to the enstatic consciousness realized in *asaṃprajñāta-samādhi*.[41] Thus, *dharmamegha-samādhi* is more or less a synonym of *asaṃprajñāta-samādhi* and can even be understood as the consummate phase of the awakening disclosed in enstasy, the final step on the long and arduous yogic journey to authentic identity and "aloneness."[42] A permanent identity shift – from the perspective of the human personality to *puruṣa* – takes place. Now free from any dependence on or subordination to knowledge or *vṛtti*, and detached from the world of misidentification (*saṃyoga*), the yogin yet retains the purified guṇic powers of virtue including illuminating "knowledge of all"[43] (due to purified *sattva*), nonafflicted activity[44] (due to purified *rajas*), and a stable body-form (due to purified *tamas*).

YS IV.30 declares: "From that [*dharmamegha-samādhi*] there is the cessation of afflicted action."[45] Hence the binding influence of the *guṇas* in the form of the afflictions, past actions, and misguided relationships is overcome; what remains is a "cloud of dharma" which includes an "eternality of knowledge" free from all impure covering (*āvaraṇa-mala*, YS IV.31) or veiling affliction and where "little (remains) to be known."[46] The eternality or endlessness of knowledge is better understood metaphorically rather than literally: it is not knowledge expanded to infinity but implies *puruṣa*-realization which transcends the limitations and particulars of knowledge (*vṛtti*).

The culmination of the yoga system is found when, following from *dharmamegha-samādhi*, the mind and actions are freed from misidentification and affliction and one is no longer deluded/confused with regard to one's true form (*svarūpa*) or intrinsic identity. At this stage of practice the yogin is disconnected (*viyoga*) from all patterns of action motivated by the ego. According to both Vyāsa[47] and the sixteenth-century commentator Vijñāna Bhikṣu,[48] one to whom this high state of purification takes place is designated as a *jīvanmukta*: one who is liberated while still alive (i.e. embodied or living liberation).

By transcending the normative conventions and obligations of karmic behavior, the yogin acts morally not as an extrinsic response and out of obedience to an external moral code of conduct, but as an intrinsic response and as a matter of natural, purified inclination. The stainless luminosity of pure consciousness is revealed as one's fundamental nature. The yogin does not act saṃsārically and ceases to act from the perspective of a delusive sense of self confined within *prakṛti's* domain. Relinquishing all obsessive or selfish concern with the results of activity, the yogin remains wholly detached from the egoic fruits of action.[49] This does not imply that the yogin loses all orientation for action. Only attachment (and compulsive, inordinate desire), not action itself, sets in motion the law of moral causation (*karma*) by which a person is confined within saṃsāric identity. The yogin is said to be non-attached to either virtue or non-virtue, and is no longer oriented within the egological patterns of thought as in the epistemically distorted condition of *saṃyoga*. This does not mean, as some scholars have misleadingly concluded, that the spiritual adept or yogin is free to commit immoral acts,[50] or that the yogin is motivated by selfish concerns.[51]

Actions must not only be executed in the spirit of unselfishness (i.e. sacrifice) or detachment, they must also be ethically sound, reasonable and justifiable. Moreover, the yogin's spiritual journey – far from being an "a-moral process"[52] – is a highly moral process! The yogin's commitment to the sattvification of consciousness, including the cultivation of moral virtues such as compassion (*karuṇā*)[53] and non-violence (*ahiṃsā*),[54] is not an "a-moral" enterprise, nor is it an expression of indifference, aloofness, or an uncaring attitude to others. Moral disciplines are engaged as a natural outgrowth of intelligent (*sattvic*) self-understanding, insight, and commitment to self-transcendence that takes consciousness out of (*ec-stasis*) its identification with the rigid structure of the monadic ego, thereby reversing the inveterate tendency of this ego to inflate itself at the expense of its responsibility in relation to others.

Having defined the "goal" of yoga as "aloneness" (*kaivalya*), the question must now be asked: What kind of "aloneness" was Patañjali talking about? "Aloneness," I suggest, is not the isolation of the seer (*draṣṭṛ*, *puruṣa*) separate from the seeable (*dṛśya*, *prakṛti*), as is unfortunately far too often maintained as the goal of yoga, but refers to the "aloneness" of the power of "seeing" (YS II.20, 25) in its innate purity and clarity without any epistemological distortion and moral defilement. The cultivation of *nirodha* uproots the compulsive tendency to reify the world and oneself (i.e. that pervading sense of separate ego irrevocably divided from the encompassing world) with an awareness that reveals the transcendent, yet immanent seer (*puruṣa*). Through clear "seeing" (*dṛśi*) the purpose of yoga is fulfilled, and the yogin, free from all misidentification and impure karmic residue (as in the former contextual sphere of *cittavṛtti*), gains full, immediate access to the world. By accessing the world in such an open and direct manner, in effect "uniting" (epistemologically) with the world, the yogin ceases to be encumbered by egoism (i.e. *asmitā* and its egoic attitudes and identity patterns), which, enmeshed in conflict and confusion and holding itself as separate from the world, misappropriates the world.

Yoga can be seen to unfold – in *samādhi* – states of epistemic oneness that reveal the non-separation of knower, knowing, and the known (YS I.41) grounding our identity in a nonafflicted mode of action. *Kaivalya* implies a power of "seeing" in which the dualisms rooted in our egocentric patterns of attachment, aversion, fear, and so forth have been transformed into unselfish ways of being with others.[55] The psychological, ethical, and social implications of this kind of identity transformation are, needless to say, immense. I am suggesting that yoga does not destroy or anesthetize our feelings and emotions thereby encouraging neglect and indifference toward others. On the contrary, the process of "cessation" (*nirodha*) steadies one for a life of compassion, discernment, and service informed by a "seeing" that is able to understand (literally meaning "to stand among, hence observe") – and is in touch with – the needs of others. What seems especially relevant for our understanding of yoga ethics is the enhanced capacity generated in yoga for empathic identification with the object one seeks to understand. This is a far cry from the portrayal of the yogin as a disengaged figure, psychologically and physically removed from the human relational sphere, who in an obstinate and obtrusive fashion severs all ties with the world. Such an image of a wise yogin merely serves to circumscribe our vision of humanity and, if anything else, stifle the spirit by prejudicing a spiritual, abstract (and disembodied) realm over and against nature and our human embodiment. In Yoga philosophy "seeing" is not only a cognitive term but implies purity of mind, that is, it has moral content and value. Nor is "knowledge" (*jñāna*, *vidyā*) in the yoga tradition to be misconstrued as a "bloodless" or "heartless" *gnosis*.

I wish to argue therefore that through the necessary transformation of consciousness brought about in *samādhi*, an authentic and fruitful coherence of self-identity, perception, and activity emerges out of the former fragmented consciousness in *saṃyoga*. If Patañjali's perception of the world of forms and differences had been destroyed or discarded, how could he have had such insight into yoga and the intricacies and subtle nuances of the unenlightened state?[56] If through *nirodha* the individual form and the whole world had been canceled for Patañjali, he would more likely have spent the rest of his days in the inactivity and isolation of transcendent oblivion rather than present Yoga philosophy to others! Rather than being handicapped by the exclusion of thinking, perceiving, experiencing, or activity, the liberated yogin actualizes the potential to live a fully integrated life in the world. I conclude here that there is no reason why the liberated yogin cannot be portrayed as a vital, creative, thoughtful, empathetic, balanced, happy, and wise person. Having adopted an integrative orientation to life, the enlightened being can endeavor to transform, enrich, and ennoble the world. I am therefore suggesting that there is a rich, affective, moral, and cognitive as well as spiritual potential inherent in the realization of *puruṣa*, the "aloneness" of the power of consciousness/seeing.

Yoga presupposes the integration of knowledge and activity; there can be no scission between *theoria* and *praxis*. The *Yoga Sūtra* is a philosophical text where *praxis* is deemed to be essential. Without actual practice the theory that informs yoga would have no authentic meaning. Yet without examination and reflection there would be no meaningful striving for liberation, no "goal," as it were, to set one's sight on. In an original, inspiring, and penetrating style, Patañjali bridges metaphysics and ethics, transcendence and immanence, and contributes to the Hindu fold a form of philosophical investigation that, to borrow J. Taber's descriptive phrase for another context, can properly be called a "transformative philosophy." That is to say, it is a philosophical perspective which "does not stand as an edifice isolated from experience; it exists only insofar as it is realized in experience."[57]

Conclusion

To conclude, it can be said that *puruṣa* indeed has some precedence over *prakṛti* in Patañjali's system, for *puruṣa* is what is ordinarily "missing" or concealed in human life and is ultimately the state of consciousness one must awaken to in yoga. The liberated state of "aloneness" (*kaivalya*) need not denote either an ontological superiority of *puruṣa* or an exclusion of *prakṛti*. *Kaivalya* can be positively construed as an integration of both principles – an integration that, I have argued, is what is most important for yoga. I have proposed that the *Yoga Sūtra* does not uphold a "path" of liberation that ultimately renders *puruṣa* and *prakṛti* incapable of "co-operating" together. Rather, the *Yoga Sūtra* seeks to "unite" these two principles without the presence of any defiled understanding, to bring them "together," properly aligning them in a state of balance, harmony, and a clarity of knowledge in the integrity of being and action.

The purified mind, one that has been transformed through yogic discipline, is certainly no ordinary worldly awareness nor is it eliminated for the sake of pure consciousness. To confuse (as many interpretations of yoga have unfortunately done) the underlining purificatory processes involved in the cessation of ignorance/afflicted identity as being the same thing as (or as necessitating the need for) a radical elimination of our psychophysical being – the prakṛtic vehicle through which consciousness discloses itself – is, I suggest, to misunderstand the intent of the *Yoga Sūtra* itself. There are strong grounds for arguing (as I have done) that through "cessation" *prakṛti* herself (in the form of the guṇic constitutional makeup of the yogin's body-mind) is liberated from the grip of ignorance. Vyāsa explicitly states (YB II.18) that emancipation happens in the mind and does not literally apply to *puruṣa* – which is by definition already free and therefore has no intrinsic need to be released from the fetters of saṃsāric existence.

Both morality and perception (cognition) are essential channels through which human consciousness, far from being negated or suppressed, is transformed and illuminated. Yoga combines discerning knowledge with an emotional, affective, and moral sensibility allowing for a participatory epistemology that incorporates the moral amplitude for empathic identification with the world, that is, with the objects or persons one seeks to understand. The enhanced perception gained through yoga must be interwoven with yoga's rich affective and moral dimensions to form a spirituality that does not become entangled in a web of antinomianism, but which retains the integrity and vitality to transform our lives and the lives of others in an effective manner. In yoga proper there can be no support, ethically or pedagogically, for the misappropriation or abuse of *prakṛti* for the sake of freedom or *puruṣa*-realization. By upholding an integration of the moral and the mystical, yoga supports a reconciliation of the prevalent tension within Hinduism between (1) spiritual engagement and self-identity within the world (*pravṛtti*) and (2) spiritual disengagement from worldliness and self-identity that transcends the world (*nivṛtti*). Yoga discerns and teaches a balance between these two apparently conflicting orientations.

This essay has attempted to counter the radically dualistic, isolationistic, and ontologically oriented interpretations of yoga presented by many scholars – where the full potentialities of our human embodiment are constrained within a radical, rigid, dualistic metaphysical structure – and propose instead an open-ended, morally and epistemologically oriented hermeneutic that frees yoga of the long-standing conception of spiritual isolation, disembodiment, self-denial, and world-negation and thus from its pessimistic image. Our interpretation does not impute that *kaivalya* denotes a final incommensurability between or dissociation of spirit and matter. While Patañjali can be understood as having adopted a provisional, practical, dualistic metaphysics, there is no proof that his system either ends in duality or eliminates the possibility for an ongoing co-operative duality. Yoga is not simply "*puruṣa*-realization"; it equally implies "getting it right with *prakṛti*."

As well as being one of the seminal texts on yogic technique and transformative/liberative approaches within Asian Indian philosophy, Patañjali's *Yoga Sūtra* has to this day remained one of the most influential spiritual guides in Hinduism. In addition to a large number of people within India, millions of Westerners are actively practicing some form of yoga influenced by Patañjali's thought clearly demonstrating yoga's relevance for today as a discipline that can transcend cultural, religious, and philosophical barriers. The universal and universalizing potential of yoga makes it one of India's finest contributions to our struggle for self-definition, moral integrity, and spiritual renewal today. The main purpose of this essay has been to consider a fresh approach in which to re-examine and reassess classical Yoga philosophy, and to help to articulate in a fuller way what I have elsewhere referred to as the integrity of the Yoga Darśana.[58] Thus, it is my hope that some of the suggestions presented here can function as a catalyst for bringing Patañjali's thought into a more fruitful dialogue and encounter with other religious and philosophical traditions both within and outside of India.

Notes

1 The system of classical yoga is often reduced to or fitted into a classical Sāṃkhyan scheme – the interpretations of which generally follow along radically dualistic lines. In their metaphysical ideas classical Sāṃkhya and Yoga are closely akin. However, both systems hold divergent views on important areas of doctrinal structure such as epistemology, ontology, ethics, and psychology, as well as differences pertaining to terminology. These differences

derive in part from the different methodologies adopted by the two schools: Sāṃkhya, it has been argued, emphasizes a theoretical or intellectual analysis through inference and reasoning in order to bring out the nature of final emancipation, while Yoga stresses yogic perception and multiple forms of practice that culminate in *samādhi*. To be sure, many followers of Yoga were closely allied with Sāmkhya both in pre-classical as well as in later periods. It is important to acknowledge, however, that in the *Mahābhārata* Yoga and Sāṃkhya are also clearly distinguished and recognized as separate schools. For more on differentiating these two Darśanas see T. S. Rukmani, "Sāṃkhya and Yoga: Where They Do Not Speak in One Voice," *Études Asiatiques*, 1999, vol. 53, pp. 733–753, and Whicher, "Classical Sāṃkhya, Yoga and the Issue of Final Purification," *Études Asiatiques*, 1999, vol. 53, pp. 779–798. Moreover, there is clear evidence throughout all four *pādas* of the *Yoga Sūtra* of an extensive network of terminology that parallels Buddhist teachings and which is absent in the classical Sāṃkhya literature. Patañjali includes several *sūtras* on the "restraints" or *yamas* (namely, non-violence [*ahiṃsā*], truthfulness [*satya*], non-stealing [*asteya*], chastity [*brahmacarya*], and non-possession [*aparigraha*]) of the "eight-limbed" path of yoga that are listed in the Acārāṅga Sūtra of Jainism (the earliest sections of which may date from the third or fourth century BCE) thereby suggesting possible Jaina influences on the Yoga tradition. The topic of Buddhist or Jaina influence on yoga doctrine (or vice versa) is, however, not the focus of this essay.

2 See, for example, Śaṅkara's (*c.* eighth to ninth century CE) use of *vyāvahārika* (the conventional empirical perspective) in contrast to *paramārthika* (the ultimate or absolute standpoint).

3 See Ian Whicher, *The Integrity of the Yoga Darśana: A Reconsideration of Classical Yoga*, Albany, NY, State University of New York Press, 1998.

4 See in particular: Georg Feuerstein, *The Philosophy of Classical Yoga*, New York, St Martin's Press, 1980, pp. 14, 56, and 108; Mircea Eliade, *Yoga: Immortality and Freedom*, trans. W. R. Trask, Princeton, NJ, Princeton University Press, 1969, pp. 94–95, 99–100; Gaspar Koelman, *Pātañjala Yoga, from Related Ego to Absolute Self*, Poona, Papal Athenaeum, 1970, pp. 224, 251; and Gerald Larson, in G. Larson and R. S. Bhattacharya (eds) *Sāṃkhya: A Dualist Tradition in Indian Philosophy*, Princeton, NJ, Princeton University Press, 1987, p. 13, who classifies Patañjali's yoga as a form of Sāṃkhya.

5 Franklin Edgerton, "The Meaning of Sāṃkhya and Yoga," *American Journal of Philology*, 1924, vol. 45, pp. 1–46.

6 As argued in Whicher, *The Integrity of the Yoga Darśana*.

7 YS I.2 (p. 4): *yogaś cittavṛttinirodhaḥ*. The Sanskrit text of the *Yoga Sūtra* of Patañjali and the YB of Vyāsa is from *Pātañjalayogadarśana, with the Vyāsa-Bhāṣya of Vyāsa, the Tattva-Vaiśāradī of Vācaspati Miśra and the Rāja-Mārtaṇḍa of Bhoja Rāja*, edited by Kāśīnātha Śāstrī Āgāśe, Poona, Ānandāśrama Sanskrit Series, 1904. The modifications or functions (*vṛtti*) of the mind (*citta*) are said to be fivefold (YS I.6), namely, "valid cognition" (*pramāṇa*, which includes perception [*pratyakṣa*], inference [*anumāna*] and valid testimony [*āgama*]), "error"/"misconception" (*viparyaya*), "conceptualisation" (*vikalpa*), "sleep" (*nidrā*), and "memory" (*smṛti*), and are described as being "afflicted" (*kliṣṭa*) or "non-afflicted" (*akliṣṭa*) (YS I.5). *Citta* is an umbrella term that incorporates "intellect" (*buddhi*), "sense of self" (*ahaṃkāra*), and "mind-organ" (*manas*), and can be viewed as the aggregate of the cognitive, conative and affective processes and functions of phenomenal consciousness, i.e. it consists of a grasping, intentional and volitional consciousness. For an in-depth look at the meaning of the terms *citta* and *vṛtti* see Ian Whicher, "The Mind (Citta): Its

Nature, Structure and Functioning in Classical Yoga," *Saṃbhāṣā*, 1997–1998, vol. 18–19, pp. 35–62, 1–50. In the first four *sūtras* of the first chapter (*Samādhi-Pāda*) the subject matter of the *Yoga Sūtra* is mentioned, defined and characterized. The *sūtras* run as follows: YS I.1: "Now [begins] the discipline of Yoga." YS I.2: "Yoga is the cessation of [the misidentification with] the modifications of the mind." YS I.3: "Then [when that cessation has taken place] there is abiding in the seer's own form (i.e. *puruṣa* or intrinsic identity)." YS I.4: "Otherwise [there is] conformity to (i.e. misidentification with) the modifications [of the mind]." YS I.1–4 (pp. 1, 4, 7, and 7 respectively): *atha yogānuśāsanam; yogaś cittavṛttinirodhaḥ; tadā draṣṭuḥ svarūpe'vasthānam; vṛttisārūpyam itaratra*. For a more comprehensive study of classical yoga including issues dealt with in this essay see Whicher, *The Integrity of the Yoga Darśana*.

8 See Ian Whicher, "Nirodha, Yoga Praxis and the Transformation of the Mind," *Journal of Indian Philosophy*, 1997, vol. 25, pp. 1–67, and Whicher, *The Integrity of the Yoga Darśana*.

9 See Whicher, "Nirodha" and *The Integrity of the Yoga Darśana*.

10 See chapter 6 in Whicher, *The Integrity of the Yoga Darśana*.

11 YS II.15 (p. 74): *pariṇāmatāpasaṃskāraduḥkhair guṇavṛttivirodhāc ca duḥkham eva sarvaṃ vivekinaḥ*. "Because of the dissatisfaction and sufferings due to change and anxieties and the latent impressions, and from the conflict of the modifications of the *guṇas*, for the discerning one, all is sorrow alone."

12 Patañjali uses the term *pratiprasava* twice, in YS II.10 and IV.34.

13 See Chris Chapple and Eugene P. Kelly, *The Yoga Sutras of Patañjali: An Analysis of the Sanskrit with Accompanying English Translation*, Delhi, Sri Satguru Publications, 1990, p. 60.

14 Georg Feuerstein, *The Yogasutra of Patañjali: A New Translation and Commentary*, Folkestone, Kent, Wm. Dawson and Sons Ltd, 1979, p. 65.

15 Cf. *Yogasūtravivaraṇa* of Śaṅkarācārya. *The complete commentary by Śaṅkara on the Yoga Sūtra-s: a full translation of the newly discovered text*. Translated by Trevor Leggett. London, Kegan Paul International, 1990, p. 195, and *Yogasūtra* of Patañjali. *Yoga-Sūtras of Patañjali with the Exposition of Vyāsa: A Translation and Commentary*, trans. by Usharbudha Arya, Honesdale, PA, Himalayan International Institute, 1986, pp. 146, 471.

16 The term *kaivalya* comes from *kevala*, meaning "alone." Feuerstein, *The Yogasutra of Patañjali*, p. 75, also translates *kaivalya* as "aloneness" but with a metaphysical or ontological emphasis that implies the absolute separation of *puruṣa* and *prakṛti*.

17 YS II.25 (p. 96): *tadabhāvāt saṃyogābhāvo hānaṃ taddṛśeḥ kaivalyam*.

18 YS II.20 and IV.18.

19 YS IV.34 (p. 207): *puruṣārthaśūnyānāṃ guṇānāṃ pratiprasavaḥ kaivalyaṃ svarūpapratiṣṭhā vā citiśaktir iti*.

20 See n. 19 above.

21 YS III.55 (p. 174): *sattvapuruṣayoḥ śuddhisāmye kaivalyam iti*. One must be careful not to characterize the state of *sattva* itself as liberation or *kaivalya*, for without the presence of *puruṣa* the mind (as reflected consciousness) could not function in its most transparent aspect as *sattva*. It is not accurate, according to yoga philosophy, to say that the *sattva* is equivalent to liberation itself. The question of the nature of the *guṇas* from the enlightened perspective is an interesting one. In the Bhagavadgītā (II.45) Kṛṣṇa advises Arjuna to become free from the three *guṇas* and then gives further instructions to be established in eternal *sattva* (beingness, light, goodness, clarity, knowledge), free of dualities, free of acquisition-and-possession, self-possessed (*nirdvandvo nityasattvastho niryogakṣema ātmavān*). It would appear from the above instructions that the nature of the

sattva being referred to here transcends the limitations of the nature of *sattva-guṇa* which can still have a binding effect in the form of attachment to joy and knowledge. It is, however, only by first overcoming *rajas* and *tamas* that liberation is possible.

22 YB III.55 (p. 175): *nahi dagdhakleśabījasya jñāne punar apekṣā kācid asti.* "When the seeds of afflictions have been scorched there is no longer any dependence at all on further knowledge."

23 Hariharānanda Āraṇya writes that in the state of *nirodha* the *guṇas* "do not die out but their unbalanced activity due to non-equilibrium that was taking place . . . only ceases on account of the cessation of the cause (*avidyā* or nescience) which brought about their contact." See H. Āraṇya, *Yoga Philosophy of Patañjali: Containing His Yoga Aphorisms with Vyāsa's Commentary*, trans. P. N. Muckerji, Albany, NY, State University of New York Press, 1983, p. 123.

24 YB IV.25 (p. 201): *puruṣas tv asatyām avidyāyāṃ śuddhaś cittadharmair aparāmṛṣṭa.*

25 YB I.41.

26 YS II.26.

27 YS III.49.

28 Vijñāna Bhikṣu insists (YV IV.34: 141) that *kaivalya* is a state of liberation for both *puruṣa* and *prakṛti* each reaching its respective natural or intrinsic state. He then cites the *Sāṃkhya Kārikā* (62) where it is stated that no *puruṣa* is bound, liberated or transmigrates. It is only *prakṛti* abiding in her various forms that transmigrates, is bound and becomes liberated. For references to Vijñāna Bhikṣu's YV I have consulted T. S. Rukmani's translation, *Yogavārttika of Vijñānabhikṣu*, 4 vols. New Delhi, Munshiram Manoharlal, 1981–1989.

29 YS I.51 and III.8; the state of *nirbīja* or "seedless" *samādhi* can be understood as the liberated state where no "seed" of ignorance remains, any further potential for affliction (i.e. as mental impressions or *saṃskāras*) having been purified from the mind.

30 RM I.1 (p. 1).

31 F. Max Müller, *The Six Systems of Indian Philosophy*, London, Longmans Green and Co., 1899, p. 309.

32 See, for example, Eliade, *Yoga: Immortality and Freedom*, Koelman, *Pātañjala Yoga*, Feuerstein, *Yoga-Sūtra of Patañjali*, and Larson and Bhattacharya, *Sāṃkhya*.

33 I am here echoing some of the points made by Chapple in his paper entitled "*Citta-Vṛtti* and Reality in the *Yoga Sūtra*," in *Sāṃkhya-Yoga: Proceedings of the IASWR Conference, 1981*, Stony Brook, NY, Institute for Advanced Studies in World Religions, 1983, pp. 103–19. See also Chapple and Kelly, *The Yoga Sutras of Patañjali*, p. 5, where the authors state: "*kaivalyam* . . . is not a catatonic state nor does it require death." SK 67 acknowledges that even the "potter's wheel" continues to turn because of the force of past impressions (*saṃskāras*); but in Yoga, higher dispassion and *asaṃprajñāta* eventually exhaust all the impressions or karmic residue. Through a continued program of ongoing purification Yoga allows for the possibility of an embodied state of freedom utterly unburdened by the effects of past actions. As such Yoga constitutes an advance over the fatalistic perspective in Sāṃkhya where the "wheel of *saṃsāra*" continues (after the initial experience of liberating knowledge) until, in the event of separation from the body, *prakṛti* ceases and unending "isolation" (*kaivalya*) is attained (SK 68). In any case, the yogic state of supracognitive *samādhi* or enstasy goes beyond the liberating knowledge of *viveka* in the Sāṃkhyan system in that the yogin must develop dispassion even toward discriminative discern-

ment itself. For more on an analysis of the notion of liberation in Sāṃkhya and Yoga see C. Chapple's chapter on "Living Liberation in Sāṃkhya and Yoga" in *Living Liberation in Hindu Thought*, ed. by Andrew O. Fort and Patricia Y. Mumme, Albany, State University of New York Press, 1996, pp. 115–134.

34 YS II.29; see the discussion on *aṣṭāṅga-yoga* in chapter 4 of Whicher, *The Integrity of the Yoga Darśana*.

35 YB II.28 (pp. 99–101).

36 YS I.48.

37 See K. Klostermaier, "Spirituality and Nature," in *Hindu Spirituality: Vedas Through Vedānta*, ed. by Krishna Sivaraman, London, SCM Press, 1989, pp. 319–337.

38 YS IV.29 (p. 202): *prasaṃkhyāne'pyakusīdasya sarvathā vivekakhyāter dharmameghaḥ samādhiḥ*.

39 YB II.15 (p. 78): *tatra hātuḥ svarūpamupādeyaṃ vā heyaṃ vā na bhavitumarhati*. "Here, the true nature/identity of the one who is liberated cannot be something to be acquired or discarded."

40 Thus the term *yoga* (like the terms *nirodha* and *samādhi*) is ambiguous in that it means both the process of purification and illumination and the final result of liberation or "aloneness." Due to Yoga's traditional praxis-orientation it becomes all too easy to reduce Yoga to a "means only" approach to well-being and spiritual enlightenment. In the light of its popularity in the Western world today in which technique and practice have been emphasized often to the exclusion of philosophical/theoretical understanding and a proper pedagogical context, there is a great danger in simply reifying practice whereby practice becomes something the ego does for the sake of its own security. Seen here, practice – often then conceived as a superior activity in relation to all other activities – becomes all-important in that through the activity called "practice" the ego hopes and strives to become "enlightened." Practice thus becomes rooted in a future-oriented perspective largely motivated out of a fear of not becoming enlightened; it degenerates into a form of selfishly appropriated activity where "means" become ends-in-themselves. Moreover, human relationships become mere instruments for the greater "good" of Self-realization. Thus rationalized, relationships are seen as having only a tentative nature. The search for enlightenment under the sway of this kind of instrumental rationality/reasoning (that is, the attempt to "gain" something from one's practice, i.e. enlightenment) never really goes beyond the level of ego and its compulsive search for permanent security which of course, according to Yoga thought, is an inherently afflicted state of affairs. To be sure, the concern of Yoga is to (re)discover *puruṣa*, to be restored to true identity thus overcoming dissatisfaction, fear, and misidentification by uprooting and eradicating the dis-ease of ignorance (*avidyā*). Yet, as Wilhelm Halbfass puts it, true identity "cannot be really lost, forgotten or newly acquired," for liberation "is not to be produced or accomplished in a literal sense, but only in a figurative sense" (*Tradition and Reflection: Explorations in Indian Thought*, Albany, NY, State University of New York Press, 1991, pp. 251, 252). Sufficient means for the sattvification of the mind are, however, both desirable and necessary in order to prepare the yogin for the necessary identity shift from egoity to *puruṣa*. By acknowledging that "aloneness" cannot be an acquired state resulting from or caused by yogic methods and techniques, and that *puruṣa* cannot be known (YB III.35), acquired or discarded/lost (YB II.15), Yoga in effect transcends its own result-orientation as well as the categories of means and ends.

41 YB I.18.

42 See Feuerstein, *The Philosophy of Classical Yoga*, p. 98.

43 YS III.49 and III.54.
44 YS IV.7; see also YS IV.30 (n. 45 below).
45 YS IV.30 (p. 202): *tataḥ kleśakarmanivṛttiḥ*. Thus, it may be said that to dwell without defilement in a "cloud of dharma" is the culminating description by Patañjali of what tradition later referred to as living liberation (*jīvanmukti*). To be sure, there is a "brevity of description" in the *Yoga Sūtra* regarding the state of liberation. Only sparingly, with reservation (one might add, caution) and mostly in metaphorical terms does Patañjali speak about the qualities exhibited by the liberated yogin. Chapple, ("Living Liberation in Sāṃkhya and Yoga," p. 116, see below) provides three possible reasons for this "brevity of description" regarding living liberation in the context of the *Yoga Sūtra* (and Sāṃkhya, i.e. the SK of Īśvara Kṛṣṇa): (1) He states: "(T)he genre in which both texts were written does not allow for the sort of narrative and poetic embellishment found in the epics and Purāṇas." (2) Perhaps, as Chapple suggests "a deliberate attempt has been made to guarantee that the recognition of a liberated being remains in the hands of a spiritual preceptor." What is to be noted here is that the oral and highly personalized lineage tradition within Yoga stresses the authority of the guru which guards against false claims to spiritual attainment on the part of others and thereby "helps to ensure the authenticity and integrity of the tradition." (3) A further reason for brevity "could hinge on the logical contradiction that arises due to the fact that the notion of self is so closely identified with *ahaṃkāra* [the mistaken ego sense or afflicted identity]. It would be an oxymoron for a person to say [']I am liberated.[']" The self (*puruṣa*) is of course not an object which can be seen by itself thus laying emphasis, as Chapple points out, on the ineffable nature of the liberative state which transcends mind-content, all marks and activity itself.
46 YS IV.31 (p. 203): *tadā sarvāvaraṇamalāpetasya jñānasyā"nantyājjñeyam alpam.*
47 See YB IV.30 (pp. 202–203): *kleśakarmanivṛttau jīvanneva vidvānvimukto bhavati.* "On cessation of afflicted action, the knower is released while yet living."
48 YV IV.30 (pp. 123–124). Elsewhere in his *Yoga-Sāra-Saṃgraha* (p. 17) Vijñāna Bhikṣu tells us that the yogin who is "established in the state of *dharmamegha-samādhi* is called a *jīvanmukta*" (*dharmameghaḥ samādhiḥ . . . asyāmavasthāyāṃ jīvanmukta ityucyate*). Vijñāna Bhikṣu is critical of Vedāntins (i.e. Śaṅkara's Advaita Vedānta school) that, he says, associate the *jīvanmukta* with ignorance (*avidyā-kleśa*) – probably because of the liberated being's continued link with the body – despite Yoga's insistence on the complete overcoming of the afflictions.
49 This is the essence of Kṛṣṇa's teaching in the Bhagavadgītā on *karmayoga*; see, for example, BhG IV.20.
50 See R. C. Zaehner, *Our Savage God*, London, Collins, 1974, pp. 97–98.
51 See B.-A. Scharfstein, *Mystical Experience*, Baltimore, Penguin Books, 1974, pp. 131–132.
52 See Feuerstein, *The Yogasūtra of Patañjali*, p. 81.
53 YS I.33 (p. 38): *maitrīkaruṇāmuditopekṣāṇāṃ sukhaduḥkhapuṇyāpuṇyaviṣayāṇāṃ bhāvanātaś cittaprasādanam.* "The mind is made pure and clear from the cultivation of friendliness, compassion, happiness and equanimity in conditions or toward objects of joy, sorrow, merit or demerit respectively."
54 YS II.35.
55 YS I.33; see n. 53 above.

56 Although the historical identity of Patañjali the yoga master is not known, we are assuming that Patañjali was, as the tradition would have it, an enlightened yoga adept.

57 John A. Taber,*Transformative Philosophy: A Study of Śaṅkara, Fichte, and Heidegger*, Honolulu, University of Hawaii Press, 1983, p. 26.

58 See Whicher, *The Integrity of the Yoga Darśana*.

4

DUELING WITH DUALISM

Revisioning the paradox of *puruṣa* and *prakṛti*

Lloyd W. Pflueger

The increasing popularity of yoga classes, videos, books,[1] and gurus in the popular culture of the West today accentuates an interesting contrast between the classical Sāṃkhya-Yoga system of Indian philosophy known from the ancient texts of the *Yoga Sūtra* (YS) of Patañjali and the *Sāṃkhya Kārikā* (SK) of Īśvarakṛṣṇa and more modern appropriations of yoga. Indeed the first usage of the term yoga in Vedic literature goes back to the Taittirīya Upaniṣad (2.4) from which time the word gains, as Eliade famously noted, a protean range of application, becoming one of the most salient characteristics of pan-Indic spirituality.[2] A wide range of yogas develop: the ascetic disciplines of the Upaniṣadic gurus, the many yogas of the Jains and Buddhists, the *yogadarśana* of the *Yoga Sūtra*, the *karma*, *jñāna*, and *bhakti* yogas of the Bhagavadgītā, and a host of theistic Śaiva and Vaiṣṇava yogas, Purānic yogas, and Vedāntic yogas of the various yoga *Upaniṣads*, and the Yogavāsiṣṭha. To this we must also add the medieval tantric yogas, *haṭhayoga* and its modern descendants listed in the yellow pages such as the Power yoga, Kripalu yoga, Iyengar yoga, Viniyoga, Ananda yoga, Vikram yoga, Transcendental Meditation etc. From the earliest time forward we have a constant revisioning of yoga. Patañjali himself seems, in his day, to have led the revisioning process: the disjointed nature of the *Yoga Sūtra* looks to many scholars like an effort to amalgamate early traditions of yogic practice from disparate sources with an underlying Sāṃkhya theory.[3] This aphoristic, enigmatic compilation, which works to collect, explain and unite techniques of spiritual practice has somehow gathered to itself over the centuries a great deal of prestige. Known as one of six orthodox Vedic viewpoints (*darśana*) and as the sister to the oldest school Sāṃkhya, the *Yoga Sūtra*, its practices and theories, seem to hang forever in the background of all future discussions of yoga, though its exact soteriology and metaphysics are honored more in the breach. Why should this be so?

The problem seems to be its unique philosophical dualism b(uncompromising and razor sharp division between conscious matter, *puruṣa* and *prakṛti.* In practice this sharp theoretic expresses itself as well in a sharp social divide: the division between the ascetic lifestyle and praxis of an elite cadre of ardent yogins reaching for the highest level of perceptual and cognitive discrimination, and the ordinary masses saddled with all the *duḥkha* of daily life and little of the time, discipline, temperament, training, or institutional support required to live such an austere vision. Patañjali's path of knowledge (*jñāna-mārga*) seems constitutionally ill-suited to real popularization. On one side we have the radical practice and dispassion (*abhyāsa* and *vairāgya*, YS 1.12), strict moral laws and disciplines (*yama* and *niyama*), the extreme refinement of mental function, and even its final extinction (*sarva-nirodha*, YS 1.51, 1.2) followed by the final dissolution of the *guṇas* (4.34 *gunānām pratiprasavaḥ*) described by classical Yoga. On the other side the simple, clear, unequivocal promise of liberation from all suffering (YS 1.3, 3.55, 4.34; SK 1 and 2). The disparity between bright promise and demanding practice seems to beg for a more comfortable revision. The history of early Buddhism and Jainism record similar difficulties in popularizing a meditation-based, ethically strict, yogic discipline which envisions a sharp split between the spiritual and the material.[4] Where do most of us, active householders, who are not ready for the *sangha* or *sannyāsa*, go for refuge?[5] The Hindu response, *par excellence*, of course, is evidenced in the Bhagavadgītā's poetic amalgam of yogas. The terms and theories of Sāṃkhya-Yoga are much in evidence, but the real thrust of the text is in reconciling (through *bhakti*) the knowledge path with the practical demands of an active life, not in promoting the strict *jñāna yoga* which Arjuna threatens to adopt by stepping down (much like Gautama Buddha) from his chariot and refusing to uphold *kṣatriya* dharma. From this time forward the promise and prestige of yogic practice, variously understood, is revisioned to meet the needs of wider groups. For example, even after centuries of revision and a fertile crop of commentaries and subcommentaries written largely by competitors (especially Vedantins of different stripes) the revision and popularization of classical Sāṃkhya-Yoga continues today. Along the way the continuity of Patañjali's fossilized school seems to have faded. No surviving institutions can convincingly claim to be in continuous line or *paramparā* from Patañjali or Īśvarakṛṣṇa and authentically represent their viewpoint.[6] Even so, practitioners of various spiritual discipline style themselves yogins, honor along the way the memory of Patañjali, and continue to blend the paths of Patañjali with those of the Bhagavadgītā and later tantric yogas. Why not? Patañjali offers philosophical building blocks and a kind of legitimacy, a base from which new spiritual creativity can flower.

Although there can be no academic problem with recognizing an efflorescent variety of yogic paths, scholars should become cautious when such varieties claim Patañjali and Īśvarakṛṣṇa as their spiritual and philosophical basis. These *darśanas*, orthodox systems of Indian philosophy, are premodern in structure, content, and practice and have a precise meaning within their original cultural context.

For scholars of the classical Sāṃkhya-Yoga tradition, modern "darśanologists," two connected problems arise. The first is the familiar problem of simply understanding the cryptic classical texts in their own contexts, embedded in a different time, language, and culture. The second, born of the dual citizenship we hold, is to seek to interpret these texts to speak to us in our own time. (I assume that the need to sell, teach, or preach a revisioned form of yoga is not the main thrust of academic scholarship.) Sympathetic scholars are naturally drawn to interpret the worldview of the classical Sāṃkhya-Yoga in relation to modern culture, its perceived needs, concepts, and presuppositions. Indeed, given the effect of our culture on our thinking it is perhaps impossible to entirely avoid such interpretation, even if one wants to. Whether from within the tradition, outside it, or somewhere in between, the question of relevance and meaning for today arises. It is here that the unique philosophical dualism of Sāṃkhya-Yoga presents a great challenge. Dinosaur bones are fascinating, even enlightening, but they may be difficult to digest. Dualism today has what we might call bad press. Mind–body dualism has fallen on hard times since its successes with Descartes and those who took up his worldview. Even the powerful dualism of God and Satan is questioned in modern theology. Einstein has made short work of the dualism of matter and energy in physics. The modern mind (and even more the postmodern) shies away from such simple bifurcations. In this cultural and intellectual context Patañjali's radical dualism of *puruṣa* and *prakṛti*, of pure consciousness and matter, though interestingly different from mind–body dualism, is neither easy for us to understand nor palatable in its implications for our modern way of life. Is there a kinder, gentler *darśana* hidden in classical Sāṃkhya-Yoga? Should we as scholars attempt to "free yoga," as Ian Whicher puts it, "of the long-standing conception of spiritual isolation, disembodiment, self-denial, and world-negation, and thus from its pessimistic image."[7] But can we honestly revision Patañjali as a liberal democrat? A public servant? A devoted family man? A fervent *bhakta*? A tantric *sadhak*? A *yogini*? A universal messiah or a mass marketing missionary? In my view the texts of the Sāṃkhya-Yoga tradition offer no support for such views. I am not opposed to criticizing Sāṃkhya-Yoga or attempting to bring it into conversation with Vedānta, with *bhakti*, or the Tantras, with existentialism or the needs of the twenty-first century. The first step, in any of this is simply to see what it is that Sāṃkhya-Yoga, in its own context, means to say.

This essay attempts to answer questions of meaning, relevance, and revisioning a bit obliquely: first by exploring the paradoxes involved in a traditional understanding of Sāṃkhya-Yoga categories of *puruṣa* and *prakṛti* as "dualism." Second, in a preliminary way we will apply this insight to the wider problem of revisioning Patañjali in the light of soteriological practice and possible relevance.

Binary opposition

First we must examine the so-called dualism of Sāṃkhya-Yoga. From the outset I presuppose that to read the *Yoga Sūtra* in context is to read it as it is often titled, as Pātañjala Sāṃkhya,[8] i.e. specifically as a form of Sāṃkhya and in the context of Īśvarakṛṣṇa's roughly contemporaneous *Sāṃkhya Kārikā*. Though there are a few philosophical differences, for example the role of Īśvara, I see the texts and systems as inextricably linked. As I understand it, the *Sāṃkhya Kārikā* examines the cosmology, epistemology, and ontology of the world of experience from inside out[9] in hopes of clarifying a liberating right apprehension of reality, and the *Yoga Sūtra* explicates the philosophical psychology of facilitating realization through meditative training. Both take with utmost seriousness the association and separation of two opposite constituent principles, *puruṣa* and *prakṛti*.[10] Both link suffering, and ignorance, to one factor alone, the association (*saṃyoga*) of matter and consciousness.[11] Both find salvation by severing that association in favor of "aloneness" of *puruṣa*.[12] (In terms of context, his *kaivalya* is strongly reminiscent of the radical *kevala jñāna* of *nāstika* Jainism with the similar split between *jīva* and *ajīva*, not to mention the split between *nirvāṇa* and *saṃsāra* in early Buddhism and the radical assertion of the *anātman* doctrine.)

Here I see no reason to debate whether Sāṃkhya-Yoga really means what it says with regard to its vision of radical dualism and the necessity of separating out matter from spirit. The soteriological reasoning is perfectly straightforward, clear-cut, unembarrassed, and logically consistent. Yes, it is a mix of what Westerners would call epistemology and ontology – a vision of the nature of the world, primarily as a world of experience. After all it is religious philosophy, in service of liberation from a problematic experience: the experience of *duḥkha*. This is not a vision which glamorizes a life of accumulating wealth, erotic joy, children, or public service. This is *mokṣa* philosophy unsuited to the goals of the householder *āśrama*.[13] Rather than restoring the homeless to homes, or finding a comfortable home in the world, like it or not, this dualism valorizes homelessness – one is to rid oneself of all desire for and all attachment to and all identification with *prakṛti* (whether gross physical or subtle physical or "mental"). Here one's only home is pure consciousness. YS 2.15 asserts:

> On account of the pain [inherent in] the impressions, [in] anxiety, and [in] the underlying process of transformation and due to the [continual] struggle among the operations of the *guṇas* – to the discriminating person the totality [of experience] is nothing but pain.

Thus the next *sūtra* advises *heyam duḥkham anāgatam*, future suffering should be avoided. The next explicitly states (YS 2.17): "The cause [of the future suffering] which should be avoided is the association (*saṃyoga*) of the seer and the seen (*puruṣa* and *prakṛti*)." Some would doubt that this is really dualism here or that the goal could actually be so cruel as to sentence the mind to dissolution and separate *puruṣa* from *prakṛti* decisively and forever. Whicher, for example, views *kaivalya* as the "expansion and enrichment of personal/empirical identity" of the yogin who "dwells in a state of balance and fulfillment serving others while feeling/being truly at home in the world."[14] Less optimistic, Vyāsa reveals the yogin to be as sensitive as an eyeball, tormented even by a light thread.[15] He notes: "The cause of that which is to be escaped is the association (*saṃyoga*) of pure consciousness and primordial matter. The absolute cessation (*atyantikī nirvṛttir*) of this association is the escape. The means of escape is right discernment (*samyag-darśanam*)."[16]

Let's have a deeper look at the nature of this *saṃyoga* between *puruṣa* and *prakṛti* just in terms of the primary texts.[17] Yoga might seem to be about uniting something, but it is really about separating something mistakenly united, the perceived association of matter and spirit. The problem here is that literally everything in the universe of experience is a thing, a form of matter, and manifest matter by definition is causally determined, impermanent, spatially finite, dynamic, plural, in need of support, emergent, composite, dependent, objective, and non-conscious.[18] *Puruṣa*, pure consciousness, to the contrary (SK 19), is established as (a) a witness, (b) eternally separate, (c) neutral, (d) the perceiver, and yet (e) a non-doer. Now this is a strange dualism indeed. What we would call mind in the West is seen here as strictly inert matter acting and interacting blindly, i.e. non-consciously (not unintelligently), with other matter in constant service of a principle which is quite unknown and essentially unknowable to it. To make matters worse, the matter that really counts, the intellectual faculty, *buddhi*, though non-conscious, seems to be conscious and more to the point consciously suffering. On the other hand *puruṣa*, eternally unchanging, a non-doer, seems to be acting, identified in some way with *buddhi*. This is a mind-boggling, mad, paradoxical dualism where everything appears to be its opposite and real suffering for unreal actors constantly spoils experience and traps the unreal actors in the realm of suffering, like so many sad bubbles trapped under water. But what is a bubble, but the absence, the antithesis of water? What harm can come to it? Beneath the ocean can it be drowned or made wet? SK 62 lets the cat out of the bag (the bubble out of the ocean?) by switching, with shades of Śaṅkara, to a higher, ultimate level of discourse:[19]

> Thus no one is bound, and certainly no one is liberated, nor does anyone really move through the cycle of rebirth; it is *prakṛti* alone in her many relations who is bound, who moves through cycles of birth and death and who is liberated.[20]

So though *puruṣa* was understood to be in danger, bound, lost as a doer and an experiencer of suffering, and though it is understood that everything from the creation of the material universe to the generation of beings is only for the reason of liberating *puruṣa* from its improper identification with matter, in actuality the whole mistake is on the side of *buddhi*, *prakṛti's* earliest, but most delicate form. The whole drama of salvation is the play of the darkening and clarification of the *buddhi*; in modern terms we have something like a computer glitch, an error in the bios software.

In itself this is an ingenious and fascinating salvation story. Imagine going to the dentist for a horrible toothache: instead of pulling your tooth he pulls your ego, your identity. There is a real surprise ending. What seems to be a play of consciousness is but a play of matter. The stakes are high, but there was never really any danger. What we have is a dualism which is paradoxically interactive. The association of *puruṣa* and *prakṛti* has two stages as it were: before manifestation, the two, both unmanifest are co-present unmanifest principles, perhaps something like what we might call virtual energy fields.

Such thinking reduces the infinite diversity of human experience to ultimate order, two opposite principles: a binary system. To have two ultimates is, in effect, just another way to have one. Non-dualism by comparison is chaos. Binary opposition is the ultimate order.

It is with binary opposition that paradox and mystery become the most pronounced. It is here that dualism is fascinating, tricky, and mysterious. Both principles are principally unmanifest. Yet when unmanifest, they are each so separate, so different, so unconnected, so unconnectable, and so alone as to create an odd *binocular monism*. What is the nature of that which is unmanifest? According to SK 10,[21] the unmanifest in binary opposition with the manifest has just the opposite qualities, thus by inference the unmanifest is: uncaused, infinite, pervasive, inactive, one, unsupported, non-emergent, without partition, and independent. In the beginning, pre-manifestation, the eye of *puruṣa* is always open, but sees nothing. The eye of *mula-prakṛti* is always closed, though full of non-conscious drive. Though Sāṃkhya-Yoga is famous for the doctrine of the so-called plurality of consciousness (*puruṣa-bahutva*), it seems clear that this unmanifest plurality is only a heuristic way to discuss the manifest plurality of *buddhis*. Numerical plurality is a logical impossibility in the unmanifest principle of consciousness, where there is no separation, no space, no time, no change, and no difference, as SK 10 asserts (the opposite of *anekam*).

Pure consciousness, though conscious, is not conscious of a thing. In layman's terms this is perhaps equivalent to being non-conscious. It is a spectator without a vision or a memory. It does not, cannot think. *Puruṣa* in its *svarūpa* is necessarily a non-dual mystery. All that can be said of it is that it is opposite to *prakṛti*, and conscious, thus not a doer, totally separate, indifferent, essentially alone. It sounds simple, but represents unfathomable value and sacred mystery.

Prakṛti is equally unmanifest in its root nature, equally mysterious. In itself, unmanifest, it is apparently seething with sameness. The *guṇas* maintain their own dynamic equilibrium, constant flow of the same balanced tension is the same as no action at all. The equilibrium, the primordial symmetry, has only one trick; it can break symmetry and evolve, displaying its full potential, the play and display of the three strands. It is also a non-dual mystery. Its blind inner drive to dynamism, to manifest itself, as it were to show itself to *puruṣa*, is a many splendored mystery. Completely different in nature, both uncaused and uncreated, they seem strangely "made for each other." Complementary opposites, in a sense they are both meaningless without each other, part of a single underlying system. The tight dualistic fit in a way prepares the philosophical ground for advaitic non-dualisms. The binary principles are made to function mysteriously together as a virtual system.

Binary function, bubbles, and the meaning of *saṃyoga*

The system features a cycle of interaction. *Puruṣa* is always conscious, always unmanifest, always static. *Prakṛti*, always non-conscious, is dynamic, fluctuating from a unmanifest dynamic equilibrium to a creative disequilibrium, evolution (*parināma*) which ultimately generates the appearance of conscious intellect (a confused *buddhi*, a wavy *citta*) and conscious identity (*ahamkāra*, *asmitā*). Here, perhaps, a bubble is a useful image: in a binary world of only two principles, the absence or contradiction of one seems to mean the presence of the other. Let's say in our limited universe there are somehow just two principles: by analogy water and air. They seem to associate, interact; the "friction" between them generates a kind of "foam," a *saṃyoga*, which seems to mix both, however briefly. The foam appears to be conscious. The foam appears to suffer. The foam forms, dissolves, and reappears. Such *saṃyoga*, neither entirely objective nor subjective, an odd mix of unmixable opposites, is the hallmark of ignorance, and pain, ordinary life.

To decisively dissolve this foam of ignorance, back into orderly water and air is the goal of Sāṃkhya-Yoga.

In a novelty shop I once found a small box with an on/off switch. Curiosity got the better of me and I switched it on: the top opened, a mechanical hand came out, reached down to the switch, turned it off again, only to retreat peacefully back inside. Sāṃkhya-Yoga seems to imply that we are caught in a similar play of opposites. The binary universe of *prakṛti* oscillates between two states: unmanifest and manifest. Whereas *puruṣa* is always conscious and always unmanifest, *prakṛti* is always dynamic, its nature is to manifest briefly and "be seen" (SK 66) and then disappear. Though the seer, pure consciousness, is always conscious, the implication seems to be that it needs *buddhi* to be conscious of anything at all, which is of course a mixed blessing. Because of the purity and uniquely "reflective" quality of *buddhi*, which enables an apparent interaction with *puruṣa*, the painful yet compelling drama of manifest existence runs its course. Ignorance, pleasure and pain, *rāga* and *dveṣa*, and other afflictions step out on the stage only to bow out, through *abhyasā* and *vairāgya*, *viveka-khyāti*, and *paravairāgya*. The good news is that these afflictions bow out at all.

It may be sheer hubris and beside the point to impute any ultimate purpose to this, or to insist that soteriology has ultimate meaning beyond the extinction of pain. Certainly aspirin finds plenty of purpose in the elimination of headaches. Why heads exist at all and fall prey to aches may be demanding too much. This is just how things are. Of course, in a sense, this does relegate the whole of creation to a colossal blunder, which when corrected, causes nothing less than the dissolution (*pratiprasava*)[22] of what was created. Both the foam and the waves disappear (at least until the next storm). If there is no clear purpose in this play, at least there is the symmetry of coming full circle.

What causes the waves? The generation of foam? The inherent interactive potential of the two principles. The metaphor in *Sāṃkhya Kārikā* is the image of the association of a blind (woman) and a lame (man).[23] They each bring something to the marriage, they seem to interact passionately and then lapse into quiescence again and again.[24] This image of return to a balanced, binary unmanifest is a kind of binary non-existence, a double *śunya* which spells infinity and freedom. No suffering. Nothing. Nobody. No problem. The bubble has burst.

Charges of world negation?

In a way this return to simplicity devalues the manifestation, but in a way it exalts it as well. There are only two states of matter, manifest and unmanifest, and only two states of consciousness by default – consciousness of nothing and consciousness (through *buddhi-s*) of creation, the generation of foam and the separation of foam again into the stillness. From the perspective of either *puruṣa* or *prakṛti* alone it is a non-dual world. When they associate in the *līlā* of *saṃyoga* the apparent world is mysteriously generated. It is repeatedly asserted that *prakṛti* exists only for the purpose of liberating *puruṣa*,[25] and yet *puruṣa*, independent and aloof, is never bound. So *prakṛti*, in the light of SK 62, must exist only for the purpose of a play, a simulation of the binding and the liberation of *puruṣa*. The high point of creation is then not so much the moment of liberation, but the moment just before, when the two principles rise to the climax of recognition: *puruṣa*, who is not only lame, immobile, but also dumb, says as it were to himself "I have seen her" and non-conscious *prakṛti* rhetorically replies, "I have been seen" (SK 66). This is, rather too anthropomorphically, perhaps the all-important moment which the *Yoga Sūtra* calls the *samādhi* of the dharma-cloud.[26] *Buddhi* has regained its complete sattvic purity, characterized by *paravairāgya*, unattached even to the highest meditative state. YS 3.55 announces: "when there is equal purity in the purity [quality of the intellect] as in pure consciousness [there is] liberation." The monsoon of dharma breaks the drought. Suffering is abolished. In a paradoxical moment matter is still manifest but in perfect association, perfect balance with consciousness. They are equally pure. *Puruṣa* for once sees the mirror-like surface of *citta* without a single wave: in some mysterious way it seems that *puruṣa* has in a way, in the only way possible, become conscious of consciousness – the glory moment which reflects the full potential of the interactive structure of reality. Matter, as it were tangled in the complexity of suffering and consciousness, is now pure and free: having been seen, it can let go of all falsely attributed consciousness and settle into sheer, non-conscious tranquillity. Consciousness has known consciousness by knowing its opposite. Matter has known itself also by realizing what it is not(!), dropping the pretense of knowledge.

What does this analysis of the *saṃyoga*, of the ignorant congress between matter and spirit, mean for a revisioning of yoga? Yes, as contemporary critics charge, human experience is ultimately devalued as painful, impermanent, and insubstantial.[27] On the other hand, paradoxically, the process of creation and dissolution is the only game in town. Bondage and liberation, like *puruṣa* and *prakṛti* (whether manifest or unmanifest), also form a binary system, a unity. The living and the non-living, consciousness and non-consciousness, are part of an interactive whole. One of the great differences between the *Sāṃkhya Kārikā* and the *Yoga Sūtra* is not only their disparity in length and style (poetry vs. prose), but also their respective specializations. *Sāṃkhya Kārikā* focuses on psychometaphysical theory, the paradoxical binary structure of the human experience world, and the *Yoga Sūtra* focuses on the meditative means to experience that binary structure. If we look at both texts we see that though liberation is the distant and lofty goal, it is the glory of the complex permutations of matter that is given the most attention in the *Sāṃkhya Kārikā* and the glory of the complex meditative states and their dazzling supernormal fruits which receives the most discussion in the *Yoga Sūtra*. There is, after all, nothing much to say about unmanifest matters. They silently take care of themselves. Both *darśanas* in effect glorify the path itself. This is not exactly world-negation, for the world itself is a mixture of two alternating principles. There is glory in the mix and glory in the unmixing. The "world" as it were has two states. Opposite values are complementary. To keep them so, each pole must remain strong. The extreme asceticism of the path, the intellectual intricacies of matter and spirit, the radical and dialectical nature of the realities involved make for a rewarding recital. It may not be a spirituality for mass consumption, but it is a strikingly rational spirituality worthy of recognition for its unique and coherent vision. By rewriting this song in a modern key, by envisioning a politically correct yoga at 400 CE, we may in fact lose the music and with it the integrity of the original vision. In Sāṃkhya-Yoga getting to the goal is more than half the fun. Languishing in the enlightened state, building perfect homes for perfect children in a perfect society is not valorized here. If *jīvan-mukti* is possible it is not more important than the continued few revolutions of a finished pot on a potter's wheel (SK 67: *saṃskāravaśāc cakrabhramivad dhṛtaśarīraḥ*). The real work is the work of treading the path to liberation. In an unexpected sense, the path can be seen as a goal in itself.

Seen in its own context the *Yoga Sūtra*, though its practice may be incompatible with most popular lifestyles, whether ancient or modern, preserves a sublime and uncompromising spiritual vision, a non-dual transcendence which (even as a distant goal) in its radical sweep revisions and enriches the meaning of life. Life need not be seen as suffering, but as progressive freedom and purity. Even so, when an interpretation compromises the final isolation of pure consciousness in *kaivalya* (YS 4.34) or Patañjali's own definition of yoga as the "extinction of the activities of the mind" (YS 1.2–3) or the ascetic rigor of the path, it trades the unique vision of classical Sāṃkhya-Yoga for a mass appeal which was likely never part of its conception.

A *darśana* which so sharply parses human experience into its binary components of matter and spirit and their complicated, paradoxical relationship must inevitably return to the simplicity of its parts. It will have few defenders of its goal since only noble silence rather than descriptive chatter can do the ultimate "aloneness" justice. This phenomenon can be seen as world-denial. Certainly the world of ordinary experience is ultimately denied for something more sublime. At the same time, in binary fashion the material world is given equal billing, and above all the path of practice, a material phenomenon of increasing *sattva*, increasing knowledge, power, virtue, and freedom is powerfully affirmed. In the *Sāṃkhya Kārikā* the intricacies of *prakṛti* and her productive, entertaining dance of liberation take center stage. In the *Yoga Sūtra* the powers and perfections of the yogin who is approaching liberation are invested with more *sūtras* than any other single topic (48 of 195). The goal in fact pales in descriptive force next to the glory of the path. Eliminative dualism cuts both ways. However thrilling the chariot of *samprajñāta samādhi*, in the end, the yogin must park it, step out of the vehicle, and rest in his real home.

Notes

1 I recently counted in the neighborhood of 1,200 titles in the area of yoga available to buy on-line from Amazon.com.
2 Mircea Eliade, *Yoga Immortality and Freedom*, Princeton, Princeton University Press, 1969, p. 101.
3 Scholars such as Deussen, Hauer, Dasupta, Rukmani, Feuerstein have argued persuasively that Patañjali represents a skillful editing together of disparate yoga traditions into one text.
4 For Jains, the split between *jīva* and *ajīva*; for Buddhists, the split between *nirvāṇa* and *saṃsāra*.
5 It strikes me that a modern analogue of this is space travel. Most of us find space travel exciting and inspiring, but alas, few of us have the qualifications, the "right stuff" to become astronauts and escape the gravity of the earth. For the immediate future flying beyond the earth's atmosphere will remain an elite calling open only to the highly trained professionals who are trained in the requisite disciplines.
6 Such as the Śaṅkarācarya *math-s* claim for Advaita Vedānta etc.
7 Ian Whicher in his contribution to this volume, p. 63. Whicher's book, *The Integrity of the Yoga Darśana*, Albany, State University of New York Press, 1998, goes into much greater detail with respect to his unique reading of yoga. Ian makes a case that in the 1,600 years since the earliest known edition of the *Yoga Sūtra* of Patañjali there has mostly been misinterpretation or misrepresentation of yoga philosophy due to inappropriate methodology. The thrust of his arguments is to make the intellectual world receptive for the expanded "universal and universalizing potential of yoga" (p. 308) such that it is no longer seen as radical, dualistic, unattractive, elitist, or impractical (p. 302).
   The errors of past interpretations of yoga include (a) misleading definition of yogic terms reducing them more to ontological categories than epistemological; (b) the emphasis of content rather than form, structure, and function; and (c) the ignoring of interpretations of yoga taught by authentic practicing yoga teachers. All of this abuse, has, he asserts, given a wrong impression that a yogin after liberation no longer experiences or engages the world, thus construing *cittavrittinirodha* as world denial and psychophysical negation (p. 306).
8 Or *Sāṃkhya-pravacana* (as Vyāsa has it labelled in his *Sāṃkhya-pravacana-bhāṣya*).
9 One of the unique features of Sāṃkhya-Yoga is the understanding which generates the physical world of gross elements and subtle elements from basic principles which are mental/psychological: *ahaṃkāra* and *buddhi*. It seems clear that this worldview was discovered through meditative procedures, which as

in the *Yoga Sūtra* increasingly quiet the operations of the *citta* from sense perception to ever more abstract capacities such as identity-sense ("I sense") and discrimination. In this worldview the universe is experience, and the building blocks of experience start with *tattva-s*, which are what we would call psychological faculties, which, getting progressively more gross, generate heavier principles, which eventually combine to make the building blocks of the external world. This is not just epistemology – our philosophical terms do not fit. It is a unique combination of ontology and epistemology, of material substance as psychological capacity, which is a clear statement that what we call matter is derivative of "mind" – even though it is no less "material" and by nature "non-conscious" and dynamic. If mind properties are not inherent in matter where could they come from? This view explains everything but consciousness itself as a material property. Only consciousness itself is "totally other," an opposite, complementary principle which is beyond the net of space and time and change. All else is a generated product of the three *guṇa-s*. Viz. SK 3.

10 SK 2, 20, 21, 45, 55, 57, 58, 65, 68 etc. YS1.2–4, 2.15–17, 2.25 etc.

11 See YS 1.3–1.4, 2.5, 2.15–16, 2.17, 2.23, 2.25–26; SK 2,11, 20, 21, 31, 55, 56–59.

12 See YS 1.2–3, 2.25–26, 3.54–55, 4.34.

13 Most yoga teachers today seem to tailor their teaching to householders – to lighten their load of stress and psychosomatic disease by a few minutes daily or weekly of yogic practices which demand little in terms of commitment or change in lifestyle. They are explicitly meant to be practiced by those living a modern Western lifestyle. They emphasize secular soteriology: ease, comfort, efficiency, and health more than religious soteriology.

14 Whicher, *Integrity*, 306.

15 Commentary on YS 2.15.

16 Ibid. *pradhāna-puruṣayoḥ saṃyogo heyahetuḥ / saṃyogasyātyantikī nirvṛttir hānam / hanopayaḥ samyag-darśanam /* World-denial has a noble history in India, the vocabulary of the Sāṃkhya-Yoga system shares a lot of concepts and terminology with that of non-orthodox Jains and Buddhists whose original solutions to the problem of *karma* and suffering share a great deal of the radical and uncompromising vision of Patañjali. The idea that one should eventually give up all for the life of the spirit – name, family, occupation, and possessions – has a curious and unique hold on the Indic mind. In the absence of a continuous tradition of Sāṃkhya-Yoga, one can, even today, point to a living tradition of *sannyāsa* and millions of wandering *sadhu-s* the embodiments of renunciation, still affirming ancient traditions of world-denial even in modern India.

The revulsion that Westerners can easily feel when encountering world-negating views becomes all the more acute when the mind or "soul" is also seemingly negated as in Sāṃkhya-Yoga or Buddhist *anātman*. Best to see all of these negations as ego-negation, or identity rectification, a turn of affairs potentially much more revolutionary than the theory of Copernicus.

17 By primary texts, of course I mean just the *Yoga Sūtra* and the *Sāṃkhya Kārikā*, though I will also refer to Vyāsa, though I do not equate him with Patañjali or give him precedence.

18 SK 10 and 11: (10) The manifest is (a) causally determined, (b) impermanent, (c) spatially finite, (d) dynamic, (e) plural, (f) in need of support, (g) emergent, (h) composite, and (i) dependent, while the unmanifest is quite the opposite. (11) Both the manifest and unmanifest matter are (a) constituted by

the three threads (*guṇa-s*), (b) indiscernible, (c) objective, (d) general, (e) non-conscious, and (f) evolutionary. Pure consciousness, *puruṣa*, is the opposite, though in some ways similar to unmanifest matter.

19 The implication is that *Sāṃkhya Kārikā* knows two levels of truth, not unlike that of later Vedanta, a *vyāvahārika* and a *paramārtika satya.*

20 SK 32: *tasmān na badhyate 'ddhā na mucyate/nāpi saṃsarati kaścit / saṃsarati badhyate mucyate ca/nānāśrayā prakṛtiḥ /*

21 SK 10: *hetumat, anityam, avyāpi, sakriyam / anekam, āśritaṃ, liṅgam, / sāvayavam paratantram vyaktam/viparitam avyaktam.* The *manifest* is (a) causally determined, (b) impermanent, (c) spatially finite, (d) dynamic, (e) plural, (f) in need of support, (g) emergent, (h) composite, and (i) dependent, while the unmanifest is quite the opposite ...

22 YS 4.34. Liberation is the dissolution of the *guṇa-s* which have become purposeless with respect to pure consciousness (*puruṣārtha-śunyam*) or the faculty of consciousness established in its own essential nature.

23 SK 21: "Ultimately the association of these two is for the sake of *puruṣa* seeing *prakṛti* [as separate and] becoming free, yet from this coming together, like that between a blind woman and a lame man, the whole of creation proceeds." Since *puruṣa* is masculine in gender and *prakṛti* feminine, the male/female "association" hangs in the background of this analogy, as it does in the analogy of a dancing girl before a king (SK 59).

24 Reminiscent of the mythology of the sporadic conjugal relations between Śiva and Pārvati.

25 SK 17, 21, 31, 36, 42, 56, 57, 58, 60, 63; YS 2.18, 2.21, 4.24, 4.34.

26 YS 4.29

27 YS 2.5. The spell of ignorance is over. Where it came from and where it went to is a mystery. Did it even really happen? Here ultimate priority remains with non-being, the unmanifest co-presence of eternally peaceful complementary, autonomous principles.

5

YOGA AND THE LUMINOUS[1]

Christopher Key Chapple

> The universe revealed through a meeting with the Light contrasts with the profane Universe – or transcends it – by the fact that it is spiritual in essence . . . The experience of Light radically changes the ontological condition of the subject by opening him to the world of the Spirit . . . a meeting with the Light produces a break in the subject's existence, revealing – or making clearer than before – the world of the Spirit, of holiness, and of freedom.
>
> Mircea Eliade[2]

> Light, most especially the camphor flame, is thus an extraordinarily potent condensed symbol of the quintessentially Hindu idea . . . that divinity and humanity can mutually become one another.
>
> C. J. Fuller[3]

Mircea Eliade wrote extensively about the centrality of light as the constant religious image appearing throughout the many traditions he studied from around the world over a period of decades. In reading the *Yoga Sūtra*, the core text of the tradition that defined Eliade as a leading scholar of the history of religions, themes of light and luminosity pervade the text, peering out in each of the book's four sections. This essay will follow Patañjali's treatment of light, lightness, and clarity as a constant root metaphor for the process of yogic attainment. In the process, I will be responding to the theme question of this book: Can yoga, as a philosophical system, be seen as providing an avenue for active engagement with the world without abrograting its goal of stilling the mind? Can *nirodha* and *kaivalyam* be seen as compatible with an ongoing relationship with the fluctuations of the mind?

One generally approaches the yoga tradition with a grounding in the second aphorism of the first section: *yogaś citta-vṛtti-nirodha*. This can be translated as "yoga is the suppression of the mind's fluctuations," leading to an overall philosophy and practice that emphasizes control and restraint. Following this experience, one is said to reside in one's own nature (*svarūpa*, I:3), an allusion to *puruṣa*, the eternally free, ever-present witness consciousness. Though this remains the definitive explanation of yoga, I would like to suggest that the living application of this experience can be understood by examining the places in Patañjali where he discusses the "shining forth" or discernment of *puruṣa* or witness consciousness. For most scholars, this event underscores the dualistic nature of the Yoga system. It is generally supposed that the world of active engagement ceases in order for the *puruṣa* to be discerned. The Sāṃkya Kārikā describes the liberation process in three phases. First, it discusses a moment of release or *kaivalyam*, in which *prakṛti*, embarrassed at being seen, runs away, leaving *puruṣa* in a state of aloneness. It then goes on to acknowledge that even after this has happened, *karma* will persist, like the turning of the potter's wheel. This is the second phase, which suggests some form of ongoing engagement with the world, but from an enlightened perspective. The third phase occurs at the time of death, when one is said to attain final severance from *prakṛti*. Knowledge (*jñāna*) is the sole tool used to enact this process. The *Yoga Sūtra*, by contrast, presents a much fuller and alluring account of the lightening process, with descriptions of many spiritual paths.

Pāda one: becoming the clear jewel

The *Yoga Sūtra*, as with most Indian philosophical texts, announces its purposes (I:1), defines its *telos* (I:2–3, as given above); and then outlines its theory of knowledge and reality (I:4–11). The description of actual yoga practice does not begin until sūtra I:12, where Patañjali, unlike Īśvarakṛṣṇa, emphasizes ongoing practice (*abhyāsa*) and the cultivation of dispassion (*vairāgya*). In the Sāṃkhya system, only knowledge (*jñāna*) leads to liberation. Patañjali puts forth practice or repetition or constant revisiting of yoga techniques combined with dispassion as the first of many effective tools for attaining the state of yoga. Furthermore, dispassion, a positive but not liberating *bhāva* in the *Sāṃkhya Kārikā*, is said itself to lend to (or proceed from, as will be discussed) the discernment of *puruṣa*: "That highest [dispassion] – thirstlessness for the *guṇas* – proceeds from the discernment (*khyāti*) of *puruṣa*" (I:16). Here we see in summary form a theme that occurs in each of the following three sections: the process of *pratiprasava* or inverse evolution, which entails, in the style of the Bhagavadgītā, first seeing things as no more than combinations of *guṇas*, then ascending from heaviness (*tamas*), through passion (*rajas*) to lightness (s… *va*), and then finally dissociating oneself even from this lightest
urity. At that moment, the goal has been attained: *prakṛti* is
vance and the witness consciousness alone stands.
al, applied terms, Patañjali describes four other instances
da of this clarified witness consciousness being revealed with-
hat the world itself dissolve, as required in Īśvarakṛṣṇa's

Sāṃkya Kārikā. The first involves the *brahmavihāras*, the famous ethical observances of friendliness, compassion, happiness, and equanimity borrowed by yoga from the Buddhist tradition (I:33). It could be argued that "clarification of the mind" refers only to an intermediary state, that this is merely a preparatory place to higher states of consciousness. However, if we look at this state in the context of the Pāli Canon, we can see that this is not the case. During his lifetime, the Buddha proclaimed that 500 of his disciples achieved liberation or *nibbāna* (*nirvāṇa* in Sanskrit) and declared them to be *arahants*. Identical with the formula given in the *Sāṃkhya Kārikā*, each *arahant* declared "I am not this, there is no self, I have nothing." Subsequent to this attainment, the Buddha described each as dwelling in the *brahmavihāra*, the abode or sanctuary of the religiously accomplished. This list of four accomplishments correlates directly with Patañjali's list of recommended attitudes found in YS 1:33: happiness for the happy, compassion for the suffering, joy for the virtuous, and equanimity toward those in error. Richard Gombrich writes that this was an assertion of the comportment of the enlightened ones, not merely a method of meditation. Gombrich states that when these four are performed, one achieves a state of releasing the mind (*ceto-vimutti*), which he asserts "is simply a term of Enlightenment, the attainment of nirvana"[4] In this state, the monk "pervades every direction with thoughts of kindness, compassion, sympathetic joy and equanimity [*mettā*, *karuṇā*, *muditā*, and *upekkhā*]."[5] Though Gombrich is writing about the Buddhist experience, the same insights might apply within Patañjali's understanding of the *brahmavihāra*. I would suggest that the practice described in YS 1:33 shows a process of active engagement whereby "clarification of mind" becomes an epithet for the applied and active insight undertaken on the part of the accomplished yogin in daily affairs.

The next reference to luminosity can be found in I:36: "Or having sorrowless illumination." Though brief, this attainment indicates that a flooding of light (*jyotis*) has occurred, through which sorrow has been expelled. Again, the Buddhist allusions in this passage are clear; the term *viśoka* carries connotations of being delivered from sorrow. This phrase also indicates a state of being or awareness that does not nihilistically deny the redeemability of that which can be perceived.

This brings me to what is perhaps my favorite *sūtra*, one that to my estimation has been both overlooked by some and misinterpreted by others:[6] "[The accomplished mind] of diminished fluctuations, like a clear jewel assuming the color of any near object, has unity among grasper, grasping, and grasped" (I.41). This *sūtra* juxtaposes two key images: the state of mind as having diminished fluctuations and the quality of a clear jewel. First, the linkage between diminished fluctuations and *cittavṛttinirodha* must be acknowledged. This *sūtra* defines the several processes for controlling the mind and achieving various forms of *samāpatti* (unity) and *samādhi* (absorption). This can be seen as not different from the process of *nirodha*, due to the direct reference to the diminishment of fluctuations. Yet this does not lead to the elimination of the mind or objects or the processes of perception. Instead, a specialized form of awareness – dare we say *puruṣa* – is revealed in which the separation between grasper, grasping, and grasped dissolves. Though Vyāsa suggests that this refers to three different foci of awareness, I would prefer to place the emphasis on the term *samāpatti*. In this state of unity (*samāpatti*), ego, senses, and objects lose their separation from one another revealing a state akin to kinesthesia, a state of being whelmed or absorbed – in short, moving into the depths of mystical at-onement. The world itself does not cease, merely the barriers that fence the self from world and world from self. This verse, embedded innocuously more than halfway through the *pāda*, defines and, in my thinking, gives high profile and importance to the processes of *samādhi* (*savitarka*, *nirvitarka*, *savicāra*, *nirvicāra*) that Patañjali describes in *sūtras* I:42–47.

The fourth image of clarity in the first *pāda* occurs at the conclusion of the discussion of the various forms of *samādhi*:

> In skill with *nivicāra*
> Clarity of authentic self occurs.
> There the wisdom bears *ṛta*
> (the peak Vedic experience) (I:47–48).

Earlier I mentioned the ascent from *tamas* through *rajas* to *sattva*. Similarly, through the *samādhis* one has ascended from unity with gross objects, first with thought and then without thought, to unity with subtle objects, presumably the *vāsanās* or residues or *saṃskāras* of past action that condition our personality and behavior. As one gains facility in this state of unity, "clarity," earlier associated with the *brahmavihāras*, and the notion of an authentic or somehow purified or elevated self arises. Again, this does not state that the world has been discarded or disengaged. In fact, the text proclaims that this accomplishment leads to a wisdom (*prajña*) through which the flow of life (*ṛtaṃ-bharā*) (the goal of the Vedic philosophy) may reach its fullness.

Pādas two and three: the seer and the shedding of light

Patañjali summarizes the Sāṃkhya system in verses 15–28 of the second *pāda* of the *Yoga Sūtra*. In the process, he emphasizes the purpose and function of the manifest world, the realm of the seen. In a nearly direct quote from the *Sāṃkhya Kārikā*, Patañjali writes:

> The seer only sees; though pure, it appears intentional. The nature of the seen is only for the purpose of that (seer). When its purpose is done, it disappears; otherwise it does not disappear due to being common to others (II:20–22).

First, I want to establish the relationship between the process of seeing, the seer, and luminosity. According to the Sāṃkhya scheme, a correspondence exists between the subtle elements, contained within the body, the sense organs manifested through the body, and the gross easements (*mahābhūtas*). The nose and smelling correspond to the Earth, the mouth and tasting correspond to water, the eyes and seeing correspond to light or *tejas*, the element that illumines and extends warmth. In the Puruṣa Sūkta of the *Ṛg Veda* the two eyes of Puruṣa correlate to the sun and the moon. The eyes of Puruṣa cast light on the world through the sun and the moon. Similarly, in the Sāṃkhya system, the function of the seer is that of casting light upon the things of the world. According to Sāṃkhya physics and metaphysics, the process of seeing takes place through the sense organs as they present their data to the witness. Paradoxically, though it cannot directly perform action, consciousness serves to illumine the external world. Without the presence of consciousness, the external world would not exist because there could be no knower. Although this may seem to be a child-like inversion of how we have come to understand physical principles, this perspective nonetheless reveals a certain wisdom: there can be no world that has meaning to me apart from my perception of it. This does not deny the reality of the external world, but underscores the importance of perspective and relationality in any endeavor or circumstance.

According to the psychology of Sāṃkhya and Yoga, the predispositions of *karma* exist in the seen, not in the seer.[7] Hence, though the limited ego claims to be the owner of personality, in fact personality and action can only emerge due to the presence of what the Chandogya Upaniṣad refers to as the "unseen seer." Everything that can be perceived is perceived for the sake of that seer, but, mistakably, the limited self assumes that the world exists for the sake of its own limited gratification, hence ensnaring the individual within its limitations. When the seen sees that "she" is not the seer, that is, when the purpose of the realm of activity is seen as providing experience to the unseen seer, then the "seen" and all the attachments it connotes, disappears. One stands alone in silence, liberated.

In this same section, Patañjali provides his own version equivalent of Īśvarakṛṣṇa's liberating knowledge (*jñāna*). Patañjali refers to this with the term *viveka*, "unfaltering discriminatory discernment," first introducing a term that receives emphasis in the third and fourth sections (III:54, IV:29), as will be discussed later.

But, as is seen in case after case in the *Yoga Sūtra*, the author is spiraling into the stratosphere, describing the highest accomplishment while still needing to include more material on method and process. The second *pāda*, in addition to its theories of *kriyāyoga* (II:1–2) and impurities (*kleśas*, II:3–14), and its summary of Sāṃkhya, also initiates its discussion of eightfold yoga, which continues into the first part of the third section. In particular, images of light appear in the two places in the second *pāda*: the accomplishment of purity (*śauca*) and the performance of breath control (*prāṇāyāma*).

Purity, of all the disciplines (*yama*) and observances (*niyama*), holds the distinction of bringing one to the point of perfect *sattva*. It is considered to be an apt preparation for "the vision of the self" and generates a more philosophically laden description than any of the other nine disciplines or observances: "From purity arises disassociation from one's own body, noncontact with others, purity of *sattva*, cheerfulness, onepointedness, mastery of the senses, and fitness for the vision of the self" (II:40–41). This discussion of purity begins with a description of the process of turning away from physical attraction, the most obvious aspect of *tamas*. With increased purity, one gains a host of benefits: increased *sattva*, a cheerful disposition, enhanced focus, mastery of the senses (which receives fuller treatment in the third *pāda*) and finally "fitness for the vision of the self." This last attainment places one again in the realm that links vision, the luminous sense, with the self. A double entendre can be found in each of these references. On the one hand, vision of the self can refer to looking at and seeing the self, which, as we still see in IV:19, cannot happen because the self can never become an object. That leaves us with the alternate reading, the other part of the double meaning: construing the compound here as a genitive *tatpuruṣa* compound, translated as "the self's vision." The practice of purity holds the allure of the physical realm in abeyance, allowing for the seer to simply see. This accomplishment is the "vision of the self," referring to a clarified process of perception rather than the notion that a self is seen as a fixed substance.

The next reference to light and luminosity occurs in the discussion of *prāṇāyāma*. The fourth state of *prāṇāyāma*, somewhat similar to the description of purity above, entails "withdrawal from external and internal conditions" (II:51). With this inwardness comes an intensification of *sattva*. Elliptically referring perhaps to visionary experiences articulated in the later *haṭhayoga* texts, Patañjali writes that "Thus, the covering of light is dissolved." This "enlightening" experience then allows for enhanced power and concentration: "And there is fitness of the mind organ for concentrations" (II:53).

Splendor and radiance can be found in the description of Patañjali's eighth limb, *samādhi*, in the third *pāda*. Echoing the earlier reference to the clear gem and to the point or moment where the purpose of the seen has been completed, Patañjali writes that "When the purpose alone shines forth as if empty of own form, that indeed is *samādhi*." When the purpose – that is, all things exist for the sake of providing experience to the seer – is known, then a crystalline luminosity, a seeing-things-as-they-really-are takes place, the quintessential poetic, mystic experience. And from the mastery of this, again recalling the description of wisdom in I:48, arises the "splendor of wisdom"

(III:5). This level of *samādhi* clearly allows for a world engaged through the aegis of wisdom.

Nine additional *sūtras* in the third section include references to light and illumination. Applying *saṃyama* on the sun brings "knowledge of the world" (III:5). By gazing upon that which the sun illuminates, one gains an understanding of the world. Moving into interior reflection on the *cakras*, concentrating on the highest *cakra*, "the light in the head" brings about "vision of the perfected ones," the *siddhas* or invisible helpmates to those who practice yoga. The next reference, in the midst of descriptions of various fabulous attainments and powers, brings us back to the philosophical purpose of the text: "When there is no distinction of intention between the pure *puruṣa* and the perfect *sattva*, there is experience for the purpose of the other (*puruṣa*); from *saṃyama* on purpose being for the self, there is knowledge of *puruṣa*" (III:35).

Again "knowledge of *puruṣa*" begs to be interpreted as "*puruṣa's* knowledge." Strictly speaking, *puruṣa* cannot possess anything, even knowledge, but this allows a process of alluding to an elevated state of consciousness without allowing anyone to claim it.

In the descriptions of light as associated with *saṃyama*, Patañjali employs three images in quick succession. The first states that the power of breath, specifically "mastery of the middle breath," yields radiance (*jvalanam*, III:40). This might refer to the physical result of being well oxygenated, when, for instance, one's cheeks become rosy after a brisk walk or some form of physical exertion. The second image talks about concentrating on the lightness of cotton (*laghu-tūla*), which allows one to move through space (*ākāśa-gamanam*, III:42). By identifying with something as flimsy as cotton, one takes on its qualities of free movement. The third image talks of moving beyond even the body toward the "great discarnate" (*mahāvideha*, III:43). This reference links to the earlier discussion rising above the manifest aspects of *prakṛti* (I:19). In the first mention of the discarnate (*videha*), a desire to become again involved with *prakṛti* lingers. In contrast, in the third section, this concentration on the discarnate results in the destruction of the covering of light (*prakāśa-āvaraṇa-kṣayaḥ*, III:43), a much more positive assessment of this yogic accomplishment. This also refers back to the prior *pāda*, where the practice of breath control also removes the covering of light (II:52).

The remainder of the third section discusses how one's *sattva* increases successively. First one masters the elements (*bhūta-jaya*, III:44). Then one attains perfection of the body (*kāya-saṃpad*, III:46). Next one rises above the body to gain mastery over the sense organs (*indriya-jaya*, III:47). This results in mastery over that which causes the world to become manifest (*pradhāna-jaya*), the latent aspect of *prakṛti* (III:48). At this level, as in the stage of *nirvicāra samādhi* mentioned in the first section, one is able to control the impulses (*saṃskāras*) that normally condition human craving and the pursuit of desire. Hence, as in the *Upaniṣads*, where one rises from the food-made body to the mind-made body to the emotion-body and finally attains the self, one first masters the relationship with the external elements, then one's body, then one's senses, including the mind, and gains control over the emotions. However, the final attainment requires an even higher level, defined as the "discernment of the difference between *sattva* and *puruṣa*." The final verses of the third section nicely underscore the need for increasing levels of lightness, until one reaches *kaivalya*:

> Only from the discernment of the difference
> between *sattva* and *puruṣa* can there be
> sovereignty over all states of being
> and knowledge of all (III:49).
> From dispassion even toward this,
> in the destruction of the seed of this impediment,
> arises perfect aloneness (*kaivalya*) (III:50).
> There is no cause for attachment and pride
> upon the invitation of those well established,
> because of repeated association with the undesirable (III:51).
> From *saṃyama* on the moment and its succession,
> there is knowledge born of discrimination (III:52).
> Hence, there is the ascertainment of two things that are similar,
> due to their not being limited (made separate) by differences
> of birth, designation, and place (III:53).
> The knowledge born of discrimination is said to be liberating,
> (inclusive of) all conditions and all times, and nonsuccessive (III:54).
> In the sameness of purity between the *sattva* and the *puruṣa*,
> there is perfect aloneness (*kaivalya*) (III:55).

Though I have discussed this portion of the text at length elsewhere,[8] let me paraphrase the trajectory of this important description of the liberative process. Liberation hinges on discerning the difference between one's best purity and the modality of pure witnessing. One cannot hang a shingle on one's purity; this leads to passion, attachment, and pride; one becomes susceptible to flattery. As one sloughs off all identification from moment to moment, one develops the critical skill of dwelling in a state of constant discrimination (*khyāti*). Hence, one keeps a constant vigil and can discern the difference between the purity attained in the state of *videha-prakṛti-laya*, the most rarefied form of *sattva* that occurs within the realm of *prakṛti*, and the witness. The two are so close. *Prakṛti* has resisted all attempts to act on prior compulsions (*saṃskāras*) and move again in the realm of attachment and passion. In dwelling in that perfect state of abeyance one becomes outwardly indistinguishable from the witnessing consciousness, but the voice that remains within *prakṛti* would continue to deny any such connection. Later commentators (Vācaspatimiśra, Vijñānabhikṣu) referred to this relationship in terms of reflection (*pratibhā*), indicating that the world reflects itself to the witness in its pure state, without any interfering patina of sullied interpretation. See Vācaspatimiśra's gloss on III:35:

> It is the sattva of the thinking-substance which reflects the Self united with this presented-idea, and which depends upon the Intelligence (*caitanya*) which has been mirrored (*chāyāpanna*) in it [as the intelligence] of the Self. Thus it exists for the sake of the Self.[9]

The fourth *pāda*: luminosity

The process of inverse evolution leading to increasing levels of luminosity is described yet again in the fourth section of the *Yoga Sūtra*. The first concept that indicates a special relationship between the purified *sattva* of *prakṛti* and the *puruṣa* is the concept of *prayojakam*, the initiator. Patañjali describes this function of *prakṛti* as "the one mind among many that is distinct from activity" (IV:5). This would probably be the intellect or *buddhi* in its most subtle form of *sattva* which we saw above as associated with *kaivalya* (III:55). All mind is in some sense active but this "one mind" is like *puruṣa* and hence pure. In the next verse, Patañjali, again elliptically, refers to an unspecified something that arises from mind that, despite its being "born" and hence in the realm of *prakṛti*, he nonetheless refers to as pure (*anāśayam*): "There, what is born of meditation is without residue" (IV:6). This reflects the theme in I:50: "The *saṃskāra* born of it obstructs other *saṃskāras*." This state of purity does not obliterate the world but in some way perhaps transforms it.

The next verse that pertains to notions of color, which can only be perceived through the sense of sight, and hence requires some form of illumination, discusses the colors of *karma*:

> The *karma* of a yogin is neither white nor black;
> that of others is threefold (IV:7).

This verse discusses what the Jains refer to as the *leśyas* or combinations of karmic impulses that obscure the luminosity (the energy, consciousness, and bliss) of the soul, referred to in Jainism as *jīva*. In Jainism, these colors range from black to blue to red to yellow to white; the perfected Jaina (*siddha*) rises above all colors in the state referred to as *kevala*. Patañjali refers to the varieties of color as mixed, and, like Jainism, suggests that the perfected one goes beyond all coloration.

Continuing the theme of colors, Patañjali later suggests that the attitude one takes toward objects depends upon the "anticipation" or projection of the mind that perceives any given object. Appealing to one of the classic proofs given in the *Sāṃkhya Kārikā* for the existence of *puruṣa*, he then states that all these changes are due to the "changelessness of their master, *puruṣa*" (IV:18). To complete this argument about the relationship between that which is objectively seen and the seer, he states that the object does not possess revelatory powers, but becomes illumined only through the presence of the seer. Only through the seer can the world be known, although the seen, particularly in its mistaken assumption of ego identity, seeks to claim all experience. Patañjali advances this argument as follows:

> An object of the mind is known or not known,
> due to the anticipation (of the mind) that colors it (IV:18).
> The fluctuations of the mind are always known
> due to the changelessness of their master, *puruṣa* (IV:19).
> There is no self-luminosity of that (*citta-vṛtti*)
> because of the nature of the seen (IV:20).

The seen can never see itself. Light ultimately comes from the highest source of illumination, which stands separate, even aloof, illuminating the things of the world through its gaze. When one sees that one does not really see, then the compulsion to grasp and cling to the ego identity ceases. Patañjali writes that "the one who sees the distinction discontinues the cultivation of self-becoming" (IV:25). Having observed and understood that the world appears to be as one assumes it to be because of the structures on one's mental conditioning, one gains the liberating perspective that allows a retreat from self-generating status quo.

The conclusion of the *Yoga Sūtra* describes this process of heightened awareness as a gradual letting go of being invested in the continuation of the world as self-construed. This results in the cryptic description of a liberated state, defined as the "cloud of *dharma samādhi*." This has been interpreted, appropriately, in many ways. On the one hand, the term *dharma* can be seen in light of its Buddhist counterpart, as a constituent of existence. This usage can also be found in the only other *sūtras* where Patañjali uses the term *dharma*. In III:13 and 14, Patañjali discusses *dharma* as the nature or essential quality of a thing, and says that things take on their particular character due to the nature of the *dharma*. In the level of *dharma megha samādhi*, this essence or nature has been purified and lightened to the point where rather than manifesting in the shape of a concrete reality, they remain as evanescent as the water vapor in a cloud, indicating that they perhaps have been resolved to their most subtle or *sāttvika* form. In terms of the technical Jaina usage of the term *dharma*, they have attained their most refined state of movement. And in the traditional, non-technical Hindu sense of *dharma*, this state might indicate that all unvirtuous activities have been overcome and that one dwells only in a *dharma* characterized by the *sattva-guṇa*. The following verse seems to support this final interpretation: "From that, there is cessation of afflicted action" (IV:30), which causes Vyāsa to state that one has attained living liberation, the only reference to this cherished state in his entire commentary.

In either case, the progression from gross to subtle culminates to completion in this last verse of the *Yoga Sūtra*. The process of outward manifestation (*pariṇāma*) has been reversed, called back to its origin. The inertia that leads to *tamas* has been reversed through the practices of yoga. The *guṇas*, even *sattva* itself, have performed their function of providing experience and liberation for the seer, the *puruṣa*, the original source of illumination, although, paradoxically, *puruṣa* never actively illumines. This returns the yoga practitioner to the state referred to in the third *sūtra* of the first *pāda*, the state of standing in *svarūpa*. This is not, however, a static state. The conclusion of the *Yoga Sūtra* does not require the cessation of all luminosity but instead avers to the notion of an ongoing presence of consciousness, referred to as *citi-śakti*, the power of higher awareness. The *Yoga Sūtra* does not conclude with a negation of materiality but with a celebration of the ongoing process of dispassionate yet celebratory consciousness:

> Indeed, in [that state of] reflection,
> for the one who has discriminative discernment
> and always takes no interest,
> there is the cloud of *dharma samādhi* (IV: 29).
> From that, there is cessation of afflicted action (IV:30).
> Then, little is to be known
> due to the eternality of knowledge
> which is free from all impure covering (IV:31).
> From that, the purpose of the *guṇas* is done
> and the succession of *pariṇāma* concluded (IV:32).
> Succession and its correlated, the moment,
> are terminated by the end of *pariṇāma* (IV:33).
> The return to the origin of the *guṇas*,
> emptied of their purpose for *puruṣa*,
> is *kaivalya*, the steadfastness in own form,
> and the power of higher awareness (IV:34).

Just as in the description of *prāṇāyāma* removing the covering of light (II:52), so also this concluding phase of yoga philosophy brings an end to all impurity (*tadā sarva-āvaraṇa-mala-apetasya*, IV:31). It does not, however, mean that the world itself ceases.

In our studies of Hindu thought, it is difficult to escape the notion, promulgated by the language of the tradition itself as well as Christian critiques of the tradition, that Hinduism denies the world. The language of the Buddha and Ramakrishna alike calls for a leaving behind of the world in search of higher values. However, does this really mean the rejection of the world? Does it mean that the world should only be condemned and shunned? Or does it mean that only the impure aspects of the world must be transcended? The concluding verses of the *Yoga Sūtra* certainly seem to allow for the engagement of a purified sense of one's place in the world, through which one is established and living in a purified consciousness, having understood and reversed the lure of the lower *guṇas*.

In recent studies of attitudes toward nature, several authors, including Callicott and Nelson, have suggested that Hindu philosophy negates the world and has helped cultivate an attitude of indifference or even contempt for nature. In a long-term study of the life and work of Sunderlal Bahuguna, a leading environmental activist in India, George James reaches quite a different conclusion about what some consider to be an ambiguous attitude toward the natural world. Referring to the Chipko movement for forest preservation, James writes:

> Chipko is unquestioningly a movement for the negation of the world. The world it negates, however, is the world of scientific forestry and of politicians, technicians, and contractors within whose knowledge nature is reduced to a commodity in a system of economic exchange that leaves the people destitute and dispossessed, that discounts their material needs and the religious life that supports them. The asceticism of Chipko is a renunciation of this world and its promises. It is also certainly correct that Hinduism inspired and grounded the Chipko movement. But the Hinduism of the Chipko activist differs widely from Callicott's characterization of Hinduism as a religion that views the empirical world as morally negligible and judges it as contemptible, because it deludes the soul into crediting appearance and pursuing false ends. For the Chipko movement, the false ends are the ends of scientific forestry: resin, timber, and foreign exhange; those of the Chipko agitation are soil, water, and pure air. The Hinduism of Chipko hears the claims of this world [of development] and, like the *jīvanmukta*, knows that they are false.[10]

Resin, timber, and foreign exchange exist in the realm of the mind's fluctuations (*citta-vṛtti*). Soil, water, and pure air can be seen in their own nature (*sva-rūpa*) by purified consciousness (*puruṣa*).

This move from the abstract theories to concrete social activist movements may seem like a bit of a leap. However, as Ortega y Gasset so beautifully articulated, we live in a world invented by our ancestors. The world of Hindu yoga, as articulated by Patañjali, has shaped many of the values and assumptions of South Asian life, including attitudes toward nature. For too long, without carefully examining the text, yoga has been characterized as a form of world-rejecting ascetiscism. Yoga does not reject the reality of the world, nor does it condemn the world, only the human propensity to misidentify with the more base aspects of the world. The path of yoga, like the Chipko movement, seeks not to deny the beauty of nature, but seeks to purify our relationship with it by correcting mistaken notions and usurping damaging attachments. Rather than seeking to condemn the world to a state of irredeemable darkness, yoga seeks to bring the world and, most importantly, the seers of the world, to a state of luminosity.

Notes

1 I am particularly grateful to Carol Rossi for her reflections on the *Yoga Sūtra* while in the gardens of Assisi, and to David Carpenter and Ian Whicher, who sparked the discussion for this collection of essays. The translations of the *Yoga Sūtras* in this chapter are largely taken from *The Yoga Sūtras of Patañjali: An Analysis of the Sanskrit with Accompanying English Translation* by Christopher Chapple and Yogi Ananda Viraj (Eugene P. Kelly, Jr), Delhi, Śri Satguru Publications, 1990.
2 Mircea Eliade, "Spirit, Light, and Seed," *History of Religions*, 1971, vol. 11, p. 2.
3 C. J. Fuller, *The Camphor Flame: Popular Hinduism and Society in India*, Princeton, Princeton University Press, 1992, p. 73.
4 Richard Gombrich, *How Buddhism Began: The Conditioned Genesis of Early Teachings*, London, Athlone Press, 1996, p. 60.
5 Ibid., p. 60.
6 Christopher Key Chapple, "Reading Patañjali Without Vyāsa: A Critique of Four Yoga Sūtra Passages," *Journal of the American Academy of Religion*, 1994, vol. 62, pp. 85–106.
7 See Gerald J. Larson, *Classical Sāṃkhya: An Interpretation of Its History and Meaning*, Delhi, Motilal Banarsidass, 1979, pp. 199–200.
8 Chapple, "Reading Patañjali Without Vyāsa."
9 James Haughton Woods, *The Yoga System of Patañjali*, Cambridge, MA, Harvard University Press, 1914, p. 264.
10 Christopher Key Chapple and Mary Evelyn Tucker, *Hinduism and Ecology: The Intersection of Earth, Sky, and Water*, Cambridge, MA, distributed by Harvard University Press for the Center for the Study of World Religions, Harvard Divinity School, 2000, p. 526.

Part II

THE EXPANDING TRADITION

6

YOGA IN ŚAṄKARAN ADVAITA VEDĀNTA

A reappraisal[1]

Vidyasankar Sundaresan

Introduction

The fundamental Advaita principle is that liberation is only through Self-knowledge, which consists of the identity of the Self with Brahman and which is obtained primarily from the *Upaniṣad*-s. The independent practice of meditation or the study of yoga doctrine is not considered as leading directly to liberation. Within modern critical scholarship, it is generally held that Śaṅkara,[2] the premier commentator of the Advaita tradition, rejects yoga[3] quite completely, and the great reliance that many neo-Vedāntins place upon the practice of yoga is therefore regarded as a significant deviation from Śaṅkara.[4]

On the other hand, even early *Upaniṣad* texts like *Kaṭha* and *Śvetāśvatara* exhibit ample influences of yoga, while there are many other *Upaniṣad*-s, typically considered to be of late origin, which are heavily colored by yoga. In addition to these, numerous independent Advaita treatises have been written over the centuries, which reveal a substantial closeness to yoga. The hagiographies of Śaṅkara, which were probably written between the thirteenth and seventeenth centuries, credit Śaṅkara with possessing numerous *yogic siddhi*-s, including that of entering another body,[5] although the same texts also give accounts of his having defeated adherents of Pātañjala yoga in debate. Mādhava's *Sarvadarśanasaṅgraha* (fourteenth century), which arranges various *darśana*-s in a hierarchical fashion, rates yoga second only to Advaita Vedānta. From a practical viewpoint, we may note that the daily life of the typical *saṃnyāsin* in the Śaṅkaran tradition incorporates a substantial amount of meditation and yoga practice, while the term *aṣṭāṅga-yoga-anuṣṭhāna-niṣṭha* is a time-honored title of the Śaṅkarācāryas of Śṛṅgeri, who head the monastic Śaṅkaran tradition in southern India.[6] The neo-Vedāntins may therefore be seen as following important historical precedents within the Advaita tradition. However, it must be noted that the statements of the traditional Śaṅkarācāryas on the place and value of yoga have been different from what is held by most neo-Vedāntins. In particular, they have never taught that the truth of non-dual Brahman needs verification through an experience of *nirvikalpa samādhi*. The previous Śaṅkarācārya of Śṛṅgeri emphasized that the goal of the true Advaita Vedāntin is to realize non-dual Brahman in all states of experience, not just in *samādhi*. The Self is seen in *nirvikalpa samādhi*, but this is nevertheless only a mental state, not to be unreservedly equated with liberation.[7] The current Śaṅkarācārya clarifies that yoga is traditionally taught, not as a route to liberation that is independent of the Veda, but as a means to cultivate the mental control that is necessary for Vedāntic study.[8]

In the commentary on *Brahmasūtra* (BS) 2.1.3, Śaṅkara provides a brief and general criticism of dualism in yoga, which is tied to his extensive criticism of the related school of Sāṃkhya. However, in his commentary on BS 1.3.33, he approvingly quotes one of the *Yogasūtra*-s (YS) dealing with *aṣṭāṅga-yoga*, affirms that the powers attainable through yoga cannot be doubted and cites an unidentified (?) *Śruti* text that extols the greatness of yoga.[9] In a later passage, under BS 2.4.12, he explicitly relies on the YS definition of the five *vṛtti*-s of the mind, which are compared with the five *prāṇa*-s.[10] He justifies this reference to YS with the comment that what is not refuted in a different system of thought is indeed acceptable. In another context, he states that acceptance or rejection of any philosophical position is in accordance with its adherence or otherwise to the Veda.[11] Thus, in the *Brahmasūtra* commentary, Śaṅkara makes it clear that his ultimate philosophical *siddhānta* is different from that of dualistic yoga, but nevertheless endorses various aspects of yoga. Given these pieces of evidence, and the explicit acknowledgement of yoga in many *Upaniṣad*-s, it is the purpose of this discussion to re-evaluate the overall place of yoga in Śaṅkara's thought.

The background of yoga in Śaṅkaran Advaita

A wide variety of views exists about the relationship between yoga and Śaṅkaran Advaita. As yoga is a dualistic school of thought, an apparent influence of yoga on independent Advaita texts is often held as sufficient reason for rejecting their traditional attribution to Śaṅkara.[12] However, Hacker holds that even among Śaṅkara's commentaries, the earlier texts reveal a significant influence of yoga, while the later texts written during a mature period reject yoga.[13] Based on his reading of the texts attributed to Śaṅkara Bhagavatpāda, Hacker deduces a chronological order of composition of Śaṅkara's commentaries, to reconstruct an intellectual transition from dualistic yoga to non-dualistic Vedānta, through Gauḍapāda's *asparśa yoga*. The problem of doctrinal overlap between yoga and Advaita

Vedānta is thereby converted to one of chronology internal to Śaṅkara's career as an author. I have argued elsewhere[14] that it is quite inconsistent to seek to explain away the influence of yoga on some of the major commentaries in this fashion, while simultaneously rejecting the authenticity of independent texts that show apparent influences of yoga. Moreover, there is no scholarly consensus on the order in which Śaṅkara may have composed the texts that are most probably genuine. For example, Biardeau[15] and Vetter[16] have each come to different conclusions as compared to Hacker. As Halbfass rightly points out:

> It requires extreme caution to identify "inconsistencies" and "contradictions" which would be illegitimate in Śaṅkara's own horizon and which would provide reliable, unambiguous clues for actual *changes* in his thought and for a development from earlier to later positions.[17]

The relationship between yoga and Advaita Vedānta therefore remains a topic that merits detailed reinvestigation.

One key instance of the influence of yoga is provided by Śaṅkara's commentary on the *Bhagavadgītā* (BhG). Mayeda comes to a thought-provoking conclusion that in this text, Śaṅkara treats *avidyā*, a key philosophical concept in his thought, as a *kleśa*, much as in the yoga school.[18] One argument that is often invoked to account for such influences is that they are forced by the source text. However, given that there is a source text behind almost every genuinely Śaṅkaran text, it becomes well nigh impossible to assume anything about what Śaṅkara might have written independently, without being forced by a source text. Moreover, Śaṅkara has often been charged with distorting the basic message of the *Gītā*, by emphasizing the ultimate renunciation of all action, rather than the diligent performance of the action that is proper to one's station. If so, it stands to reason that Śaṅkara could have equally well interpreted the text in accordance with his supposed rejection of yoga. That he does not do so indicates that the influence of yoga on this commentary may not be altogether forced by BhG itself.

In this essay, I intend to focus largely on core issues, and will therefore limit my discussion to a few selected texts. In addition to YS, BS and BhG, I will primarily draw upon the *Bṛhadāraṇyaka Upaniṣad* (BU), Vyāsa's *Yogasūtra Bhāṣya* (YSBh) and Śaṅkara's *Bhāṣya*-s on BU, BhG and BS (abbreviated as BUBh, BGBh and BSBh). I will occasionally refer to *Chāndogya Upaniṣad* (CU), *Taittirīya Upaniṣad* (TU) and Śaṅkara's corresponding *Bhāṣya*-s (CUBh and TUBh), as also to *Upadeśasāhasrī* (US).[19] The last is perhaps the only independent text that is accepted to be authentic, both within the Advaita tradition and by critical scholarship. In addition to these, I will cite relevant portions of Sureśvara's

Bṛhadāraṇyaka Upaniṣad Bhāṣya Vārttika (BUBhV) and *Naiṣkarmyasiddhi* (NS). I will not attempt to discuss Śaṅkara's possible authorship of a *vivaraṇa* on YSBh, as that is a topic meriting an independent investigation in its own right.

In the following discussion, I will be paying much attention to BGBh and BUBh, for the following reasons. Śaṅkara is, by definition, the author of BSBh, but it is by no means correct to assume that that text fully exhausts the range of his thought. Other commentaries do have fresh perspectives to offer. In my opinion, the traditional importance of BhG as the premier *Smṛti* text is reflected in the fact that Śaṅkara quotes frequently from it, in addition to writing a commentary on it. Moreover, internal evidence in BGBh indicates that it was probably written after BSBh.[20] As for BUBh, Daniel Ingalls[21] observed, and I can only concur, that it is a more original text than BSBh, inasmuch as it breaks new ground where BSBh seems to stick closely to Śaṅkara's predecessors in the Vedānta tradition. The importance of BUBh is also underscored by Sureśvara's composition of a *Vārttika* on it. Sureśvara has been noted as being very faithful to Śaṅkara,[22] although he explicitly disagrees with his teacher on some issues. It would be reasonable to assume that Sureśvara's thought builds upon that of the mature Śaṅkara, but Sureśvara's works have seldom been employed to define or resolve critical issues with respect to Śaṅkara's thought. What may appear as an internal contradiction in Śaṅkara's thought may perhaps be better resolved by turning to Sureśvara, rather than by appealing to some speculative reconstruction of internal chronology, or to pedagogical technique.[23] The issue I will primarily discuss is the following. How does yoga figure in the works of Śaṅkara and Sureśvara? Do these authors completely reject yoga, or do they accommodate it in some sense within Advaita Vedānta?

An important point that needs to be first clarified is that depending on the context, a number of meanings may be attached to Śaṅkara's usage of the word yoga. At numerous places in BS and BSBh, yoga refers not to a distinct school of thought but only to appropriate usage of the norms of interpretation.[24] In other instances, yoga refers to the union of two or more entities that would otherwise be distinct. Conversely, the word *viyoga* is used to refer to the separation of entities that are usually joined together.[25] In TU 2.4, yoga is the self (*ātman*) of the *vijñānamaya* sheath. Śaṅkara interprets this usage of yoga as a reference to sound reasoning (*yukti*) and resolution or collectedness (*samādhāna*).[26] Obviously, one cannot interpret the word yoga uniformly across all these instances. More explicit references to terms like *citta-vṛtti*, *dhyāna*, *dhāraṇā* and *samādhi* should be sought.

Similar caution needs to be exercised with respect to *sāṃkhya* and to the combination *sāṃkhya-yoga*. For example, in BGBh, *sāṃkhya* often merely means *jñāna-yoga*, the path of knowledge, followed by those who have renounced the world, seeking to be established in Brahman. The word *sāṃkhya* then becomes almost synonymous with *vedānta*, and indeed, in BGBh 18.13, Śaṅkara explicitly equates the two terms.[27] Correspondingly, yoga stands for *karma-yoga*, the path of detached action. This distinction simply follows that made in the source text (BhG 3.3) itself. Thus, when Śaṅkara says that yoga is preliminary to *saṃnyāsa*, e.g. in BGBh 5.1, he refers only to *karma-yoga*, and should not be mistaken as completely rejecting yoga in these contexts. However, at other places in BGBh, Śaṅkara sees reason to distinguish between practitioners of yoga and performers of detached action.[28] Such elasticity in terminology, based on the range of meanings of the word yoga, should not be misinterpreted as indications of internal contradictions in Śaṅkara's thought.

Śaṅkara and Sureśvara on *citta vṛtti nirodha*

Śaṅkara makes a key reference to *citta vṛtti nirodha* in BUBh 1.4.7, where he elaborates at great length why the *Upaniṣad*-s do not enjoin meditation on Brahman. In this discussion, he states that *citta vṛtti nirodha* is also not enjoined upon the seeker of liberation. While this seemingly rejects the usefulness of yoga and meditation for the Advaita Vedāntin, it must be noted that in addition to yoga and Advaita, there is a substantial component of Pūrva Mīmāṃsā to this argument, which needs to be properly understood. The Mīmāṃsā school of thought regards the epistemological validity of scripture as being vested primarily in its injunctive capacity. Accordingly, Vedic statements that enjoin or prohibit action are of central importance, while sentences that merely convey factual or other information are secondary to injunctions (*vidhi*)[29] and prohibitions (*pratiṣedha*). Śaṅkara, however, holds that Self-knowledge is fundamentally opposed to action, so that it is impossible for scripture to enjoin any action as a means to liberation. For Śaṅkara, the epistemological validity of the *Upaniṣad*-s lies not in their enjoining or prohibiting actions, but in the fact that these texts convey valid Self-knowledge.

This fundamental point of difference between Pūrva Mīmāṃsā and Uttara Mīmāṃsā (Vedānta) forms the immediate background for the discussion about *citta vṛtti nirodha* in BUBh 1.4.7. The major argument offered by Śaṅkara's opponent here is that liberation is a result of meditation on Brahman, and that correspondingly, the *Upaniṣad*-s contain an initial injunction (*apūrva vidhi*) to meditate on Brahman. This position is allied with what is called *prasaṃkhyāna vāda* and with *jñāna-karma-samuccaya vāda*.[30] Śaṅkara's primary response to this is that the Self always exists and is never a result, so that there can be no initial injunction for any action in regard to liberation.[31] The results of action are bound to be transitory, so that any kind of liberation that is obtained through action would eventually come to an end. Śaṅkara agrees that the ritual portion of the Veda is injunctive in nature, but rejects this possibility for the *Upaniṣad*-s.[32] The opponent then responds that if Self-knowledge cannot be enjoined, then *citta vṛtti nirodha*, i.e. the cessation or control of mental transformations, must be enjoined. This may be different from the Self-knowledge conveyed by scripture, and is prescribed in another school (*tantrāntara*).[33] This is obviously a reference to the classical school of yoga, particularly to YS 1.2. Śaṅkara disagrees and responds that scripture teaches nothing other than Self-knowledge, i.e. the essential identity of the Self with Brahman, as the means to liberation.[34]

This argument has been the topic of much discussion, but two of its key features have not been adequately appreciated. The first is that the major thrust of this argument is not against yoga, but primarily against a Pūrva Mīmāṃsā-based interpretation of the *Upaniṣad*-s. The second is that the opponent's argument assumes that *citta vṛtti nirodha* is different from Self-knowledge. Consequently, the rest of the discussion in BUBh 1.4.7 has been largely ignored (e.g. Hacker[35]). Most remarkably, Śaṅkara goes on to state that having gained the Self-knowledge taught in scripture, the steady recollection of such Self-knowledge (*ātma-vijñāna-tat-smṛti-saṃtāna*) is the only means (*ananya-sādhana*) to *citta vṛtti nirodha*.[36] This is a crucial statement about the goal of yoga practice and the means to it. In Śaṅkara's view, Self-knowledge and *citta vṛtti nirodha* are far from being quite different entities. To restate his position briefly, in the absence of a firm grounding in scripture, efforts to cease mental activity (*citta vṛtti nirodha*) will not reveal anything about Brahman. On the other hand, after the knowledge taught in scripture, that the Self is Brahman, has been properly grasped, its steady recollection naturally culminates in *citta vṛtti nirodha*. Thus, the process of gaining Self-knowledge and ideally maintaining it leads to the cessation of mental transformations. This is unsurprising, inasmuch as true Self-knowledge puts an end to *all* actions, including mental ones, but it is noteworthy that the term *citta vṛtti nirodha* is used here. Śaṅkara concludes BUBh 1.4.7 by telling us why he considers the steady recollection of Self-knowledge to be important. Even after the rise of right knowledge (*samyag-jñāna*), an assertion of a tendency towards action, generated by the previously operative *karma*, may remain stronger than the tendency towards knowledge, i.e. towards transcending action. To counter this, a steady recollection of Self-knowledge (*ātma-vijñāna-smṛti-saṃtati*) is to be maintained, bolstered by renunciation (*tyāga*) and dispassion (*vairāgya*). Therefore, the *Upaniṣad*-s may be interpreted in terms of a restrictive injunction (*niyama vidhi*) for recollecting Self-knowledge.[37] This conclusion must be compared with the earlier statement that the steady recollection of Self-knowledge results in *citta vṛtti nirodha*.

From a Mīmāṃsā perspective, it might be argued that Śaṅkara's admission of a *niyama vidhi*, after having rejected the very possibility of an *apūrva vidhi*, is self-contradictory. However, it should be remembered that, according to Śaṅkara, the rise of Self-knowledge need not coincide with the death of the body, which continues so long as the momentum of *prārabdha karman* lasts. One who truly knows the Self will naturally remember it constantly, so that the steady recollection of Self-knowledge cannot be enjoined as an *apūrva vidhi*.[38] Moreover, once one knows that one is Brahman, there is no longer an individual on whom injunctions would be binding. Nevertheless, so long as life continues in the body, the mind and intellect continue to operate. Therefore, Śaṅkara does acknowledge the means to be adopted to mitigate the effects of prior *karman*, and recommends the steady recollection of Self-knowledge along with renunciation and dispassion. Calling this a *niyama vidhi* is probably only a concession to the exegetical concerns of pre-Śaṅkaran Vedāntins, but note that the end result of following this *niyama* is nothing other than *citta vṛtti nirodha*.

This remarkable confluence of fundamental issues involved in yoga, Mīmāṃsā and Vedānta is consistently seen in Śaṅkara's works. In BUBh 1.4.7, Śaṅkara quotes the sentence *vijñāya prajñāṃ kurvīta* (BU 4.4.21) as an example of a restrictive injunction for the steady recollection of Self-knowledge. In BUBh 4.4.21, he mentions the basic qualifications necessary for the traditional student of the *Upaniṣad*-s, and quotes *Muṇḍaka* 2.2.6 (*aum ity evaṃ dhyāyata ātmānam*), to advise meditation on *auṃ*.[39] Note that in BSBh 2.3.39, Śaṅkara says that *samādhi* is taught as the means to know the Self, quoting the same *Muṇḍaka* statement as above, along with CU 8.7.1 (*so'nveṣṭavyas sa vijijñāsitavyaḥ*) and BU 2.4.5 (*ātmā vā are draṣṭavyaś śrotavyo mantavyo nididhyāsitavyaḥ*). In CUBh, he interprets CU 8.7.1 as a restrictive injunction.[40] Note also that wherever Śaṅkara interprets a text as containing a *niyama vidhi*, the content of this restrictive injunction involves meditation on *auṃ* or the steady recollection of Self-knowledge, which culminates in *citta vṛtti nirodha*. An explicit reference to yoga is also found in BUBh 4.4.2, where the context is that of the cycle of death and rebirth. Here, Śaṅkara observes that one who wishes to overcome this cycle and realize the sovereignty of the Self should practice *yogadharma* and *parisaṃkhyā* meditation.[41] This may be compared with BGBh 2.40, where *dharma* stands for *yogadharma*, which protects from the fear of birth and death. It is interesting to note in this connection that in BGBh 2.39, the word yoga stands not only for *karma*-yoga but also *samādhi-yoga*, to be performed after discarding pairs of opposites.[42] This acknowledgement of yoga practice in BUBh seems to have been largely ignored within modern scholarship. Note also that while BUBh 4.4.2 merely mentions the term *parisaṃkhyā*, US II.3 gives details of the *parisaṃkhyāna* meditation, which is taught to seekers of liberation, who desire to reduce the effects of prior merit and demerit and prevent further accumulation of both.[43] Another largely unknown reference to yoga is in BSBh 3.2.24. Here Śaṅkara explicitly says that although the

Self can only be described as "not this, not this," *yogin*-s nevertheless do see the Self, by means of devotion (*bhakti*), meditation (*dhyāna*) and dedication (*praṇidhāna*). Not surprisingly, in US I.12.5–6,[44] Śaṅkara says that the best *yogin* is one who truly knows pure seeing (*dṛśi*) as apart from that which is seen (*dṛṣṭa*).[45]

In BUBhV, Sureśvara provides a number of additional arguments against a strictly injunctive interpretation of scripture. Where Śaṅkara allows for the possibility of a restrictive injunction (*niyama vidhi*), Sureśvara clarifies that even this admission is made only to show that injunctions lack force when it comes to Self-knowledge. He notes that others interpret the *Upaniṣad*-s in terms of an excluding injunction (*parisaṃkhyā vidhi*), but points out that neither a *niyama* nor a *parisaṃkhyā* injunction can control passion (*rāga*), whereas dispassion (*vairāgya*) is a prerequisite for Self-knowledge. In NS 1.88, he allows for the alternatives of both kinds of *vidhi*-s, and says that the only means to the true Self is the rejection of the not-Self.[46] In BUBhV 4.4.21, Sureśvara says that meditation on *auṃ* is to be done after the renunciation of all *karman*. This leads to Self-knowledge, as conveyed through the *Upaniṣad mahāvākya*-s. NS 1.51 and verse 1093 in BUBhV 4.4.22 both reproduce BhG 6.3, where one who aspires to yoga while performing *karman* is contrasted with one who scales the peak of yoga, after withdrawing from *karman*.[47] In the NS passage that immediately follows this quotation, Sureśvara explicitly says that *yogābhyāsa* is to be taken up after the renunciation of all *karman*. This results in the mind being turned inwards, which is a prerequisite for understanding the true meaning of the *mahāvākya*-s. Note that as NS is an independent Vedānta treatise, we may take this text as representing Sureśvara's own views as accurately as US represents that of Śaṅkara. We may also note that in NS 1.47, Sureśvara says that the *citta* needs to be purified of the impurities (*mala*) of *rajas* and *tamas*, which is reminiscent of YSB 1.2.[48] Taking these texts together, *yogadharma* in BUBh and *yogābhyāsa* in NS are perhaps inclusive of or synonymous with meditation on *auṃ*, as mentioned in both BUBh and BUBhV. Thus, both Śaṅkara and Sureśvara clearly recommend meditative practices and yoga for the *mumukṣu*, the one who seeks Self-knowledge. After the rise of Self-knowledge, its steady recollection, which does not require any effort, naturally culminates in *citta vṛtti nirodha*. Finally, note that as in US I.12.6 and I.13.26, where Śaṅkara refers to one who knows the Self as the best of *yogin*-s, Sureśvara's salutation in NS 4.76 refers to the process by which Śaṅkara obtained Self-knowledge as yoga.[49]

Now, it is generally thought that Śaṅkara rejects yoga quite completely, at least in his mature texts, if not in the earlier ones. Seen in the light of the above discussion, this seems to be a grave misunderstanding of Śaṅkara's position on yoga and meditation. When Śaṅkara rejects the contention that *citta vṛtti nirodha* is enjoined on one who seeks liberation, his argument is primarily against viewing it as an injunction. He also rejects the notion that *citta vṛtti nirodha* is quite different from Self-knowledge, and states that the steady recollection of Self-knowledge leads to *citta vṛtti nirodha*. He also tells us why such recollection is necessary after the rise of Self-knowledge. This gives us an answer, at least partially, to the question of how exactly the ideal *jīvanmukta*, one who truly knows the Self, behaves. The state where one abides in one's own Self (*svātmany eva avasthānam*) is obviously one in which a steady remembrance of Self-knowledge is maintained. As Śaṅkara himself admits that this steady recollection leads to *citta vṛtti nirodha*, it may as well be described in terms of YS 1.3 (*tadā draṣṭuḥ svarūpe'vasthānam*). Thus, BUBh 1.4.7 and related texts show that in the final analysis, Advaita Vedānta and yoga have a lot in common and even converge in one sense. Śaṅkara consistently upholds Self-knowledge as the only means to liberation, and rejects the doctrines of the multiplicity of *puruṣa*-s and of *prakṛti* as an independent ontological principle. Nevertheless, Śaṅkara and Sureśvara take a highly nuanced attitude towards yoga. While being clearly informed by the epistemological status of scripture, the practice of yoga is seen as preparatory to Self-knowledge, and the steady recollection of Self-knowledge is affirmed as resulting in the goal of yoga. Clearly, there has been a significant accommodation of yoga within Advaita, even in the early development of this Vedāntic *darśana* in the hands of Śaṅkara and Sureśvara.

Moreover, contrary to the usual scholarly assumption that yoga has influenced only post-Śaṅkaran Vedānta, and especially so in recent times, a close relationship must have existed between even pre-Śaṅkaran Vedānta and yoga. The context in BUBh 1.4.7 is one of meditation on the Self, but this does not force Śaṅkara to refer either generally to yoga or specifically to *citta vṛtti nirodha*. We need not assume that the opponent, who explicitly refers to a *tantrāntara*, is totally imaginary, introduced by Śaṅkara solely in order to make a point about yoga, and we may conclude that the *prasaṃkhyāna vādin* must have been very significantly indebted to yoga. The only scenario that suggests itself is that some pre-Śaṅkaran Vedāntins must have sought to syncretize a Vedānta (Uttara Mīmāṃsā) doctrine out of elements of yoga and Pūrva Mīmāṃsā, by viewing the goal of yoga in terms of injunctions defined according to Pūrva Mīmāṃsā.[50] Śaṅkara rejects this attempt at syncretism primarily because of his fundamental differences with Pūrva Mīmāṃsā, in contrast to which, his attitude towards yoga is quite positive. Thus, he strongly rejects the notion that *citta vṛtti nirodha* is enjoined, but independently states that it is attained through Self-knowledge. Clearly, yoga has never been far from pre-Śaṅkaran and Śaṅkaran Vedānta. If YS 1.2 (*yogaś citta vṛtti nirodhaḥ*) is taken as the quintessential definition of yoga, then what BUBh 1.4.7 tells us about its relation to Self-knowledge is highly remarkable.

One possible counter-argument to the above discussion would be to hold that it is uncharacteristic of Śaṅkara, the author of BSBh, to give importance to yoga, and that we must therefore question whether some entirely different author wrote BUBh. Another possible argument is that BUBh was originally written by Śaṅkara, the author of BSBh, but modified in later times. Accordingly, it might be thought that the BUBh statements about *citta vṛtti nirodha* are due to some person other than Śaṅkara. However, this would have to presume that BSBh itself has never been modified in the course of its own transmission within the same tradition that has transmitted the other texts. Thus, when pushed to a logical extreme, such an argument about authenticity attributes the textual transmission with self-contradictory traits of absolute fidelity with respect to BSBh and high variability with respect to the rest. If the authenticity of even such an important text as BUBh may be thus questioned, we must then wonder whether each commentary attributed to Śaṅkara was written by a different author. In the absence of any serious effort to prepare critical editions of Śaṅkara's principal commentaries, such arguments would merely prejudge the issue, while masking serious lacunae in the academic understanding of Śaṅkara's thought.

On the other hand, the very structure of the argument in BUBh 1.4.7, pitted against a Mīmāṃsā-based interpretation of the *Upaniṣad*-s, implies that this is one of the earliest features of Advaita. However, the Mīmāṃsā emphasis of this argument has resulted in Śaṅkara's comments about yoga and meditation coming to be partly ignored and partly misunderstood. If we are to take it that Śaṅkara is indeed the author of BUBh, we must significantly revise scholarly assumptions and conclusions regarding yoga and meditation in Śaṅkaran Advaita. BUBh 1.4.7 contains an important argument that mediates scriptural knowledge of Brahman and the state of personal certitude of being Brahman, showing us the true sense in which Śaṅkara interprets the *Upaniṣad*-s. In Śaṅkara's view, his opponent both misunderstands the nature of *citta vṛtti nirodha* and mistakenly applies Pūrva Mīmāṃsā principles to an exegesis of the *Upaniṣad*-s. When Śaṅkara holds that meditation or *citta vṛtti nirodha* is not enjoined, his stand is simply that there is no possibility of an initial injunction in this regard. This does not mean that meditation on Brahman is strictly prohibited. Both injunction and prohibition presume an agent, who can be ordered to do or not to do, but the real Self is quite unconnected with action. The argument that *citta vṛtti nirodha* may be different from Self-knowledge but nevertheless enjoined upon the seeker of liberation is flawed, because nothing other than Self-knowledge leads to liberation. Moreover, rather than being something quite different from Self-knowledge, *citta vṛtti nirodha* is achieved only through a steady recollection of Self-knowledge. At a fundamental level, knowledge is completely different from action. Injunctions and prohibitions apply to actions, but knowledge cannot be enjoined or prohibited. According to Śaṅkara, Self-knowledge is not and cannot be enjoined, but liberation is through Self-knowledge, the steady recollection of which is necessary to counter *prārabdha karman*. The Self always exists, is always liberated, and does not act, so that it is impossible to enjoin either liberation or any means to it. This does not mean that liberation is impossible, but only that it is never a result of action. Similarly, when Śaṅkara says that *citta vṛtti nirodha* is not enjoined, this does not mean that *citta vṛtti nirodha* is itself rejected in his thought.

Importantly, as it is held that the steady recollection of Self-knowledge requires no effort, the nature of the true Self as a non-agent is not compromised. Nevertheless, it should be remembered that the nature of the Self as a non-agent has to be realized by the same person who has habitually identified with action and the fruits of action. Śaṅkara and Sureśvara hold that precisely because men generally consider themselves to be doers of actions, scripture enjoins (in the technical Mīmāṃsā sense of *vidhi*) the renunciation of action upon those who seek liberation.[51] This is seen as a prerequisite for correctly understanding the meaning of the term *tvam* in the great sentence *tat tvam asi*. Thus, the path of action is at best a preliminary discipline, which is renounced on the path to Self-knowledge and also rendered meaningless after the rise of Self-knowledge. In contrast, the practice of yoga is recommended after the total renunciation of all action, in order to prepare the aspirant for the rise of proper Self-knowledge as taught in the great sentences of the *Upaniṣad*-s, and *citta vṛtti nirodha* is affirmed as the natural result of Self-knowledge and its steady recollection. Thus, the path leading from *pravṛtti* (action in the world) to *nivṛtti* (withdrawal from the world) passes through yoga, and the life of *nivṛtti* naturally culminates in the goal of yoga.

The eight limbs of yoga in Śaṅkara's commentaries

The rest of this discussion will explore how Śaṅkara conceives of yoga as mediating the transition from action to knowledge. We have already seen on p. 103 that following BhG 3.3, Śaṅkara makes a key distinction between *karma-yoga* and *jñāna-yoga*. Those who follow the latter path, the one of knowledge, are directly liberated. For the others, throughout BGBh, Śaṅkara charts out a consistent course towards liberation. *Karma-yoga* lies in doing works with an attitude of dedication to the Lord, which results in the mental purification that is necessary for proper knowledge. Following this, action is to be renounced, and one should then seek to remain established in knowledge. In other words, *karma-yoga*, which involves the performance of actions, albeit without attachment to its fruits, eventually leads to *jñāna-yoga*, which requires the renunciation of all action, and thereby to liberation.[52] Perhaps the most important references for our purposes occur in BGBh, which describes how *dhāraṇā-yoga*, *dhyāna-yoga* and *samādhi-yoga* are involved in moving from *karma-yoga* to *jñāna-yoga*. As Sureśvara quotes BhG 6.3 in both BUBhV and NS, in order to position *yogābhyāsa* between the renunciation of action and the rise of Self-knowledge, BGBh 6.3 becomes a natural and appropriate starting point for our purposes.

Śaṅkara states that according to BhG 6.3, the performance of detached action leads to an aspiration for yoga, but in order to scale the peak of yoga, one must gradually, but completely, withdraw from all action. It is interesting to note that for Śaṅkara, the word yoga here primarily indicates *dhyāna-yoga*. In BGBh 2.46, the performance of action is compared to the water in a well or a tank, in contrast to the abundant flood that is the state of abiding in Self-knowledge. Nevertheless, prior to acquiring the competence to abide in that state, the performance of action is necessary. In BGBh 4.38, Śaṅkara interprets the word yoga as consisting of both *karma-yoga* and *samādhi-yoga* and tells us that the competence to obtain knowledge is obtained by the seeker of liberation (*mumukṣu*) through perfection in yoga. In BGBh 4.39, 5.27 and in his introduction to chapter six, Śaṅkara tells us that the right vision (*samyag-darśana*) of Self-knowledge liberates immediately, and that *dhyāna-yoga* is an integral part (*antaraṅga*) of this right vision. The performance of action is only an external limb (*bahiraṅga*) of *dhyāna-yoga* itself, and is to be performed by one who is unable to remain established in *dhyāna-yoga*.[53] Such references, many of which are sprinkled throughout BGBh, are indicative of the importance that Śaṅkara gives to *dhyāna-yoga*, which is placed higher than *karma-yoga* in his scheme. We must also note that he does not ignore the role of the limbs of yoga that are preparatory to *dhyāna* and *samādhi*. The following discussion provides an overview of what may be gleaned in this regard from Śaṅkara's primary commentaries. In the process, I will take a course dictated by the internal logic of what Śaṅkara says about *samyag-darśana*, rather than attempting to follow the order of the limbs of yoga in YS 2.29. Thus, after discussing *yama* and *niyama*, I will take up *dhāraṇā*, *prāṇāyāma*, *pratyāhāra*, *āsana*, *dhyāna* and *samādhi*, in that order.

As Śaṅkara points out at numerous places in BGBh, ignorance (*avidyā*) is removed through right vision. No effort is necessary to know the Self, which is self-evident. BGBh 18.50 echoes the BUBh stance that Self-knowledge is not enjoined, but acknowledges that effort is necessary to repudiate the superimposition of the not-Self on the Self.[54] It may be noted that properly discerning the Self from the not-Self is the essence of the *parisaṃkhyāna* meditation that Śaṅkara teaches independently in US II.3.[55] In BGBh 2.58–68, he states that even the wisdom born out of this discernment is apt to be destroyed by the attachment of the mind to sense-objects, so that stability in this wisdom needs to be secured, by first learning to control the senses.[56]

To this end, Śaṅkara frequently mentions the qualities to be cultivated by the seeker of liberation, which may be compared to *yama* and *niyama* in yoga. In the second chapter of BGBh, he points out that these qualities are taught as means to liberation, precisely because they characterize one who is steadfast in wisdom (*sthitaprajña*).[57] The traits said to be necessary for the student of Vedānta have normative status in the classical Śaṅkaran tradition. In addition to a desire for liberation (*mumukṣutva*), these include discernment (*viveka*), dispassion (*vairāgya*) towards the fruits of actions in this world and the next, tranquillity of mind (*śama*), self-control (*dama*), withdrawal from sense-objects (*uparati*), endurance (*titkṣā*), faith (*śraddhā*) and collectedness or resolution (*samādhāna*). This list is derived primarily from BU 4.4.23 and BhG 18.42, but from a purely practical viewpoint, it would seem that the practice of yoga is absolutely necessary for cultivating and strengthening these qualities. It also seems to me that such a perspective has already been taken into account in BhG itself, and in Śaṅkara's commentary on it. Throughout BGBh, and particularly in BGBh 13.7–11, he gives specific details of the qualities necessary in one who desires to know the Self. He prefaces his comments on these verses by saying that these qualities are means to knowledge, and that the *saṃnyāsin* who is intent on them is thereby established in knowledge. He concludes with a statement that although these qualities are only *yama*-s and *niyama*-s, they are justifiably exalted as being equal to knowledge, inasmuch as they lead to and co-operate with the direct cause of Self-knowledge.[58]

Now, it is well known that *yama* and *niyama* are the first two limbs of *aṣṭāṅga-yoga*. Among the *niyama*-s listed in YS 2.29–32, *tapas* (penance), *svādhyāya* (self-study) and *īśvara-praṇidhāna* (meditation on the Lord) are also mentioned in YS 2.1 as constituting *kriyā-yoga*. I will briefly discuss the role given to these three in the Vedāntic texts. *Tapas* and *svādhyāya* are given key importance in TU 1.9, and consequently in TUBh too. In BGBh 4.28, *svādhyāya* is explained as the prescribed study of the scriptures, beginning with the *Ṛg Veda*. Three kinds of *tapas*, physical, verbal and mental, are described in BhG 17.14–16. Some of these are directly mentioned as *yama*-s and *niyama*-s in YS, although not subsumed under the category of *tapas*. In BhG, qualities like *śauca* (cleanliness), *ahiṃsā* (non-violence) and *brahmacarya* (continence) are described as physical *tapas*. Speaking the truth (*satya*) in an inoffensive (*anudvegakara*) manner is verbal *tapas*, while mental calmness (*manaḥ-prasāda*), gentleness (*saumyatva*), silence (*mauna*) and self-control (*ātma-vinigraha*) constitute mental *tapas*. Śaṅkara's comments in BGBh 17.15–16 are most interesting. His example of a true and inoffensive utterance is the sentence, "remain calm, pursue your studies (*svādhyāya*) and practice yoga; thus will good accrue to you." He explains the terms *saumyatva* and *ātmavinigraha* in BhG 17.16 as *saumanasya* and *mano-nirodha* respectively.

The use of the terms *saṃyama* and *vṛtti* in his explanation of the word *mauna* is also noteworthy.[59] Note that it is Śaṅkara who has introduced such technical yoga terms, as also an explicit reference to yoga in his commentary on these verses. The easy explanation for this is to consider Śaṅkara as being circumscribed by the influence of yoga in his source text. I would, however, like to redirect attention to (a) his explicit statement in BUBh 4.4.2 about *yogadharma* and (b) his positive quotation of YS with respect to *svādhyāya* in BSBh 1.3.33. In TUBh 3.6, Śaṅkara says that one who desires to know Brahman should perform *tapas*, which is the means to cultivate *samādhāna*. This statement occurs at the conclusion of Śaṅkara's discussion, as the final lesson to be drawn from TU 3.1–6. Thus, Śaṅkara particularly emphasizes the sentence, *sa tapo'tapyata*, which occurs repeatedly in TU 3.1–6. It is therefore noteworthy that in TU 2.4, where yoga is the self of the *vijñānamaya* sheath, Śaṅkara has already interpreted yoga as *samādhāna*.[60]

While *tapas* and *svādhyāya* are thus given an important place in Śaṅkara's thought, much more can be said about his statements on Īśvara. Here, I will restrict my discussion to Śaṅkara's basic conception of Īśvara and the level of familiarity with YSBh that he exhibits in this connection. All schools of Vedānta consider omniscience as one of the primary attributes of Īśvara, and would therefore agree with YS and YSB in this respect. Unlike in yoga, however, Śaṅkara does not consider Īśvara to be a special (*viśeṣa*) kind of *puruṣa*. In Advaita Vedānta, Īśvara is *saguṇa* Brahman, the lord of *prakṛti*, which consists of the three *guṇa*-s and which is equated with *māyā* and said to be characterized by *avidyā*.[61] In BGBh 13.19, both *prakṛti* and *puruṣa* are the two *prakṛti*-s of Īśvara, which are beginningless (*anādī*), and through which Īśvara causes the origin, sustenance and dissolution of the universe. Indeed, the very overlordship (*īśvaratva*) of Īśvara subsists in this twofold *prakṛti*.[62] This view is based on BhG 7.4–5, where two natures (*prakṛti*-s) of the Lord are described. The lower nature is called *māyā-śakti*, consisting of the transformations of *prakṛti*, as is familiar from Sāṃkhya texts and YSBh, but the higher nature is the *jīva*, i.e. *puruṣa*. BhG and BGBh 7.4–5 connect this description of the higher nature with Upaniṣadic doctrine, according to which Īśvara sustains the world by entering it in the form of the *jīva*.[63]

Śaṅkara tells us in BSBh that Īśvara has a causal role in all actions of the *jīva*, although the absolute dependence of the *jīva* on Īśvara may not ordinarily be obvious. Indeed, the ability of the *jīva* to do actions (*kartṛtva*) and to enjoy their fruits (*bhoktṛtva*), which characterizes bondage, itself derives from Īśvara. The attainment of liberation, through the knowledge that the Self is unconnected with actions and their fruits, also occurs only through the grace (*anugraha*) of Īśvara.[64] Śaṅkara's introduction to the fifteenth chapter of BGBh tells us that this grace (*prasāda*) is obtained through *bhakti-yoga*. We must also note that according to Śaṅkara, *karma-*

yoga involves not only detachment towards the fruits of actions, but also total dedication to Īśvara while performing actions. Inasmuch as the obtaining of knowledge may be seen as the fruit of *karma-yoga*, even the attachment to this fruit must be given up, while remaining grounded in dedication to the Lord.[65] In this sense, *bhakti-yoga* is an essential aspect of *karma-yoga*, while also being necessary for the transition to gaining Self-knowledge and *jñāna-yoga*.

In this context, the meditation on *praṇava* (the sound *auṃ*) that is frequently prescribed gains in significance. Meditation on *auṃ* is an extremely important feature of both yoga and Vedānta. Again BhG acts as a mediating text, as BhG 8.13 mentions that one who utters *auṃ* and remembers Kṛṣṇa during one's last moments reaches the highest goal. In his commentary on this verse, Śaṅkara reveals a clear familiarity with, or perhaps even verbal dependence on, YS and YSBh 1.27–28, where contemplation of the *praṇava* as the symbol of Īśvara is described. Thus, he refers to *vācaka-rūpa*, *abhidhāna-bhūta* and *tad-artha-bhūta*, but note that BhG 8.13 itself does not force a commentator to use these terms.[66]

More generally, the source-texts of Vedānta, the principal *Upaniṣad-s*, teach many different kinds of meditation on *auṃ*. The most relevant one for our discussion is found in texts such as *Praśna* 5.1–2, which teaches the typical Vedāntic methodology of meditation on Īśvara, involving the three constituent units (*mātra*-s) of *auṃ*, i.e. the *a-kāra*, *u-kāra* and *ma-kāra*.[67] This is different from the mental repetition of the syllable that is involved in *japa* (YS 1.28). Śaṅkara quotes this *Praśna* text regarding meditation on the units of *auṃ* in both BGBh 8.12–13 and BSBh 1.3.13, and says that this is to be followed by those of slow and middling intellects. Its result is the attainment of the world of (*saguṇa*) Brahman, on the path of gradual liberation (*krama-mukti*), and it eventually leads to right vision (*samyag-darśana*).[68] I will discuss below the details of this meditation as described in BGBh.

According to Śaṅkara, the entire eighth chapter of BhG teaches *dhāraṇā-yoga* through meditation on the *auṃkāra*. BGBh 8.10–12 reveal remarkable influence of *yogic* thinking. As YS 3.1–6 tell us, *dhāraṇā* involves binding the mind to one place, while *saṃyama* involves all three of *dhāraṇā*, *dhyāna* and *samādhi*, and is applied in stages. Thus, where BhG 8.10 refers to the power of yoga, Śaṅkara interprets this power as being characterized by the steadiness of mind born out of the accumulated impressions (*saṃskāra*) of *samādhi*. He also refers to controlling the *citta* within the lotus of the heart, causing the *prāṇa* to rise up, through the channel (*nāḍī*) that rises upward, by mastering it in stages (*bhūmijaya-krama*), and then fixing it between the eyebrows (*bhruvor-madhye*). It should be noted that none of these details is found in BhG 8.10, the verse being commented upon, except for the reference to the midst of the eyebrows. It is Śaṅkara who brings in the other references, particularly the one about controlling the *citta* in the heart and mastering the breath in stages. Immediate comparisons with YS 3.1, where *dhāraṇā* is defined in terms of binding the *citta* in one place, and with YS and YSBh 3.5–6 suggest themselves.[69] Similarly, BhG 8.12 refers to fixing the breath in the crown of the head, and BGBh 8.12 again refers to the channel that rises upwards. The eighth chapter of BhG goes on to correlate the meditation on *auṃkāra*, as described in BhG 8.13, with the path of light, which leads to immortality and non-return, as opposed to the lunar path, which leads to rebirth. These are obviously references to what are called *devayāna* and *pitṛyāna* in the *Upaniṣad*-s, but note that many later commentators introduce references and terminology specific to Kuṇḍalinī yoga into this chapter of BhG. As far as Śaṅkara is concerned, rather than turning to Kuṇḍalinī yoga or Tantra, it is certain that he implicitly refers to the principal *Upaniṣad*-s here. CU 8.6.6 refers to the one channel that rises upward, leading to immortality, as opposed to the hundred others that lead to rebirth. In CUBh 8.6.5–6, Śaṅkara says that meditation on Brahman through *dhyāna* on the *auṃkāra* eventually leads to immortality through this upward rising channel, while the other bodily channels lead to rebirth.[70] We may compare these statements of CUBh and BGBh with the conclusion of BSBh 4.4.22, that those who depart on the *devayāna*, through the upward rising bodily channel, attain the world of Brahman, and do not return to the cycle of rebirths, as they eventually attain right vision (*samyag-darśana*). Thus, what BGBh calls *dhāraṇā-yoga* is remarkably congruent with what Śaṅkara says about *krama-mukti* in his other commentaries.[71] Note also that under BhG 8.24, where the path of light is described, he explicitly states that those who already have the right vision are immediately liberated (*sadyo-mukti*), and there is no question of any further going and coming anywhere.[72] In a remarkable parallel to yoga (where *dhāraṇā* leads to *dhyāna*), we are told that *dhāraṇā-yoga* leads by stages to *samyag-darśana*, of which *dhyāna-yoga* is an integral part. The association of what Śaṅkara calls *dhāraṇā-yoga* in BGBh with the *devayāna* in BSBh attests to the very ancient origin of this meditation on *auṃ*.

The above description of *dhāraṇā-yoga* leads naturally to *prāṇāyāma* and *pratyāhāra*, inasmuch as it is based on the control of *prāṇa* and withdrawal of the senses from their objects. YS 2.53 tells us that *prāṇāyāma* makes the mind competent for *dhāraṇā*. The principal *Upaniṣad*-s also frequently refer to the *prāṇa*-s, but a full investigation of Śaṅkara's commentaries on these texts will have to remain outside the scope of this discussion. It is perhaps sufficient to note here that Śaṅkara provides specific details of *prāṇāyāma* in BGBh 4.29, where he introduces technical terms such as *pūraka*, *recaka* and *kumbhaka*, which are not used in BhG. These terms are familiar to us from late texts, but not from YS or YSBh themselves.[73] As for *pratyāhāra*, the limb of yoga that follows *prāṇāyāma*, it seems to be explicitly mentioned only in BGBh 4.28, as far as my investigations indicate. Here, *prāṇāyāma* and *pratyāhāra* are both said to characterize yoga, which is conceived of as sacrifice. Note that BhG 4.28 itself does not explicitly refer to *pratyāhāra*. We will see in the following discussion that in his descriptions of *dhyāna-yoga*, Śaṅkara always mentions withdrawal of the senses from their objects, although without using the term *pratyāhāra*. We have already seen that at various contexts, BGBh frequently refers to control of the senses, using forms of the verb *vaśī-kṛ*, which reminds one of YS 2.55.[74]

Śaṅkara describes *āsana* in relation to *dhyāna* and *samādhi*, in BSBh 4.1.7–11. *Upāsana* or *dhyāna*, which is the flow of identical thoughts, is to be carried out in a seated posture. The reason given is that the mind gets distracted while standing, walking or running, and one is apt to fall asleep while lying down. Therefore, an investigation into subtle issues is possible only in a seated posture. The goal is to achieve focused concentration (*ekāgratā*) and firmness of mind (*acalatva*). There are no restrictions on the place and time where *dhyāna* is to be carried out, nor on the direction to be faced while seated, the only guiding criterion being the ease with which mental concentration is achieved. As part of this discussion, where the *sūtra* appeals to *Smṛti* authority, Śaṅkara quotes BhG 6.11 and also refers to the *yogaśāstra* where *padma* and other *āsana*-s are described.[75] In the sixth chapter of BhG, which is called *dhyāna-yoga*, Śaṅkara says that this yoga is characteristic (*lakṣaṇa*) of the right vision (*samyag-darśana*) of the Self, the fruit of which is liberation. We have already seen that throughout BGBh, Śaṅkara describes *dhyāna-yoga* as an integral part (*antaraṅga*) of *samyag-darśana*. BGBh 6.11 says that *āsana* is the first among the means to this yoga. The seat should be made of *kuśa* grass, covered with hide and then with cloth, in the reverse order of what is mentioned in BhG 6.11. We may note that a little later in the same chapter, Śaṅkara quotes an unknown *yogaśāstra* text, with respect to the amount of food that is prescribed for *yogin*-s.[76] Thus, Śaṅkara does not neglect to offer practical comments on the regulations of the aspiring *yogin*, and the characteristics of the perfected *yogin*, such as how to lay down a seat for meditation, the proper posture for meditation and the food intake required for bodily maintenance. These cannot be viewed as being forced by the source text, as Śaṅkara provides details over and above what is mentioned in BhG itself.

As in BSBh, in BGBh 12.3 and BGBh 13.24 too, Śaṅkara defines *upāsana* or *dhyāna* as a long-lasting flow of identical thought or an uninterrupted stream of thought, comparable to the steady flow of oil. The technical terms he uses are *samāna-pratyaya-pravāha* and *avicchinna-pratyaya*.[77] We have already seen that BGBh 6.3, from which we began this part of this discussion, tells us that *karma-yoga* gradually leads to *dhyāna-yoga*. More extensive details are given in the sixth chapter of BGBh, but we must remember that Śaṅkara also tells us that *karma-yoga* eventually leads to *sāṃkhya-yoga*. How then are *dhyāna-yoga* and *sāṃkhya-yoga* related?

BGBh 13.24 tells us that these are alternative means (*upāya-vikalpa*) to the vision of the Self (*ātma-darśana*). In this passage, Śaṅkara tells us that *dhyāna* involves one-pointed and uninterrupted thought, preceded by withdrawal of the senses from their objects and into the mind. As in BGBh 2.58, where the *sthitaprajña* is described, instead of *pratyāhāra*, the term that Śaṅkara uses for withdrawal of the senses is derived from a related verb, namely *upasaṃhṛ*. This *dhyāna* purifies the internal organ and prepares it for seeing the Self. Alternatively, the Self may be seen through the *sāṃkhya* contemplation, which consists of properly differentiating between the not-Self, consisting of the three *guṇa*-s (*sattva*, *rajas* and *tamas*), and the Self, the witness, who is different from the three *guṇa*-s. On the other hand, Śaṅkara reiterates that *karma-yoga* leads to the vision of the Self, not independently, but by leading to mental purity and finally to knowledge.[78] We must remember that according to BGBh 6.3, *dhyāna* involves gradual withdrawal from the performance of actions, while according to BGBh 3.3, *sāṃkhya* is closely associated with *saṃnyāsa* and sharply distinguished from the performance of actions. The element of choice between *sāṃkhya* and *dhyāna* in BGBh 13.24 seems to be closely associated with the choice regarding when to renounce action – directly from the student or householder stages or in a specific sequence, from student to householder to forest-dweller to monk. Direct *saṃnyāsa* provides the sharp contrast between action and renunciation while the sequential progression in stages represents the gradual withdrawal from action.

To summarize the preceding discussion, Śaṅkara incorporates *yama*, *niyama*, *āsana*, *prāṇāyāma*, *pratyāhāra*, *dhāraṇā* and *dhyāna* at various places in his major commentaries. Among these, *yama* and *niyama* are the basic requirements of one who seeks liberation, as well as the qualities that characterize the man of knowledge. *Prāṇāyāma* and *pratyāhāra* are particularly associated with yoga conceived of as sacrifice, and technical terms associated with the former are described in some detail. *Dhāraṇā* is used in a specific sense, in the context of a meditation on *auṃ* involving the bodily channels, and based on control of the senses and the *prāṇa*-s. This is associated with the path of light on which a knower of *saguṇa* Brahman departs from this world and does not return to rebirth. *Dhyāna-yoga* is frequently mentioned as an integral part of *samyag-darśana*, which liberates immediately, and which involves neither a departure to a different world nor return to rebirth. As *dhyāna* is necessarily preceded by withdrawal of the senses from their objects, *pratyāhāra* is implicitly assumed, although Śaṅkara tends to use terms derived from *upasaṃhṛ* more often. As for *āsana*, even in BSBh, we have an explicit affirmation that it is necessary for *upāsana* or *dhyāna*, and that different postures are taught in the yoga texts for this purpose. *Dhyāna* is described as one of the means by which a vision of the Self is obtained, an alternative means being the *sāṃkhya* reasoning.

The eighth limb of yoga, namely *samādhi*, is used by Śaṅkara in a variety of meanings, parallel with the multivalent usage of yoga itself. We have already seen that in BSBh 2.3.39, *samādhi* is said to be taught as the means to the Self, and associated with meditation on *auṃ*, while BGBh 8.10 refers to *samādhi* in the context of *dhāraṇā-yoga* and meditation on *auṃ*. We have also seen that BGBh 2.39 and 4.38 mention *samādhi-yoga* separately from *karma-yoga*. In BGBh 2.53–54, Śaṅkara equates *samādhi* with the Self, in which the internal organ rests in stillness, without distractions (*vikṣepa*) and without any mental constructions (*vikalpa*). In the same passage, *samādhi* is also equated with the wisdom of discernment, while the *sthitaprajña*, who knows that he is the highest Brahman, is described as one who has obtained this wisdom through *samādhi*.[79] It bears reiteration that throughout BGBh, Śaṅkara emphasizes that the marks of the liberated person are what are taught as means to liberation.[80] Thus, beginning with *yama-niyama* and ending with *samādhi*, every limb of yoga has a place in Advaita Vedānta, initially as things to be accomplished by the seeker of liberation and ultimately as characterizing one who is established in Self-knowledge. This is in perfect accord with Śaṅkara's stance in BUBh 1.4.7, that the steady recollection of Self-knowledge leads to *citta vṛtti nirodha*.

Conclusion: re-examining *samādhi* and yoga in BSBh

We may now briefly revisit what Śaṅkara says about *samādhi* and yoga in BSBh. To begin with, we may note that in BSBh 2.3.39, Śaṅkara does not say that *samādhi* is enjoined as the means to liberation. However, he does tell us that scriptural passages regarding meditation on *auṃ* (*Muṇḍaka* 2.2.6), about seeing, hearing, thinking of and meditating on the Self (BU 2.4.5) and about investigating and knowing Brahman (CU 8.7.1) teach *samādhi*. BSBh 2.3.40 takes note of the contention that *samādhi* is enjoined, and refutes it, on the grounds that the Self is not an agent. Scripture takes into account that people presume themselves to be doers of actions, and consequently enjoins or prohibits actions, but it does not teach that the real Self is an agent.[81] Agency is superimposed on the Self through the adjunct (*upādhi*) of the internal organ (*buddhi*). We must remember that according to Śaṅkara and Sureśvara, precisely because of this state of affairs, scripture enjoins nothing other than the eventual renunciation of action upon the seeker of liberation. As in BUBh 1.4.7, the thrust of the discussion in BSBh is also not against yoga or *samādhi*, but against the Mīmāṃsā-related argument that liberation is to be achieved through enjoined action. Thus, BSBh 2.3.39 affirms that *samādhi* is taught as the means to the Self that is spoken of in the *Upaniṣad*-s, while BSBh 2.3.40 refutes that this as an injunction, because such a notion falsely presumes that the Self is intrinsically a doer of action.

This brings us to BS and BSBh 2.1.3, where it is said that the criticisms of Sāṃkhya throughout the preceding portions of BSBh also serve to criticize yoga, inasmuch as both schools share many points in common. It must be noted that in addition to the *Upaniṣad* sentences quoted in BSBh 2.3.39, Śaṅkara refers to passages from *Śvetāśvatara* and *Kaṭha Upaniṣad*-s that mention *sāṃkhya* and yoga. According to Śaṅkara, yoga is specifically mentioned in BS 2.1.3 because among all the *Smṛti* traditions, Sāṃkhya and yoga are closest to the *Upaniṣad*-s and are accepted by those who follow the Vedic tradition. He then quotes a sentence, *atha tattva-darśanābhyupāyo yogaḥ*, attributing it to a *yogaśāstra*. This reads like a *sūtra* from a yoga text, which is perhaps no longer extant. Śaṅkara comments that the proponents of the Sāṃkhya and yoga schools are dualists who postulate an independent *prakṛti* or *pradhāna* as the material cause of the universe. Nevertheless, the doctrines of these two *Smṛti*-s are only partially opposed to the teachings of the *Upaniṣad*-s. Śaṅkara acknowledges that those teachings of Sāṃkhya and yoga that do not contradict the *Upaniṣad*-s are perfectly acceptable. The followers of Sāṃkhya accept that the *puruṣa* is intrinsically pure and unconnected to action, while followers of yoga accept the path of *nivṛtti* that is taught in the *Upaniṣad*-s as the means to know the Self. Consequently, as far as Vedāntins are concerned, *sāṃkhya* is *jñāna* and yoga is *dhyāna* that are both in accordance with the *Upaniṣad*-s.[82] This is quite consistent with BGBh 13.24, where Śaṅkara describes *sāṃkhya-yoga* and *dhyāna-yoga* as alternative means to the vision of the Self.

Scripture plays a central role in Śaṅkara's thought, as he holds that it is the source of Self-knowledge. As an exegete, Śaṅkara makes a special effort to criticize Sāṃkhya and yoga in order to highlight the points on which these schools differ from Vedānta, but this is precisely because he himself views these schools as being closely related to Vedānta. It is pertinent to recall here that YS 1.7 lists *āgama* as the only acknowledged source of valid knowledge other than perception and inference, and that Śaṅkara quotes YS 1.6 with approval in BSBh 2.4.12. Thus, even while criticizing yoga, BSBh acknowledges the relevance of *sāṃkhya* and yoga and their roles as means (*upāya*) to obtain knowledge. According to Śaṅkara, scripture teaches us that the Self is Brahman, which always exists and is not something to be accomplished through action. On the other hand, one who seeks liberation has to first know one's own Self as Brahman, and then remain established in Brahman. Inasmuch as liberation is something that is sought after, this vision needs to be obtained, if only in a figurative sense of the word. Śaṅkara does acknowledge that effort may be necessary to remove the ignorance that blocks this right vision of the Self. What is taught as the means to the right vision is nothing other than the set of qualities that characterize one who already has the right vision. As we have seen in our extensive examination of BGBh, yoga plays a key role in the effort to cultivate these qualities.

From the perspective of one who seeks liberation, we may note that Śaṅkara firmly grounds his thought in the Brahminical milieu of *saṃnyāsa*. The transition from action to renunciation involves yoga in the following manner. After the stage of the student (*brahmacārī*), one who is competent for *jñāna-yoga* can directly renounce the world and become a *saṃnyāsin*.[83] This option is associated with *sāṃkhya-yoga* in BGBh 3.3. In this context, we may note that Śaṅkara teaches *parisaṃkhyāna* meditation in BUBh 4.4.2 and in US II.3. One who is not mentally equipped to renounce at this early stage becomes a householder (*gṛhastha*). If he seeks liberation, he must enter the path of *karma-yoga*, by performing actions with detachment and with dedication to the Lord. This leads to mental purity and prepares the aspirant for embarking upon Self-knowledge. Nevertheless, action is only an outer limb of *dhyāna-yoga*, which is an integral part of the right vision (*samyag-darśana*) that liberates immediately (*sadyo-mukti*). Therefore, the householder is to perform action only so long as he finds himself unable to remain established in *dhyāna-yoga*. The ability to remain thus established is necessarily to be tested through repeated practice or *abhyāsa*. The householder may then progress onto the stage of the forest-dweller (*vānaprastha*), which ultimately leads to *saṃnyāsa*. As BhG 6.25 tells us, the path of *dhyāna-yoga* can be a gradual process, as one has to withdraw from action slowly, aided by a resolute intellect. Additionally, the householder has the option to directly renounce the world, given the right conditions, and enter the path of *jñāna-yoga*. If one's intellect is not well equipped for the rigour of Self-knowledge, meditation on *auṃ* may be carried out, conceiving of *auṃ* as the symbol of the Lord, and by focusing one's concentration on ascending through the upward rising channel. This is *dhāraṇā-yoga*, which leads to liberation in stages or *krama-mukti*, by first leading to the world of *saguṇa* Brahman and eventually to *samyag-darśana*. Whether Self-knowledge is obtained through *dhyāna-yoga* or *sāṃkhya-yoga*, BGBh 2.54–72 advise that one must maintain the state of Self-knowledge, without being led astray by the senses. The state of abiding in Self-knowledge, or *jñāna-niṣṭhā*, is quite akin to *yogic* meditation, as described in the BGBh discussion of the *sthitaprajña*, who obtains his wisdom through *samādhi*. BSBh 2.3.39 tells us that the *Upaniṣad*-s teach *samādhi* in order to know the Self, and BGBh often describes *dhyāna-yoga* as an integral part of right knowledge. In addition, we may note the frequent usage of the term *saṃyama* in BGBh, which as YS 3.4 tells us, consists of *dhāraṇā*, *dhyāna* and *samādhi* together. The other limbs of yoga, i.e. *yama*, *niyama*, *āsana*, *prāṇāyāma* and *pratyāhāra* (or as Śaṅkara might call it, *upasaṃhāra*) are described at appropriate places, as preparatory to *dhāraṇā*, *dhyāna* and *samādhi*. BUBh 1.4.7 provides us with the reason why one who knows the Self should ideally maintain *jñāna-niṣṭhā*. The steady recollection of Self-knowledge, which naturally culminates in *citta vṛtti nirodha*, bolstered by renunciation and dispassion, is necessary to counter the effects of *prārabdha-karman*, which continues in its momentum even after the rise of Self-knowledge.

Apart from these doctrinal considerations, we have seen that Śaṅkara often shows deep familiarity or even verbal dependence on YS and YSBh, in addition to other ancient yoga texts, in his commentaries on the source texts of Vedānta. His references to yoga in BGBh sometimes far exceed what BhG itself requires, while he quotes YS at least twice with approval in BSBh. He repeatedly affirms *dhyāna-yoga* as an integral part of the liberating vision, and does not hesitate to describe the liberated being as the best of *yogin*-s. He acknowledges in BUBh that *citta vṛtti nirodha* is a natural aspect of the state of remaining established in Self-knowledge. Śaṅkara's attitude towards yoga is perhaps best reflected by Sureśvara, his direct disciple, who recommends *yogābhyāsa* after the renunciation of all *karman*. We must also note that Toṭaka, the author of *Śrutisārasamuddharaṇa*, traditionally said to be another direct disciple of Śaṅkara, uses the term *citi-śakti*,[84] which is familiar to us from YS and YSBh, but not common in the works of Śaṅkara. Maṇḍana Miśra, a contemporary of Śaṅkara and an important Advaita Vedāntin in his own right, uses the term *dṛk-śakti* in his *Brahmasiddhi*, in a manner that seems indebted to YS and YSBh, although he does not explicitly refer to yoga or *yogin*-s.[85] The chronological closeness of these other authors to Śaṅkara, along with the explicit reliance of the pre-Śaṅkaran *prasaṃkhyāna vādin* on yoga, indicates that a close relationship with yoga did not have to be freshly introduced into Advaita Vedānta during either the fourteenth century or the twentieth. Moreover, in all of Śaṅkara's commentaries examined here, there is a consistent intertwining of aspects of yoga and Pūrva Mīmāṃsā in the context of meditation on Brahman, along with an absolute rejection of Mīmāṃsā principles and significant acceptance of yoga concepts. It is putting the cart before the horse, so to speak, to assume that influences of yoga in Śaṅkaran Advaita Vedānta may be explained away by appealing to changes in Śaṅkara's thought over time.

In conclusion, it seems to me that Śaṅkara is being vastly misunderstood with respect to yoga and meditation, both by modern critical scholarship and by non-traditional interpreters of Vedānta. Nowhere does Śaṅkara reject yoga as completely as academic scholarship is inclined to believe. Neither does he give room to believe that the existence of Brahman is to be "verified" through an experience of *nirvikalpa samādhi*. For Śaṅkara, scripture is the only valid source of knowledge of Brahman, and knowledge is the only direct means to liberation. Nevertheless, liberation entails that one should know with absolute certainty, in one's own experience, that Brahman is one's own Self. I have not discussed the role of the *guru* in this connection, but it goes without saying that Śaṅkara sees the *guru* as being absolutely necessary to impart valid Self-knowledge. The vision of the Self within one's own cognitive experience is obtained through either *dhyāna-yoga* or *sāṃkhya-yoga*, while the steady recollection of Self-knowledge effortlessly leads to *citta vṛtti nirodha*. Thus, even in classical Advaita, yoga has a significant place, both in the process of gaining Self-knowledge and in the state of remaining established in Self-knowledge. That *samādhi* or *citta vṛtti nirodha* is not enjoined is a consequence of Śaṅkara's rejection of the Mīmāṃsā principle of injunction with respect to liberation. It is not a rejection of yoga on the road to liberation.

Notes

1 This essay is dedicated to my guru, Svāmī Śrī Bhāratī Tīrtha, the contemporary Śaṅkarācārya of Śṛṅgeri Śāradā Pīṭham, as also to the memories of my father, M. Sundaresan, and his guru, Svāmī Śrī Abhinava Vidyātīrtha of Śṛṅgeri.

2 Śaṅkara is here taken as the author of commentaries (*Bhāṣya*-s) on the source texts of Vedānta, namely, the *Brahmasūtra*, *Bhagavadgītā* and the principal *Upaniṣad*-s. It is usually taken as axiomatic in critical scholarship, that the same author wrote all these commentaries.

3 In this essay, yoga (plain text, capital Y) refers to the classical school derived from Patañjali, while yoga (italicized text, small y) is used in all other contexts. A similar convention holds for *sāṃkhya* and *vedānta*.

4 Although most contemporary interest in Advaita Vedānta and yoga tends to be derived from the influence of neo-Vedāntins (see, for example, Michael Comans, "The Question of the Importance of Samādhi in Modern and Classical Advaita Vedānta," *Philosophy East & West*, 1993, vol. 43, pp. 19–38, and Andrew O. Fort, *Jīvanmukti in Transformation: Embodied Liberation in Advaita and Neo-Vedanta*, Albany, NY, State University of New York Press, 1998), I would like to clarify here that my interest in the subject stems largely from my inherited familial connection with the monastic institutions of the classical Advaita tradition, as also my independent studies of Śaṅkara's texts.

5 Cf. YS 3.38, *bandha-kāraṇa-śaithilyāt pracāra-saṃvedanāc ca cittasya para-śarīrāveśaḥ*.

6 This title may perhaps be traced to the legacy of Vidyāraṇya, who was the head of the Śṛṅgeri monastery in the fourtheenth century, and who recommends the practice of *aṣṭāṅga-yoga*, quoting extensively from Patañjali's *Yogasūtra*-s in his *Jīvanmuktiviveka*. See Andrew O. Fort, "On Destroying the Mind: The Yogasūtras in Vidyāraṇya's Jīvanmuktiviveka," *Journal of Indian Philosophy*, 1999, vol. 27, pp. 377–395.

7 See R. M. Umesh, *Yoga, Enlightenment, and Perfection of Abhinava Vidyatheerth Mahaswamigal*, Chennai, Sri Vidyatheerth Foundation, 1999, p. 183.

8 See Andrew Fort, *Jīvanmukti in Transformation: Embodied Liberation in Advaita and Neo-Vedanta*, Albany, NY, State University of New York Press, 1998, p. 170.

9 *api ca smaranti, "svādhyāyād iṣṭa-devatā saṃprayoga" ityādi. yogo'py aṇimādy aiśvarya-prāpti-phalakas smaryamāṇo na śakyate sāhasa-mātreṇa pratyākhyātum. śrutiś ca yoga-māhātmyaṃ prakhyāpayati, "pṛthvy-ap-tejo'nila-khe samutthite pañcātmake yoga-guṇe pravṛtte na tasya rogo na jarā na mṛtyuḥ prāptasya yogāgnimayaṃ śarīram" iti* – commentary on BS 1.3.33 (p. 208).

10 BS 2.4.12 compares the five *prāṇa*-s to the five *vṛtti*-s of the mind – *pañca-vṛttir manovad vyapadiśyate*. The fivefold list of *prāṇa*, *apāna*, *vyāna*, *udāna* and *samāna* is perhaps too well known to need much explanation, but in his

commentary, Śaṅkara has to explain the term "like the mind" (*manovat*). He discounts the *Bṛhadāraṇyaka* text describing desire, intent etc. as transformations of the mind, because this list does not yield the number five. Interestingly, he concludes with a reference to YS 1.6 – *"paramatam-apratiṣiddham anumataṃ bhavati" iti nyāyād iha api yogaśāstra-prasiddhā manasaḥ pañca vṛttayaḥ parigṛhyante, "pramāṇa-viparyaya-vikalpa-nidrā-smṛtayaḥ"* – commentary on BS 2.4.12 (p. 510).

11 *śruty anusāra-ananusāra-viṣaya-vivecanena ca sanmārge prajñā saṃgrahaṇīyā* – commentary on BS 2.1.1 (p. 285).

12 See Karl Potter (ed.) *Advaita Vedānta up to Śaṅkara and His Pupils*, Delhi, Motilal Banarsidass, 1981.

13 See Wilhelm Halbfass (ed.) *Philology and Confrontation: Paul Hacker on Traditional and Modern Vedanta*, Albany, NY, State University of New York Press, 1995, pp. 101–134.

14 See V. Sundaresan, "What Determines Śaṅkara's Authorship? The Case of the Pañcīkaraṇa," *Philosophy East & West*, 2002, vol. 52, pp. 1–35.

15 Madeleine Biardeau, "Quelques Réflections sur L'apophatisme de Śaṅkara," *Indo-Iranian Journal*, 1959, vol. 3, pp. 81–101.

16 Tilmann Vetter, *Studien Zur Lehre Und Entwicklung Śaṅkaras*, Vienna, The De Nobili Research Library, 1976.

17 Halbfass, *Studies in Kumārila and Śaṅkara*, Reinbek, Inge Wezler, 1983, p. 39.

18 Sengaku Mayeda, *A Thousand Teachings: The Upadeśasāhasrī of Śaṅkara*, Albany, NY, State University of New York Press, 1992.

19 Following Mayeda, *A Thousand Teachings*, the verse portion of US is numbered I and the prose chapters are numbered II. In addition to these texts, Śaṅkara's *Kaṭha Upaniṣad* commentary contains many references to yoga, which have already been discussed in comparison with relevant portions of BSBh and BUBh by Comans, "The Question of the Importance of Samādhi."

20 For example, where the path of light is mentioned in BhG, Śaṅkara says, *devatā eva mārga-bhūtā iti sthito'nyatra* – BGBh 8.24 (p. 291). The word *anyatra* clearly points to the discussion of the *devayāna* and BhG 8.23–24 in BSBh 4.2.21, as BhG itself does not refer to the *devatā*-s.

21 Daniel Ingalls, "Śaṅkara's Arguments Against the Buddhists," *Philosophy East & West*, 1954, vol. 3, pp. 291–306.

22 See Potter, *Advaita Vedānta.*

23 Mayeda, *A Thousand Teachings*, points to an apparent conflict between rejecting *prasaṃkhyāna vāda* in US I.18 and simultaneously teaching a meditation called *parisaṃkhyāna* in US II.3, and thinks that Śaṅkara sacrifices theoretical consistency in favour of effective pedagogy. Comans, "Śaṅkara and the Prasaṅkhyānavāda," *Journal of Indian Philosophy*, 1996, vol. 24, pp. 49–71, discusses the details of *prasaṃkhyāna vāda*, while Sundaresan, "On Prasaṃkhyāna and Parisaṃkhyāna: Meditation in Advaita Vedānta, Yoga, and Pre-Śaṅkaran Vedānta,"*The Adyar Library Bulletin*, 1998, vol. 62, pp. 51–89, argues that there is no basic contradiction involved between rejecting *prasaṃkhyāna vāda* and independently recommending *parisaṃkhyāna* meditation.

24 *jīva-mukhyaprāṇa-liṅgān neti cen na, upāsā-traividhyād āśritatvad iha tad yogāt* – BS 1.1.31 (p. 87). Here, yoga means that it is appropriate to interpret *prāṇa* as Brahman (not the *jīva*) in some *Upaniṣad* passages.

25 *asminn asya ca tad yogaṃ śāsti* – BS 1.1.19 (p. 57). Here, the reference is to the union of the *vijñānātman* in the *paramātman*. The word *viyoga* is used in BUBh 3.9.28.7 – *śarīra-viyogo hi mokṣa ātyantikaḥ.*

26 *tasya śraddhaiva śiraḥ ... yoga ātmā* – TU 2.4. *yogo yuktis samādhānam* – TUBh 2.4 (p. 66).

27 *jñātavyāḥ padārthās saṃkhyāyante yasmin śāstre tat sāṃkhyaṃ vedāntaḥ ... tasminn ātmajñānārthe sāṃkhye kṛtānte vedānte proktāni* – BGBh 18.13 (p. 563).

28 *loke'smin dvividhā niṣṭhā purā proktā mayā'nagha jñāna-yogena sāṃkhyānāṃ karma-yogena yoginām* – BhG 3.3. Śaṅkara explains, *sāṃkhyānāṃātmānātma-viṣaya-viveka-vijñānavatāṃ brahmacaryāśramād eva kṛtasaṃnyāsānāṃ vedānta-vijñāna-suniścitārthānāṃ paramahaṃsa-parivrāja-kānāṃ brahmaṇy eva avasthitānāṃ niṣṭhā proktā. ... karma eva yogaḥ karma-yogaḥ ... yogināṃ karmiṇāṃ niṣṭhā proktā* (p. 101). For a distinction between *yogin*-s and doers of actions, see BGBh 8.23 – "*yogina*" *iti yoginaḥ karmiṇaś ca ucyante, karmiṇas tu guṇataḥ, "karma-yogena yogināṃ" iti viśeṣaṇāt* (p. 290). Śaṅkara frequently refers to BhG 3.3 in order to argue against combining the paths of knowledge and action throughout one's life.

29 Three different kinds of *vidhi*-s are pertinent to this discussion. The original or initial injunction (*apūrva vidhi*) enjoins a new action upon the ritual agent. The restrictive injunction (*niyama vidhi*) prescribes the way(s) in which a given action is to be performed, out of two or more possible ways of doing it. The excluding injunction (*parisaṃkhyā vidhi*) approaches this issue from the opposite direction, and lists the way(s) in which a given action should *not* be done.

30 The difference between the *prasaṃkhyāna vādin* and the *jñāna-karma-samuccaya-vādin* is as follows. The former says only that meditation (*prasaṃkhyāna*) has to be done till the *Ātman* is experienced (*prasaṃkhyānam ataḥ kāryaṃ yāvad ātmā anubhūyate* – US I.18), but the latter holds that knowledge is to be combined with action all through one's life (*yāvaj-jīvam*).

31 Interestingly, Śaṅkara holds that if scripture enjoins anything at all as a means to liberation, it is *śama*, mental calmness, and *saṃnyāsa*, the renunciation of action. Śaṅkara takes CU 3.14.1, *sarvaṃ khalv idaṃ brahma tajjalān iti śānta upāsīta* for explanation in BSBh 1.2.1, and says, *śama-vidhi vivakṣayā brahma nirdiṣṭam* (p. 97). In BUBh 4.4.22, he interprets the verb *pravrajanti* as *pravrajeyuḥ*, calling it a *vidhi*. See also note 39 below, and the introduction to chapter 3 of BGBh – *sarvopaniṣatsv itihāsa-purāṇa-yogaśāstreṣu ca jñānāṅgatvena mumukṣos sarvakarma-saṃnyāsa-vidhānād āśrama-vikalpa-samuccaya-vidhānāc ca śruti-smṛtyoḥ* (p. 95). Note that Śaṅkara includes *yogaśāstra*-s among the texts cited here, and also refers to a *vidhāna* (i.e. a *vidhi*). The term *āśrama-vikalpa-samuccaya* refers to the element of choice between entering *saṃnyāsa* from any of the preceding *āśrama*-s (*vikalpa*) and going through the four *āśrama*-s in sequential order (*samuccaya*). Śaṅkara always argues for choice in the matter of when to take up *saṃnyāsa*, although most *Smṛti* authorities, including Manu, argue strongly in favor of the sequential order.

32 *na ca "ātmetyevopāsīta" ity apūrva vidhiḥ ... na ca "ekam evādvitīyaṃ brahma" ityādi vākyeṣu vidhir avagamyate* – BUBh 1.4.7 (pp. 134–138).

33 *nirodhas tarhy arthāntaram iti cet. athāpi syāc citta-vṛtti-nirodhasya veda-vākya-janita-ātma-vijñānād arthāntaratvāt. tantrāntareṣu ca kartavyatayā avagatatvād vidheyatvam iti cet* – *pūrvapakṣa* in BUBh 1.4.7.

34 *na. mokṣa-sādhanatvena anavagamāt. na hi vedānteṣu brahmātma-vijñānād anyat parama-puruṣārtha-sādhanatvena avagamyate* – Śaṅkara's response to the above argument.

35 See Halbfass, *Philology and Confrontation*, p. 107.

36 *ananya-sādhanatvāc ca nirodhasya. na hy ātma-vijñāna-tat-smṛti-saṃtāna-vyatirekeṇa citta-vṛtti-nirodhasya sādhanam asti. abhyupagamya idam uktam.*

na tu brahma-vijñāna-vyatirekeṇa anya-mokṣa-sādhanam avagamyate – BUBh 1.4.7 (p. 138). A form of the verb *abhi* + *upa* + √*gam* is used here, which is often employed for tentatively admitting an opponent's position as part of a *reductio ad absurdum* argument. However, note that Śaṅkara simply makes an independent comment about *citta vṛtti nirodha* here, without admitting any part of his opponent's stance and without proving any self-contradiction.

37 *yady apy evaṃ śarīrārabdhakasya karmaṇo niyata-phalatvāt, samyag-jñāna prāptāv apy avaśyaṃ bhāvinī pravṛttir vāṅ-manaḥ-kāyānām. labdha-vṛtteḥ karmaṇo balīyastvāt. mukteṣv ādi pravṛttivat. tena pakṣe prāptam jñāna-pravṛtti-daurbalyam. tasmāt tyāga-vairāgyādi-sādhana-balāvalambena ātma-vijñāna-smṛti-saṃtatir niyantavyā bhavati, na tv apūrvā ... prāpta-vijñāna-smṛti-saṃtāna-niyama-vidhy-arthāni "vijñāya prajñāṃ kurvīta" ityādi vākyāni* – BUBh 1.4.7 (pp. 140–141).

38 *ātma-vijñāna-smṛti-saṃtater arthata eva bhāvān na vidheyatvam* – BUBh 1.4.7 (p. 134).

39 The quotation, *vijñāya prajñāṃ kurvīta*, in BUBh 1.4.7 (note 37 above) is from BU 4.4.21, the commentary on which says, *prajñā-kāraṇa sādhanāni saṃnyāsa-śama-dama-uparama-titikṣā-samādhānāni kuryād ity arthaḥ ... ātmaikatva-pratipādakās svalpāś śabdā anujñāyante, "aum ity evaṃ dhyāyatha ātmānam, anyā vāco vimuñcatha" iti* (p. 684). This quotation about meditation on *auṃ* is from Muṇḍaka Upaniṣad 2.2.5–6.

40 *aupaniṣad-ātma-pratipatti-prayojanas samādhir upadiṣṭo vedānteṣu, "ātmā vā are draṣṭavyaś śrotavyo mantavyo nididhyāsitavyaḥ," "so'nveṣṭavyas sa vijijñāsitavyaḥ," "aum ity evaṃ dhyāyatha ātmānam" iti ...* – BSBh 2.3.39 (p. 469). CUBh 8.7.1 states, *anveṣṭavyo vijijñāsitavya iti ca eṣa niyama vidhir eva* (p. 472), while CUBh 8.6.6 refers to meditation on *auṃ* (see note 70 below).

41 *svātantryārthaṃ yogadharmānusevanaṃ parisaṃkhyābhyāsaś ca ... kartavya iti* – BUBh 4.4.2 (p. 647).

42 BhG 2.40 ends, *svalpam apy asya dharmasya trāyate mahato bhayāt*. BGBh says, *dharmasya yogadharmasya ... trāyate ... bhayāt saṃsāra-bhayāj janma-maraṇādi-lakṣaṇāt. yoge ... dvandva-prahāṇapūrvakam īśvarārādhanārthe karma-yoge karmānuṣṭhāne samādhi-yoge ca* – BGBh 2.39 (pp. 62–63).

43 *mumukṣūṇām upātta puṇyāpuṇya kṣapaṇa-parāṇām apurvānupacayārtināṃ parisaṃkhyānam idam ucyate* – US II.3.1. See Mayeda, *A Thousand Teachings*, pp. 251–254 and Sundaresan, "On Prasaṃkhyāna and Parisaṃkhyāna." See also note 23 above.

44 Mayeda, *A Thousand Teachings*, pp. 129–135.

45 *api ca enam ātmānaṃ nirasta-samasta-prapañcam avyaktaṃ saṃrādhana-kāle paśyanti yoginaḥ. saṃrādhanaṃ ca bhakti-dhyāna-praṇidhānādy-anuṣṭhānam* – BSBh 3.2.24 (pp. 601–602). *dṛśeś cchāyā yadārūḍhā mukhacchāyeva darśane paśyaṃs taṃ pratyayaṃ yogī dṛṣṭa ātmeti manyate. taṃ ca mūḍhaṃ ca yady anyaṃ pratyayaṃ vetti no dṛśeḥ sa eva yogināṃ śreṣtho netaras syān na saṃśayaḥ* – US I.12.5–6. Compare with *pratyaya* and terms deriving from root *dṛś* in yoga, particularly YS 2.20–21 – *draṣṭā dṛśi-mātraś śuddho'pi pratyayānupaśyaḥ, tadartha eva dṛśyasyātmā*. See also US I.13.25d-26ab – ... *ṛṣir mukto dhruvo bhavet. kṛtakṛtyaś ca siddhaś ca yogī brāhmaṇa eva ca.*

46 *vidhayas tu kathaṃ rāgaṃ nirudhyanta iti bhaṇyatām na hi te parisaṃkhyārthā nāpi caite niyāmakāḥ* – introduction to BUBhV, verse 412 (p. 91). ... *pratyag-jñāne nirudhyante citta-tad-vṛttayo yataḥ. abhyupetyaitad asmābhir ucyate sambhavād iti* – BUBhV 1.4.7, verses 850–851 (p. 398), and *uktaṃ ca nyāyam āpekṣya niyamo'tyanta durlabhaḥ vidher daurbalya siddhyartham ato bhāṣyakṛd uktavān* – verse 931 (p. 408). *vidhy abhyupagame'pi nāpūrva-vidhir*

ayam. ata āha, niyamaḥ parisaṃkhyā vā vidhy artho'pi bhaved yataḥ anātmādarśanenaiva parātmānam upāsmahe – NS 1.88 (p. 63).

47 *"āruruksor muner yogaṃ karma kāraṇam ucyate yogārūḍhasya tasyaiva śama" eveti ca smṛtiḥ ... mumukṣutvaṃ tatas tad-upāya-paryeṣaṇaṃ tatas sarva-karma-tat-sādhana-saṃnyāsas, tato yogābhyāsas, tataś cittasya pratyak-pravaṇatā, tatas "tat tvam asy" ādi vākyārtha parijñānaṃ, tato'vidyocchedas, tataś ca svātmany eva avasthānam* – NS 1.51–52 (pp. 36–37). The quotation described as *smṛti* in the above passage is from BhG 6.3.

48 *cittaṃ ... apaviddha rajas-tamo-malaṃ prasannam* – NS 1.47 (p. 34). Compare *tamasā anuviddhaṃ ... anuviddhaṃ rajomātrayā ... rajo-leśa-malāpetam* – YSB 1.2 (p. 6).

49 *viṣṇoḥ pādānugāṃ yāṃ nikhila-bhava-nudaṃ śaṅkaro'vāpa yogāt* – NS 4.76 (p. 268). See note 45 above, for references to *yogin*-s in US.

50 Note that *prasaṃkhyāna* occurs once in YS 4.29 (*prasaṃkhyāne'py akusīdasya sarvathā-viveka-khyāter dharmamegha-samādhiḥ*) and frequently in YSBh, to refer to the fire that burns *kleśa*-s. The term also occurs in a discussion of *adhyātma-vidhi* and *yogaśāstra* in *Nyāyabhāṣya* 4.2.46 – *yogaśāstrāc ca adhyātmavidhiḥ pratipattavyaḥ. sa punas tapaḥ prāṇāyāmaḥ pratyāhāro dhyānaṃ dhāraṇeti. indriya-viṣayeṣu prasaṃkhyānābhyāso rāga-dveṣa-prahāṇārthaḥ. upāyas tu yogācāra-vidhānam iti* (p. 1095). Note that there is a reference to *tapas*, but none to *yama*, *niyama*, *āsana* and *samādhi* in the above list. Halbfass (1991) notes about *prasaṃkhyāna*, "It appears that this method was adopted and perhaps reinterpreted by certain Vedāntins who employed it as a technique to realize the meaning of the Upaniṣadic 'great sayings' (*mahāvākya*)." For more about the philosophical position called *prasaṃkhyāna vāda*, see Comans (1996) and Sundaresan (1998).

51 *tvam-arthasya avabodhāya vidhir apy āśritaḥ* – NS 3.126 (p. 233). See also note 31 above.

52 *paraṃ niḥśreyasaṃ ... sarva-karma-saṃnyāsa-pūrvakād ātma-jñāna-niṣṭhā-rūpād dharmād bhavati ... abhyudayārtho'pi yaḥ pravṛtti-lakṣaṇo dharmaḥ . .. īśvarārpaṇa-buddhyā anuṣṭhīyamānas sattva-śuddhaye bhavati ... jñāna-niṣṭhā-yogyatā-prāpti-dvāreṇa jñānotpatti-hetutvena ca* – BGBh, Śaṅkara's introduction (pp. 1–4). *"īśvarāya karmāṇi karomi ..." ityevaṃ samāhitaḥ ... śāntiṃ ... āpnoti ... sattva-śuddhi jñāna-prāpti sarva-karma-saṃnyāsa jñāna-niṣṭhā krameṇa* – BGBh 5.12 (p. 195).

53 *ārurukṣoḥ ... anārūḍhasya dhyāna-yoge'vasthātum aśaktasyaiva ity arthaḥ ... kim ārurukṣoḥ? yogam. yogārūḍhasya punas tasyaiva śama upaśamas sarva-karmabhyo nivṛttiḥ kāraṇam. ... yāvad yāvat karmabhya uparamate, tāvat tāvat ... jitendriyasya cittaṃ samādhīyate* – BGBh 6.3 (p. 220). *vijñāna-phalaṃ sarvatas saṃplutodaka-sthānīyam ... prāk jñāna-niṣṭhādhikāra-prāpteḥ karmaṇy adhikṛtena kūpa-taḍāgādy-artha-sthānīyam api karma kartavyam* – BGBh 2.46 (p. 68). See note 42 above for *samādhi-yoga* in BGBh 2.39. *karma-yogena samādhi-yogena ca saṃsiddhas saṃskṛto yogyatām āpannas san mumukṣuḥ* – BGBh 4.38. *samyag-darśanāt kṣipram eva mokṣo bhavati* – BGBh 4.39 (pp. 176–177). *samyag-darśana-niṣṭhānāṃ saṃnyāsināṃ sadyo-muktir uktā ... dhyāna-yogaṃ samyag-darśanasya antaraṅgam* – BGBh 5.27 (p. 210). *samyag-darśanaṃ praty antaraṅgasya ... dhyāna-yogasya bahiraṅgaṃ karma iti, yāvad dhyāna-yogārohaṇa asamarthas tāvad ... kartavyaṃ karma* – BGBh 6.1 (p. 213).

54 *ātma-viṣayaṃ jñānaṃ ca na vidhātavyam. kiṃ tarhi? nāma-rūpādy-anātmā-adhyāropaṇa-nivṛttir eva kāryā, na ātma-caitanya-vijñānaṃ kāryam ... avidyā-adhyāropita-nirākaraṇa-mātraṃ brahmaṇi kartavyaṃ, na tu brahmav-ijñāne yatnaḥ. atyanta-prasiddhatvāt* – BGBh 18.50 (p. 601).

55 See Mayeda, *A Thousand Teachings*, pp. 251–254; and Sundaresan, "On Prasaṃkhyāna and Parisaṃkhyāna."

56 *samyag-darśanātmikāyāḥ prajñāyās sthairyaṃ kartavyam ... ādāv indriyāṇi svavaśe sthāpayitavyāni* – BGBh 2.59. *indriyāṇāṃ hi yasmāc caratāṃ svasvaviṣayeṣu ... pravṛttaṃ mana asya yater harati prajñām ātmānātma-vivekajām nāśayati* – BGBh 2.67 (pp. 79–85).

57 *sthitaprajña-lakṣaṇaṃ sādhanaṃ ca upadiśyate. sarvatraiva hy adhyātma-śāstre kṛtārtha-lakṣaṇāni yāni tāny eva sādhanāny upadiśyante, yatna-sādhyatvāt* – BGBh 2.55 (p. 76). See also note 80 below.

58 *yasmin sati tajjñeya-vijñāne yogyo'dhikṛto bhavati, yatparas saṃnyāsī jñānaniṣṭha ucyate, tam amānitvādi-gaṇaṃ jñāna-sādhanatvāt jñāna-śabda-vācyam ... nanu yamā-niyamāś-ca amānitvādayaḥ ... naiṣaḥ doṣaḥ. jñāna-nimittatvāj jñāna ucyata iti hy avocāma. jñāna-sahakāri-kāraṇatvāc ca* – BGBh 13.7–12 (pp. 425–430).

59 *svādhyāyo yathāvidhi ṛgādy-abhyāsaḥ* – BGBh 4.28 (p. 169). *satyaṃ vākyam anudvegakaraṃ ... tapo vāṅmayaṃ, yathā "śānto bhava vatsa, svādhyāyaṃ yogaṃ ca anutiṣṭha, tathā te śreyo bhaviṣyati" iti ... saumyatvaṃ yat saumanasyam āhuḥ ... antaḥkaraṇasya vṛttiḥ. maunaṃ vāk-saṃyamo'pi manaḥ-saṃyama-pūrvakaḥ ... mano-nirodhas sarvatas sāmānyarūpa ātma-vinigrahaḥ* – BGBh 17.15–16 (pp. 538–539). Compare *sattva-śuddhi-saumanasya-ekāgrya-indriyajaya-ātma-darśana-yogyatvāni ca* – YS 2.41. See note 9 above, for the YS quotation regarding *svādhyāya* in BSBh 1.3.33.

60 *brahma vijijñāsunā bāhyāntaḥkaraṇa samādhāna lakṣaṇam ... tapaḥ-sādhanam anuṣṭheyam* – TUBh 3.6 (p. 105). See note 26 above for TUBh 2.4.

61 *kleśa-karma-vipākāśayair aparāmṛṣṭaḥ puruṣa-viśeṣa īśvaraḥ, tatra niratiśayaṃ sarvajña-bījam* – YS 1.24–25. BGBh 9.10 says, *dṛśi-mātra-svarūpeṇa avikriyātmanā adhyakṣeṇa ... māyā triguṇātmikā avidyā-lakṣaṇā prakṛtis sūyate* (p. 303). Compare *dṛśi-mātra* here with YS 2.20–21 (note 45 above).

62 *na vidyate ādir yayos tāv anādī ... prakṛti-dvayavattvam eva hi īśvarasya īśvaratvaṃ, yābhyāṃ prakṛtībhyām īśvaro jagad-utpatti-sthiti-pralaya-hetuḥ* – BGBh 13.19 (p. 442).

63 *prakṛtir me mama aiśvarī māyā-śaktir aṣṭadhā bhinnā bhedam āgatā ... aparā na parā nikṛṣṭā aśuddhā anarthakarī saṃsāra-bandhanātmikā iyam ... anyāṃ viśuddhāṃ prakṛtiṃ mama ātma-bhūtāṃ viddhi me parāṃ prakṛṣṭāṃ jīva-bhūtāṃ kṣetrajña-lakṣaṇāṃ prāṇa-dhāraṇa-nimitta-bhūtāṃ ... yayā dhāryate jagad antaḥ praviṣṭayā* – BGBh 7.4–5 (pp. 254–255).

64 *sataḥ parasmād ātmanaḥ karmādhyakṣāt sarvabhūtādhivāsāt sākṣiṇaś cetayitur īśvarāt tad anujñayā kartṛtva-bhoktṛtva-lakṣaṇasya saṃsārasya siddhiḥ, tad-anugraha-hetukenaiva ca vijñānena mokṣa-siddhir bhavitum arhati ... yadyapi ca loke kṛṣyādiṣu karmasu na īśvara-kāraṇatvaṃ prasiddhaṃ, tathāpi sarvāsv eva pravṛttiṣv īśvaro hetukarteti śruter avasīyate ... karoty eva jīvaḥ. kurvantaṃ hi tam īśvaraḥ kārayati ... atyanta paratantratvāj jīvasya* – BSBh 2.3.41–42 (pp. 476–477).

65 *yasmād mad-adhīnaṃ karmiṇāṃ karma-phalaṃ, jñāninām ca jñāna-phalam, ataḥ bhakti-yogena māṃ ye sevante te mama prasādāt jñāna-prāpti-krameṇa guṇātītāḥ mokṣaṃ gacchanti ... ato bhagavān ātmanas tattvaṃ vivakṣur uvāca* – BGBh 15.1 (p. 490). *Yogasthas san kuru karmāṇi kevalam īśvarārthaṃ ... phala-tṛṣṇā-śūnyena kriyamāṇe karmaṇi sattva-śuddhi-jā jñāna-prāpti-lakṣaṇā siddhis, tad-viparyaya-jā asiddhis, tayos siddhy-asiddhyor api samas tulyo bhūtvā kuru karmāṇi ... samatva-buddhi-yuktam īśvarārādhanārthaṃ karma* – BGBh 2.48–49 (p. 70).

66 *aum ity ekākṣaraṃ brahma vyāharan mām anusmaran yaḥ prayāti tyajan dehaṃ sa yāti paramāṃ gatim* – BhG 8.13. *parasya brahmaṇo vācaka-rūpeṇa*

... *brahmaṇo'bhidhāna-bhūtam auṃkāraṃ vyāharann uccārayan tad-artha-bhūtaṃ mām īśvaram anusmarann anucintayan* – BGBh 8.12–13 (pp. 281–283). Compare *tasya vācakaḥ praṇavaḥ, taj japas tad artha bhāvanam*, and *praṇavasya japaḥ praṇava-abhidheyasya ca īśvarasya bhāvanā* – YS and YSBh 1.27–28 (pp. 64–65).

67 Meditation on the "partless" fourth is taught in the *Māṇḍūkya Upaniṣad* and *Kārikā*-s, and associated with realizing *nirguṇa* Brahman, and with immediate liberation (*sadyo-mukti*) or living liberation (*jīvan-mukti*).

68 *trimātreṇa-auṃkāreṇa-ālambanena paramātmānam abhidhyāyataḥ phalaṃ brahmaloka-prāptiḥ krameṇa ca samyag-darśanotpattir iti krama-mukty-abhiprāyam etat* – BSBh 1.3.13 (p. 164). *parabrahma-prāpti-sādhanatvena manda-madhyama-buddhīnāṃ vivakṣitasya auṃkārasya upāsanaṃ kālāntare mukti-phalam uktaṃ ... pratipatty-upāya-bhūtasya auṃkārasya kālāntara-mukti-phalam upāsanaṃ yoga-dhāraṇā-sahitaṃ vaktavyaṃ ... iti* – BGBh 8.12 (p. 282).

69 *yogasya balaṃ yogabalaṃ samādhija-saṃskāra-pracaya-janita-citta-sthairya-lakṣaṇaṃ ... hṛdaya-puṇḍarīke vaśīkṛtya cittaṃ tata ūrdhvagāminyā nāḍyā bhūmijaya-krameṇa bhruvor madhye prāṇam āveśya sthāpayitvā ... saṃyamanaṃ kṛtvā ... hṛdaya-puṇḍarīke nirudhya nirodhaṃ kṛtvā ... vaśīkṛtena manasā* – BGBh 8.10–12 (pp. 280–282). Cf. YS 3.1 – *deśa-bandhaś cittasya dhāraṇā*. Also compare *bhūmijaya-krama* and *saṃyama* with YS 3.4–6 – *trayam ekatra saṃyamaḥ, taj-jayāt prajñālokaḥ, tasya bhūmiṣu viniyogaḥ*, and *saṃyamasya jitabhūmer yā anantarā bhūmis tatra viniyogaḥ ... jitottara bhūmikasya ca na adharabhūmiṣu paricittajñādiṣu saṃyamo yuktaḥ* – YSBh 3.6 (p. 255).

70 *śataṃ caikā ca hṛdayasya nāḍyas tāsāṃ mūrdhānam abhiniḥsṛtaikā tayordhvam āyann amṛtatvam eti viṣvaṅṅ anyā utkramaṇe bhavanti* – CU 8.6.6. The same verse is also found in *Kaṭha* 6.16. CUBh 8.6.5–6 says, *vidvān yathokta-sādhana-sampannaḥ ... auṃkāreṇa ātmānaṃ dhyāyan ... kālena ... brahmalokaṃ gacchati ... viṣvaṅṅ nānāgatayas tiryag visarpiṇy anūrdhvagāś ca anyā nāḍyo bhavanti saṃsāra-gamana-dvāra-bhūtā, na tv amṛtatvāya* (pp. 469–470).

71 *nāḍī-raśmi-samanvitena arcirādi-parvaṇā devayānena pathā ye brahmalokaṃ śāstrokta-viśeṣaṇaṃ gacchanti ... te taṃ prāpya na candralokād iva bhukta-bhogā āvartante ... samyag-darśana-vidhvasta-tamasāṃ ... siddhaiva anāvṛttiḥ. tad āśrayaṇenaiva hi saguṇa-śaraṇānām apy anāvṛttis siddhir iti* – BSBh 4.4.22 (p. 861). *aṣṭame nāḍī-dvāreṇa dhāraṇā-yogas saguṇa uktaḥ. tasya ca phalam agny-arcirādi-krameṇa kālāntare brahma-prāpti-lakṣaṇam eva anāvṛtti-rūpaṃ nirdiṣṭam* – BGBh, introduction to chapter 9 (p. 295).

72 *tasmin mārge gacchanti ... brahmopāsana-parāḥ ... "krameṇa" iti vākya-śeṣaḥ. na hi sadyo-mukti-bhājāṃ samyag-darśana-niṣṭhānāṃ gatir āgatir vā kvacid asti. "na tasya prāṇā utkrāmanti" iti śruteḥ, brahma-saṃlīna-prāṇā eva te ... brahma-bhūtā eva te* – BGBh 8.24 (p. 291). See also note 20 above.

73 YS 2.49 and 2.53 read, *tasmin sati śvāsa-praśvāsayor gati-vicchedaḥ prāṇāyāmaḥ* and *dhāraṇāsu ca yogyatā manasaḥ*. BhG and BGBh 4.29 say, *apāne juhvati prāṇaṃ prāṇe'pānaṃ tathāpare prāṇāpāna-gatī ruddhvā prāṇāyāma-parāyaṇāḥ. apāne apāna-vṛttau juhvati ... prāṇaṃ prāṇa-vṛttiṃ pūrakākhyaṃ prāṇāyāmaṃ kurvanti ... prāṇe'pānaṃ tathā ... recakākhyaṃ ca prāṇāyāmaṃ kurvanti ... prāṇāpāna-gatī ... ruddhvā nirud-dhya ... kumbhakākhyaṃ prāṇāyāmaṃ kurvanti* (p. 169). Note that *pūraka*, *recaka*, *kumbhaka*, *prāṇāyāma* and *pratyāhāra* occur in *Viṣṇu Purāṇa* 5.10.14–16, and also that BGBh 3.37 quotes *Viṣṇu Purāṇa* 6.5.74–78.

74 *prāṇāyāma-pratyāhārādi-lakṣaṇo yogo yajño yeṣāṃ te yoga-yajñāḥ* – BGBh 4.28 (p. 169). See also notes 56 and 69 above and 78 below, for BGBh references to control of the senses, and cf. *tataḥ paramā vaśyatendriyāṇām* – YS 2.55.

75 BS 4.1.7–11 read, *āsīnas saṃbhavāt, dhyānac ca, acalatvam cāpekṣya, smaranti ca, yatraikāgratā tatrāviśeṣāt.* Śaṅkara explains, *āsīna evopāsīta ... upāsanaṃ nāma samāna-pratyaya-pravāha-karaṇam. na ca tad gacchato dhāvato vā saṃbhavati. gatyādīnāṃ citta-vikṣepakatvāt. tiṣṭhato'pi deha-dhāraṇe vyāpṛtaṃ mano na sūkṣma-vastu-nirīkṣaṇa-kṣamaṃ bhavati. śayānasyāpy akasmād eva nidrayā abhibhūyeta. āsīnasya evaṃjātīyako bhūyān doṣas suparihara iti saṃbhavati tasyopāsanam. api ca dhyāyaty artha eva yat samāna-pratyaya-pravāha-karaṇam. ... āsīnaś ca anāyāso bhavati. ... acalatvam āpekṣya dhyāyati-vādo bhavati. ... ata eva padmakādīnām āsana-viśeṣāṇām upadeśo yogaśāstre. ... yatra ekāgratā tatraiva ity etad eva darśayati* – BSBh 4.1.7–11 (pp. 782–785).

76 *samyag-darśanam anūdya tat phalaṃ mokṣa abhidhīyate ... samyag-darśana-niṣṭhas sa yogī parama utkṛṣṭaḥ ... yathoktasya samyag-darśana-lakṣaṇasya yogasya* – BGBh 6.31–33 (pp. 240–241). See also note 53 above. *pratiṣṭhāpya sthiram acalam ātmana āsanam ... cailājinakuśottaram ... pāṭhakramād viparīta atra kramaḥ* – BGBh 6.11. *Yogaśāstre paripāṭhāt ... "ardhaṃ sa-vyañjanānnasya tṛtīyam udakasya ca vāyos saṃcaraṇārthaṃ tu caturtham avaśeṣayet"* – BGBh 6.16 (pp. 226–231).

77 *yathā-śāstram upāsyasyārthasya viṣayīkaraṇena sāmīpyam upagamya taila-dhārāvat samāna-pratyaya-pravāheṇa dīrgha-kālaṃ yad āsanaṃ tad upāsanam ācakṣate* – BGBh 12.3 (p. 387). *taila-dhārāvat santata avicchinna-pratyayo dhyānaṃ* – BGBh 13.24 (p. 452). See note 75 above.

78 *atra ātma-darśane bahava upāya-vikalpā ime dhyānādaya ucyante – dhyānenātmani paśyanti kecid ātmānam ātmanā anye sāṃkhyena yogena karma-yogena cāpare – ... dhyānaṃ nāma śabdādibhyo viṣayebhyaś śrotrādīni karaṇāni manasy upasaṃhṛtya, manaś ca pratyak-cetayitari, ekāgratayā yac cintanaṃ, tad dhyānaṃ ... tena dhyānena ātmani buddhau paśyanty ātmānaṃ pratyak-cetanam ātmanā svenaiva pratyak-cetanena dhyāna-saṃskṛtena antaḥkaraṇena kecid yoginaḥ ... sāṃkhyaṃ nāma "ime sattva-rajas-tamāṃsi guṇāḥ mayā dṛśyāḥ, ahaṃ tebhyo'nyas tad-vyāpāra-sākṣi-bhūto guṇa-vilakṣaṇa ātmā," iti cintanaṃ, eṣas sāṃkhyo yogaḥ ... karmaiva yoga īśvarārpaṇa-buddhyā anuṣṭhīyamānaḥ ... yoga ucyate guṇataḥ. tena sattva-śuddhi-jñānotpatti-dvāreṇa ca* – BhG and BGBh 13.24 (p. 452). See also BGBh 2.58 – *jñāna-niṣṭha indriyāṇi indriyārthebhyas sarvaviṣayebhya upasaṃharate* (p. 79).

79 *yadā ... niścalā vikṣepa-calana-varjitā satī samādhau, samādhīyate cittam asminn iti samādhir ātmā ... acalā, tatrāpi vikalpa-varjitā ... tadā ... yogam avāpsyasi viveka-prajñāṃ samādhiṃ prāpsyasi ... labdha-samādhi-prajñasya lakṣaṇa-bubhutsayā ... sthitaprajñasya iti - sthitā pratiṣṭhitā "aham asmi paraṃ brahma" iti prajñā yasya sa sthitaprajñas tasya* – BGBh 2.53–54 (pp. 74–75). See Comans, "The Question of the Importance of Samādhi," for an earlier discussion of *samādhi* in other works of Śaṅkara.

80 See, for example, *jīvanneva guṇān atītya amṛtam aśnuta iti ... uktaṃ yāvat yatna-sādhyaṃ tāvat saṃnyāsino'nuṣṭheyaṃ guṇātītatva-sādhanaṃ mumukṣoḥ. sthirībhūtaṃ tu sva-saṃvedyaṃ sad guṇātītasya yater lakṣaṇaṃ bhavati iti* – BGBh 14.21–26 (pp. 482–486). See notes 54–58 above, for related references from other chapters in BGBh.

81 See note 40 above for BSBh 2.3.39, and note that Śaṅkara uses the word *upadiṣṭa*, with respect to *samādhi*, without referring to *vidhi* here. BSBh 2.3.40 says, *nanu mokṣa-sādhana-vidhānān mokṣas setsyati, na. sādhanāyat tasya anityatvāt. api ca nitya-śuddha-mukta-ātma-pratipādanāt mokṣa-siddhir abhi-*

matā, tādṛg ātma-pratipādanaṃ ca na svābhāvike kartṛtve'vakalpeta, tasmād upādhi-dharmādhyāsenaiva ātmanaḥ kartṛtvam, na svābhāvikam ... vidhi-śāstraṃ tāvad yathā-prāptaṃ kartṛtvam upādāya kartavya-viśeṣam upadiśati. na kartṛtvam ātmanaḥ pratipādayati. na ca svābhāvikam asya kartṛtvam asti brahmātmatvopadeśād ity avocāma. tasmād avidyā-kṛtaṃ kartṛtvam upādāya vidhi-śāstraṃ pravartiṣyate.... samādhy-abhāvas tu śāstrārthavattvenaiva parihṛtaḥ. yathā-prāptam eva kartṛtvam upādāya samādhi-vidhānāt. tasmāt kartṛtvam apy ātmana upādhi-nimittam eveti sthitam (pp. 470–474).

82 *etena yogaḥ pratyuktaḥ* – BS 2.1.3. *etena sāṃkhya-smṛti-pratyākhyānena yoga-smṛtir api pratyākhyātā ... kimarthaṃ punar atidiśyate? asti hy atra abhyadhikāśaṅkā. samyag-darśanābhyupāyo hi yogo vede vihitaḥ, "śrotavyo mantavyo nididhyāsitavya" iti ... yogaśāstre'pi "atha tattva-darśanābhyupāyo yoga" iti samyag-darśanābhyupāyenaiva yogo'ṅgīkriyate.... arthaikadeśa-saṃpratipattāv apy arthaikadeśa-vipratipatteḥ ... sāṃkhya-yoga-smṛtyor eva nirākaraṇe yatnaḥ kṛtaḥ. sāṃkhya-yogau hi paramapuruṣārtha-sādhanatvena loke prakhyātau śiṣṭaiś ca parigṛhītau.... nirākaraṇaṃ tu, na sāṃkhya-smṛti-jñānena veda-nirapekṣeṇa yoga-mārgeṇa vā niḥśreyasam adhigamyata iti.... vaidikam eva tatra jñānaṃ dhyānaṃ ca sāṃkhya-yoga-śabdābhyām abhilapyete pratyāsatter ity avagantavyam. yena tv aṃśena na virudhyete tena iṣṭam eva sāṃkhya-yoga-smṛtyos sāvakāśatvam. tad yathā, "asaṅgo hy ayaṃ puruṣa" ity evam ādi śruti-prasiddham eva puruṣasya viśuddhatvaṃ nirguṇa-puruṣa-nirūpaṇena sāṃkhyair abhyupagamyate. tathā ca yogair api, "atha parivrāḍ vivarṇa-vāsā muṇḍo'parigraha" ity evam ādi śruti-prasiddham eva nivṛtti-niṣṭhatvaṃ pravrajyādy upadeśena anugamyate* – BSBh 2.1.3 (pp. 287–289).

83 Śaṅkara's vigorous arguments in favor of becoming a *saṃnyāsin* from the *brahmacārī* stage itself have continued to be influential in the monastic tradition. While it is possible for a householder to become a *saṃnyāsin*, the heads of the traditional *maṭha*-s, especially in southern India, have typically been those who renounce at a young age, without passing through the stage of the householder. This practice is followed in Dvaita Vedānta also, the monastic tradition of which is historically an offshoot of the Advaita monastic tradition. In Viśiṣṭādvaita Vedānta, on the other hand, there is strong opposition to the tradition of renouncing the world from the *brahmacārī* stage, while the sequential progression through the householder stage and finally to *saṃnyāsa* is privileged.

84 *citi-śakti-guṇaḥ kim ahaṃkaraṇaṃ ... iti cintyam idaṃ ... yatibhiḥ* – *Śrutisārasamuddharaṇa*, verse 21 (p. 19). See also Toṭaka's usage of *dṛśi-mātra* and *dṛśi-rūpa* – *dṛśi-mātram avehi sadāham iti* – verse 159 (p. 104), and *dṛśi-rūpam-anantam-ṛtaṃ tad asi* – verse 170 (p. 111). Note that like Śaṅkara and Sureśvara, Toṭaka also argues vigorously against injunctive interpretations of the *Upaniṣad*-s.

85 Allen Thrasher, *The Advaita Vedānta of Brahma-Siddhi*, Delhi, Motilal Banarsidass Publishers, 1993, pp. 8 and 68–70.

7

LOSING ONE'S MIND AND BECOMING ENLIGHTENED

Some remarks on the concept of yoga in Śvetāmbara Jainism and its relation to the Nāth Siddha tradition

Olle Qvarnström

In contrast with Mīmāṃsā philosophy, for which ritual activity alone (*kriyāmātra*) was of paramount importance, early Śvetāmbara Jainism in the final analysis regarded all forms of activity (*āraṃbha/karma*) as an impediment to reaching the state of liberation.[1] Activity was divided into three modalities: mental, verbal and physical. These were collectively designated yoga, reflecting, on the one hand, the operations of the mind (*manas*), sense of speech (*vāc*) and body (*kāya*), and, on the other, the three kinds of vibration (*spanda*) of the Self (*jīva*). Viewed from the former perspective, these three forms of activity caused an influx (*āsrava*) of subtle matter into the Self (*jīva*) which then translated into different forms of *karma*, bringing Self and matter (*ajīva*) together and causing the former to vibrate. Viewed from the latter perspective, the Self was the agent of these three forms of activity, as well as of the influx of matter and the production of *karma*, since as a part of cyclic existence (*saṃsāra*) it had always been connected with matter and in human embodiment vibrated in three different ways correlated to the activity of the body, mind and the senses.[2] Ultimately, through meditation (*dhyāna*) the influx of matter could be stopped and the destruction of accumulated *karma* achieved. Through this artificial device, the natural process of karmic maturation, whereby *karma* was automatically annihilated, was deliberately enhanced by creating a state of non-activity (*ayogatā*).[3] Such a state was, therefore, the final objective of meditation and, through repeated practice, resulted in the destruction of *karma* and consequently in the attainment of enlightenment and omniscience (*sarvajña*), followed by release from karmic bondage (*nirvāṇa*) and final liberation (*mokṣa*).

The path of liberation (*mokṣamārga*), including the process of meditation, may therefore be portrayed as a path from activity to non-activity, or in the terminology of early Jainism, from yoga to *ayoga(tā)*. Such a path was codified by Umāsvāti in his post-canonical *Tattvārtha Sūtra* (AD 150–350). This text was the first attempt to systematize Jaina canonical teachings into a philosophical system (*darśana*) and holds the same position in Śvetāmbara Jainism as that of the *Yoga Sūtra* in the yoga tradition.[4] The path as described by Umāsvāti consisted of two main aspects: moral (*karma*) and cognitive (*jñāna*).[5] The former dealt with the cultivation of activity, limiting the production of especially inauspicious *karma*; the latter with the annihilation of activity, involving the inhibition (*saṃvara*) of the influx of matter (*āsrava*)[6] as well as the partial (*nirjarā*) and complete annihilation of already amassed karmic matter (*mokṣa*).[7] These two aspects, *karma* and *jñāna,* were mutually complementary and presupposed a third aspect, faith or confidence in the teaching and its propagators, the Jinas. Both mendicant and lay religion included all three aspects, but only the adherents of the former – with a few exceptions – were able to reach the permanent state of no activity or liberation which lay at the end of a path consisting of fourteen steps (*guṇasthāna*).[8] The annihilation of activity, the result of meditation, was understood by the canonical scriptures as well as the *Tattvārtha Sūtra* and subsequent tradition as a gradual process resulting in the "cessation of [the activity of] the mind" (*cittaniroha/cittanirodha*).[9] Given the conditions of the individual practitioner, meditation was thus, as far as it was physically possible, instrumental in bringing mental activity, and connected with it, verbal and physical activity, to a standstill for a limited period of time, erasing karmic matter from the Self. Through repeated practice, all *karma* was completely eradicated and a state of non-activity permanently established.[10] This state was gradually implemented as the lay person and mendicant proceeded along their respective paths.[11] Its final realization was, however, in the main reserved for the latter and was divided into four consecutive states, corresponding to the effects resulting from the four varieties of what was labelled pure meditation (*śukladhyāna*). Of these four consecutive states, two were of prime importance. The first prime state emerged from the successful performance of the second variety of pure meditation and consisted in the cessation of the activity of the mind (*cittanirodha*) as the so-called destructive (*ghātiyā*) *karmas* along with the passions were abolished. This was a state of enlightenment and omniscience[13] as the Self was totally isolated from destructive *karmas* defiling and obstructing its inherent qualities (*guṇa*). The second prime state resulted from the performance of the fourth variety of pure meditation and was achieved by eliminating non-destructive *karmas* (*aghātiyā*) and making it impossible for new *karma* to cling to the passion-free (*vītarāga*) Self.[12] This state was characterized by permanent release from karmic bondage (*nirvāṇa*) immediately followed by liberation (*mokṣa*), the Self leaving the body and ascending to the abode of the liberated (*siddhaloka*) at the apex of the inhabited universe (*lokākāśa*).[13] The unenlightened person (*chadmastha*) qualified for pure meditation sought, therefore, to permanently establish a non-active state of mind in which the Self (*jīva*) cognized reality directly rather than via the mind (*manas*). Having "lost his mind," the omniscient mendicant continued his practice striving for the termination even of physical activity.[14]

According to early Śvetāmbara Jainism as codified by the *Tattvārtha Sūtra,* the term *yoga* thus had the basic meaning of "activity," both related to the Self and to the body, including the mind and the senses. As this activity, along with passions, connected the Self with matter, the term yoga also acquired the derived meaning of "connection" or "juncture."[15] The path and its constitutive exercises, however, did not go under the name of yoga, nor did its *telos*. Consequently, the mendicant who followed the path was not referred to as a *yogin*, nor was his role model, the Jina. On the contrary, the mendicant who had reached the state in which the function of the mind was completely annihilated was entitled *sayogin* or *sayogakevalin* (one who possesses enlightenment or omniscience while in the state of activity), whereas the mendicant who had entered the state where all activity, mental, verbal and physical, had come to an end was called *ayogin* or *ayogakevalin.*[16] Compared to the terminology used within the classical yoga tradition, the terminal points of the Jaina path were described in opposite terms. If Umāsvāti and Patañjali shared the notion of *cittanirodha*, both as embodying the key element in the process of liberation and the state of liberation itself, they nevertheless had formed distinctive identities.

From Umāsvāti and the early systematizers to the medieval period the semantic range of the term *yoga* was widened, as one can see from a large number of texts written during the latter period by Śvetāmbara authors. The first conspicuous landmark in this process is found in the works of one of the two perhaps most prominent of all representatives of Śvetāmbara Jainism, the eighth century philosopher Haribhadra.[17] Instead of exclusively organizing the Jaina path of liberation according to the fourteen *guṇasthānas* or the threefold divison into faith, knowledge and conduct, as in the case of the *Tattvārtha Sūtra*, Haribhadra employs the eight limbs (*aṣṭāṅga*) of the *Yoga Sūtra* (II.29) as an organizing principle in an attempt to synthesize the soteriological paths of three distinctive yoga systems, including that of Patañjali, with Jainism.[18] Consequently, the word *yoga* was used as a designation for the entire Jaina soteriological path. In the same vein, the term *yoga* was equated by Haribhadra not only with mental, verbal and physical activity, connecting the Self with matter, as in early Jainism, but with a specific "activity which connects one with liberation" (*mukkheṇa joyaṇāo jogo*).[19] Elaborating on the different meanings of the word *yoga*, Haribhadra declared that "the highest form of yoga among all yogins is thus without yoga (*ayoga*). It is characterized by total abandonment since it connects [a yogin] with liberation."[20] The observance of the path was termed *yogācāra* and the followers, i.e. the Jaina mendicants, *yogins*.[21] The final goal of the path was, however, still designated *ayoga*.

The next notable extension of the semantic range of the term *yoga* is found in the writings of the other major representative of Śvetāmbara Jainism, Hemacandra (AD 1089–1172). In addition to the various connotations ascribed to the term by Haribhadra, whose scholarly production was familiar to Hemacandra,[22] the word *yoga* is in the opening verse of Hemacandra's magnum opus, the *Yogaśāstra*,[23] used in an honorific epithet applied to the last saviour or Jina, Mahāvīra: Yoginātha, "the Lord of Yogins." Furthermore, *yoga* is used as a synonym for the three main divisions or jewels (*ratnatraya*) of Jainism: correct faith, knowledge and conduct, and is also compared to a "yogic dance" (*yaugaṃ tāṇḍavaḍambaram*).[24] Classical Hīnayāna and Mahāyāna Buddhism seem to have been more cautious in using terms like *yoga* and *yogin* to denote its three jewels, the Buddha, the mendicants of the congregation (*saṅgha*) and the teaching (*dharma*), as these terms probably were seen as having too strong denotations to the Brāhmaṇical tradition. Nonetheless, we occasionally find passages in which, for example, a bodhisattva is given the epithet *yogin*.[25] Tantric Buddhism, however, frequently employs terms such as *yogeśvara* for the Buddha.

Based on a limited reading of the works of Umāsvāti, Haribhadra and Hemacandra, we may conclude that the term *yoga* had one and the same basic meaning in early as well as in medieval Śvetāmbara Jainism, namely, activity. In a negative sense it denoted that influx of karmic matter which together with the passions united the Self with matter; in a positive sense it signified (with Haribhadra and Hemacandra) that teaching and its constitutive exercises which ultimately brought about liberation.

The extension of the semantic range of the word *yoga* demonstrates a process where Jaina ideas and practices were framed in novel terms and organizational structures and where hitherto relatively insignificant practices were brought to the fore. Instead of, for example, designating the Jaina teaching *jainaśāsana* or *jainadarśana*, it was labelled yoga and organized under eight "limbs" in texts which carried *Yoga-* as the first element in the title and which saw meditation and auxiliary practices, such as *āsana*, as paramount to the mortification of the body etc. Instead of merely referring to Jaina mendicants as *sādhus*, *munis* etc., they were also called *yogins*, and in addition to giving the Jaina saviours the epithet *Jina* or *Tīrthaṅkara*, they were now also referred to as *yogināthas*. This change of nomenclature mirrors a historical development consisting, *inter alia*, in the increased influence of classical and post-classical yoga on all religio-philosophical systems (*darśana*). This influence was both of a rhetorical nature and included the integration of previously unknown practices.[26] It was, therefore, a decisive step when medieval *paṇḍits* and custodians of the Śvetāmbara Jaina tradition, such as Haribhadra and Hemacandra, incorporated these new elements and reformulated and restructured their dogma in order to participate in the pan-Indian debate on yoga as well as to contribute to the preservance and expansion of their faith.[27]

In order to further demonstrate this influence of classical and tantric yoga on Śvetāmbara Jainism, viewed from the perspective of the path of liberation gradually bringing all activity to cease, we shall once more have a look at the *Yogaśāstra*. This text did not only contribute historically to the unity and survival of Jainism, but is still used today as a normative account for all Śvetāmbara Jainas in India and abroad. Hemacandra opens and concludes the final chapter of this text, which also bears the (for our purposes) suitable title *Yogopaniṣad*, by declaring that he, in the preceeding eleven chapters, had truthfully summarized the canonical and traditional teachings as known to him through his own reading and his teacher (*guru*). In the twelfth and final chapter, however, his aim is to describe reality according to his own experience (*svasaṃvedana*). This statement inevitably brings to mind the career of Hemacandra, covering an initial phase as a Jaina monk (*sādhu*) and teacher (*sūri*), followed by an extensive period as a monk-scholar at the court of Kumārapāla and his predecessor Jayasiṃha Siddharāja, and possibly ending with a phase dominated by religious practice or yoga guided by his own claim that meditation is paramount, and that everything else is simply textual details (*granthavistara*).[28] This tallies with the reasoning of Haribhadra in his *Yogadṛṣṭisamuccaya,* where it is said that one should first observe the teachings (*dharma*) which are laid down in the canonical scriptures and the authoritative traditional texts, then one should thoroughly examine these, and finally one should personally assimilate the highest knowledge through meditative insight, thus transcending the first two.

The fundamental doctrine in the twelfth chapter of the *Yogaśāstra* is that, through practice (*abhyāsa*) and indifference (*audāsīnya*) or passionlessness, the mind (*manas/antaḥkaraṇa*) should be brought under control. From being scattered (*vikṣipta*), partly controlled (*yatāyāta*) and collected (*śliṣṭa*), it should be fully immersed (*sulīna*) into the supreme reality (*paratattva*) of the Self (*ātman*). This state is characterized as a state of non-mind, using terms like *amanaska*, *amanaskatā*, *vimanaska* and *unmanībhāva*, a state gradually reached through meditation, restraining verbal, mental and bodily activity.[29]

The *Yogaśāstra* XII.22–25 reads:

> He who is seated in a comfortable posture in a secluded, extremely pure [and] pleasant location, who has all the limbs loosened from

the tip of the toe to the top of the head, who while perceiving a beautiful form, listening to soft speech which is agreeable to the mind, smelling fragrant plants, tasting sweet flavour [or] touching soft objects, does not restrain the activity of the mind, who once and for all has destroyed all erroneous opinions, who possesses indifference (*audāsīnya*), who has completely suppressed all mental and physical activities [and] who has obtained the state of identity with the [supreme reality], [that] mendicant (*yogin*) will quickly accomplish the state of no-mind (*unmanībhāva*). [Ergo, just as there is absorption (*laya*) into the supreme reality (*paratattva*) for he who possessess indifference (*audāsīnya*), there is also absorption into the state of no-mind.]

Further (*Yogaśāstra* XII.33–36, 53):

The Self, which is permanently immersed in indifference (*audāsīnya*), which has completely abandoned all effort [and] which has cultivated supreme bliss, does not employ the mind anywhere. The mind, which once [for all] is overlooked by the Self, does not [in turn] control the senses [and] consequently, the senses do not engage even in their own objects. When the Self does not set the mind in motion and the mind does not set the senses in motion, at that time, separated from both sides [– the Self and the senses –] the mind undergoes annihilation (*vināśa*) by itself. When all [the activities of the mind, such as thinking (*cintā*) and rememberance (*smṛti*)],[30] have completely perished (*naṣṭa*) and [the mind] has dissolved (*yāte vilayam*) entirely, [just as a fire covered by ashes and then saturated with a current of water], reality [in the form of the knowledge of the Self, free from karma], fully comes forth, like a lamp which is placed in a sheltered spot./. . ./When the [mind] exists, it grasps an object even from a distance, [such as a tiger or a woman], which [then] gives it displeasure or pleasure. When the mind does not exist, however, even [an object] which is close [to the mind] is not at all received [as either pleasant or unpleasant]. Certainly, how can there not be desire to serve good teachers which is a cause of the attainment of the state of non-mind (*unmanībhāva*) for men who have understood [correctly] in this way?

The examples could be multiplied, but in substance the description of the meditative process conforms with the earliest definition of yoga found in the Kaṭha Upaniṣad[31] and systematized in the *Yoga Sūtra,* a text familiar to Hemacandra.[32] Consequently, one almost agrees with our two paragons of Śvetāmbara Jainism that, as far as the theory and practice of yoga is concerned, it is basically a matter of terminological differences (*saṃjñā-bheda*) and development of details (*granthavistara*).[33] The basic doctrine of yoga presented in the twelfth chapter of the *Yogaśāstra* is apparently not specific to Jainism, Śvetāmbara or Digambara,[34] but shared by most Indian religious traditions. What is interesting, however, is the distinctive terminology used by Hemacandra which not only bears witness to classical yoga, but leads us to historically unexploited areas as well as to contemporaneous tantric doctrines.

Turning to history, we are reminded of *Ṛg Veda* X.129 where "the one" (*tad ekam*), beyond existence (*sat*) and non-existence (*asat*) were differentiated due to mind (*manas*) and desire (*kāma*).[35] "The one" was later, most probably, identified with the highest reality of the *Upaniṣads*, *brahman* or *puruṣa*, and characterized, among other things, as "non-mind" (*amanas*).[36] The Maitrī Upaniṣad (VI.20, 34) declares that the supreme state (*paraṃ padam*) arises when the mind is bereft of desire (*kāma*), motionless (*suniścala*), and thus has reached the state of no-mind (*amanībhāva*), the fluctuations (*vṛtti*) of the mind being destroyed. The same idea and terminology are then repeated in later *Upaniṣads*.[37] Naturally, we also find it in systematic Vedānta texts, such as the *Gauḍapādīyakārikā*[38] and the *Upadeśasāhasrī*.[39] It is also prevalent in Buddhism and Hinduism. The Dīghanikāya, for example, teaches that liberation (*nibbāna*) comes about through the supression of consciousness (*viññānassa nirodhena*), indicating a state devoid of bodily, mental and verbal activity,[40] and the *Bhagavadgītā* (VI.20) concludes that when the mind is checked and comes to rest one finds content in the Self.

Leaving history, the first impression of a text that Hemacandra calls a "personal description" is that it in fact does not bear any traces of an informal narrative. Quite the contrary, it breathes classification and a consistent technical terminology, probably revealing a hitherto unknown influence on mainstream Śvetāmbara Jainism. Recent scholarship has shown that certain meditative practices, as well as the associated terminology, found in chapters 7 to 10 of the *Yogaśāstra*, most probably originate from the Trika of "Kashmiri" Śaivism as codified in texts such as the *Tantrāloka* of Abhinavagupta.[41] The terminology used in the twelfth chapter of the *Yogaśāstra* is, however, neither found in this text (except for a few occurances),[42] nor in the *Jñānārṇava*, a Digambara work which most likely constituted the source from which Hemacandra gathered his information about Trika Śaiva meditative practices.[43] Rather than looking for an answer to our terminological search within the intellectual world of Hemacandra, we should therefore perhaps search in his immediate physical and religious surroundings.

From inscriptions it is established that the dominating branch of Śaivism in Gujarat during the time of Hemacandra was Pāśupata, but we also know that other groups, such as the Kaula, Kāpālika, Rahamāna and

Ghaṭachaṭaka, existed. All these Śaiva denominations were opposed to the Śvetāmbara Jainas and are, for example, said to have called on their former co-religionist Kumārapāla to express their dissatisfaction with the moral prohibitions imposed on them as a result of the king's conversion to Jainism.[44] What is intriguing is that two of these groups, the Pāśupata and Kāpālika, formed part of the so-called Nāth Sampradāya, which was established in the twelfth or thirteenth century in western India.[45] The followers of this religious order, the Nāth Siddhas, or more correct, their predecessors in whatever form they may have had, may have been alluded to by Hemacandra, since they were generally called "Kānphaṭas" ("Split Eared"), thus reminding us of the expression in the *Yogaśāstra*, "He whose ears have not been pierced by the needle of the syllables yoga" (*aviddhakarṇo yo yoga ity akṣaraśalākayā*).[46] The Nāth Siddhas or the Kānphaṭas were first of all practitioners of *haṭhayoga*, and their doctrine was codified in texts such as the *Amanaskayoga*. Interestingly enough, the Śvetāmbara Jainas and the Kānphaṭas shared the same cult centers. The focal point of Kānphaṭa activity in western India was Girnar in Gujarat. Crags located at this mountain, as well as at Mt Abu in Rajasthan, formed the scene of Nāth practice, which apart from *haṭhayoga* also included alchemy.[47] As is well known, these two mountains constituted important religious sites for the Jainas as well, and Girnar was visited by Hemacandra in the company of his royal employers, Jayasiṃha Siddharāja and Kumārapāla.[48] The two mountains were also associated with the twenty-second and twenty-third Tīrthaṅkaras, Nemī and Pārśva, both of whom were honored with temples situated at these locations, where the Jainas, like the Nāth Siddhas, also seem to have been engaged in alchemical practices.[49] The two Jaina Tīrthaṅkaras were further transformed by the Nāth tradition into sons of Matsyendra, its legendary founder, who is said to have initiated them and made them the founders of the Nīmnāthi- and Pārasnāthi-panths, two Jaina suborders of the Nāth Sampradāya.[50] Jaina temples and Nāth Siddha crags together with polemical writings and other evidence, point at a close relationship between Jainas and Kānphaṭas. Apart from the few hints occurring in the *Yogaśāstra* – the designation of Mahāvīra as *yoginātha*, the teaching as a yogic dance, and figuratively calling the followers "split-eared" – this is further substantiated by the fact that the Jainas and the Nāth Siddhas occupied substantially the same area in the old town of Bombay, the Pūe Dhūni (Paidhoni). Here the Jainas had a temple sheltering a statue of Ghorajīnāth![51]

The question now presents itself as to what type of relation existed between the Śvetāmbara Jainas and the Kānphaṭas, and whether or not Hemacandra was in contact with some kind of embryonic *haṭhayoga*/Nāth tradition existing prior to the formation of the religious order (*sampradāya*), and which, for one or the other reason, may have influenced his narration in chapter 12 of the *Yogaśāstra*. Gathering from later polemics between the Śvetāmbara Jainas and the Nāth Siddhas,[52] together with the doctrinal content of the above-mentioned text, presupposing that it contains an earlier ideological stratum, a common doctrinal basis is unthinkable. On the other hand, the two religious groups most likely shared various (tantric) practices, except for those of a sexual nature which were reprehensible to the Jainas.

Apart from similarities of religious *praxis*, which to a great extent are of a pan-Indian nature and from which it therefore is difficult to draw any conclusions, we are left with terminological correspondences. Jambuvijaya[53] has provided the textual material for a comparison based on which we may conclude that the key terms, on which the entire philosophy of texts like the *Amanaskayoga* hinges, are also found and consistently used in the twelfth chapter of the *Yogaśāstra*. It is therefore plausible to assume that, since these terms, like *amanaska*(*tā*), *vimanaska*, *unmanībhāva* – not the basic idea behind them – are not found in consistent use in any texts known to me prior to the *Amanaskayoga* and other texts belonging to the same tradition,[54] with the exception of stray references in Brāhmaṇical and Buddhist texts, and since these terms are not attested in the Śvetāmbara Jaina tradition prior to the twelfth chapter of the *Yogaśāstra,* we may at least for now posit that Hemacandra borrowed these from some source which came to be part of the Nāth Sampradāya established a century or so after his death. Not to rule out personal motives, this case is thus similar to that of Trika Śaivism, providing a nomenclature (and organizational structure) for meditative practices in the *Yogaśāstra* without interfering with fundamental Śvetāmbara doctrines laid out in Umāsvāti's *Tattvārtha Sūtra*. Furthermore, the purpose behind such a rhetorical device and its target groups is also the same in these two cases. Firstly, the *Yogaśāstra* was written at the request of a king who despite his conversion to Śvetāmbara Jainism never completely left his Śaiva faith.[55] Second, the contemplated addressee of this epitome did not consist of a certain Śaivite of noble descent only. It was also meant to address the majority of the population of Gujarat, who belonged to various Śaivite denominations; as well as the scholars of those days with whom Hemacandra was in close contact.

Granted that such a terminological borrowing actually took place, we may thus through further research on the Śvetāmbara Jaina tradition in western India also improve our knowledge of the emergence, spread and influence of the Nāth Sampradāya. In contrast to classical Jainism and its understanding of the term *amanaska* as an irrational being not yet having acquired a mind,[56] the same word was now used to denote the highest ideal of Jainism, thereby adopting a linguistic usage prevalent among the Nāth Siddhas of Gujarat but with deep historical roots.

Notes

1 Although Kumārila, according to Mādhava, on his deathbed admitted that the Jainas after all did contribute some insights (see *The Sarvadarśanasaṃgraha, or, Review of the different systems of Hindu philosophy*, trans. by E. B. Cowell and A. E. Gough, London, Kegan Paul, Trench, Trübner & Co., 1904, p. 84, n. 9), the ideological opposition between Jainas and Mīmāṃsākas is apparent throughout the religious history of India. This is illustrated, for example, in the *Ārhatadarśana* chapter of the *Sarvadarśanasaṃgraha*. On Kumārila's critique of the Buddhist and Jaina notions of omniscience, see e.g. the *Ślokavārttika* I.1.2 and K. B. Pathak, "Kumārila's Verses Attacking the Jaina and Buddhist Notions of an Omniscient Being," *Annals of the Bhandarkar Oriental Research Institute,* 1930–1931, vol. 12, pp. 123–131. On the Jaina criticism of the Mīmāṃsākas and the defence of personal omniscience, see e.g. Haribhadra's *Sarvajñasiddhi* and *Śāstravārtāsamuccaya.*

2 *Tattvārthasūtra* (TAS) with *Svopajña Bhāṣya* (SB) VI.1–5, VIII.1; see W. J. Johnson, *Harmless Souls: Karmic Bondage and Religious Change in Early Jainism with Special Reference to Umāsvāti and Kundakunda*, Delhi, Motilal Banarsidass, 1995, pp. 14ff., Paul Dundas, *The Jains*, London, Routledge, 1992, pp. 84–85, and Nathmal Tatia, *Studies in Jaina Philosophy*, Banaras, Jain Cultural Research Society, 1951, pp. 252–254. The *Svopajña Bhāṣya* was believed by the Śvetāmbara tradition to be the sūtras and commentary by Umāsvāti himself.

3 On the deliberate (*sakāma*) enhancement of karmic maturation, see TAS/SB IX.3, 19ff.; on *ayogatā/ajogatta,* see *Uttarādhyayanasūtra* XXIX.37 (referred to by Johannes Bronkhorst, *The Two Traditions of Meditation in Ancient India*, Stuttgart, Steiner Verlag Wiesbaden, 1986, p. 32). For an in-depth study of Jaina karma theory, see Kristi L. Wiley, "*Āghatiyā Karmas*: Agents of Embodiment in Jainism," PhD dissertation, University of California at Berkeley, 2000.

4 See P. S. Jaini, *The Jaina Path of Purification*, Berkeley, University of California Press, 1979, p. 81. For a review of the evidence surrounding the question of the affiliation, identity, time, authorship etc. of Umāsvāti, see Johannes Bronkhorst, "On the Chronology of the Tattvārtha Sūtra and Some Early Commentaries," *Wiener Zeitschrift für die Kunde Südasiens und Archiv für Indische Philosophie,* 1985, vol. 29, pp. 155–184.

5 Cf. O. Qvarnström, "Stability and Adaptability: A Jain Strategy for Survival and Growth," *Indo-Iranian Journal*, 1998, vol. 41, pp. 33–55, and the introduction to Qvarnström, *The Yogaśāstra of Hemacandra. A Twelfth Century Handbook on Śvetāmbara Jainism*, Cambridge, MA, Harvard University Press, 2002, pp. 1–14.

6 TAS/SB IX.

7 TAS/SB X.

8 The layman's path as originally described in the canonical *Upāsakadaśāḥ* consisted of eleven *pratimās*. These were modelled on the fourteen *guṇasthānas* of the mendicant. See Jaini *Jaina Path of Purification*, p. 186; and R. Williams, *Jaina Yoga. A Survey of the Mediaeval Śrāvakācāras*, London, Oxford University Press, 1963, pp. 173–181.

9 See *Uttarādhyayanasūtra* XXIX.25 (quoted by Bronkhorst, *Two Traditions*, p. 36: *egaggamaṇasannivesaṇayāe ṇaṃ cittanirohaṃ karei*). See also TAS/SB IX.27 (quoted by the autocommentary, the *Svopajñavṛtti*, ad *Yogaśāstra* IV.115). Cf. *Yoga Sūtra* I.2, III.12. For a historical and philosophical analysis of the term "nirodha" as used in Indian philosophical texts (except for Jaina), see Frederich Smith, "Nirodha and the Nirodhalakṣaṇa of Vallabhācārya,"

Journal of Indian Philosophy, 1998, vol. 26, pp. 489–551, and Paul Griffiths, *On Being Mindless: Buddhist Meditation and the Mind-Body Problem*, La Salle, IL, Open Court, 1986. Cf. also Ian Whicher, "Nirodha, Yoga Praxis and the Transformation of the Mind," *Journal of Indian Philosophy*, 1997, vol. 25, pp. 1–67.

10 TAS/SB IX.27, 37ff. It may be inferred from the insurmountable requirements related to the performance of *śukladhyāna,* including the possession of a perfect *physique* (*uttamasaṃhanana*) and knowledge of the (lost) Pūrva scriptures, that external ascetism (*bahistapas*) in the form of fasting, etc. has been the dominating practice from earliest times to the present day (see *Yogaśāstra* XI.1–4; Dundas, *The Jains*, pp. 143–146). This is also reflected in the polemics between the Jainas and the Buddhists where they accused each other of being too occupied with physical and mental activity, respectively (Bronkhorst, *Two Traditions*, pp. 10–11, 24–26, 28, n. 8).

11 On the path of the lay person and the mendicant, see note 8 on p. 139.

12 TAS/SB VIII.7–14; IX.39–43.

13 TAS/SB X.5.

14 Cf. Vyāsa ad *Yoga Sūtra* I.1, 2, 18 (on *saṃprajñāta-/asaṃprajñāta-* or *sabīja-/nirbīja-samādhi*); Ian Whicher, "The Final Stages of Purification in Classical Yoga," *The Adyar Library Bulletin,* 1997, vol. 61, pp. 1–44.

15 Cp. Johnson, *Harmless Souls*, pp. 14ff. with Kristi Wiley, "Karmic Bondage and Kaṣāyas: A Re-Examination of 'Umāsvāti's Jainism'," in V. P. Jain (ed.) *Proceedings of the International Seminar on Umāsvāti and His Works*, Delhi, Bhogilal Leherchand Institute of Indology, forthcoming.

16 See TAS/SB ad IX.42–43, 49.

17 Haribhadra wrote four major works on yoga: *Yogadṛṣṭisamuccaya, Yogaviṃśikā, Yogabindu*, and *Yogaśataka,* all of which have been translated by K. K. Dixit. Haribhadra also composed a summary (*samāsena*) of yoga entitled *Yogabheda* forming chapter XIV of his *Ṣoḍaśakaprakaraṇa.*

18 See Chris Chapple, "Haribhadra's Analysis of Pātañjala and Kula Yoga in the *Yogadṛṣṭisamuccaya*," in John Cort (ed.) *Open Boundaries: Jain Communities and Culture in Indian History*, Albany, NY, State University of New York Press, 1998, pp. 15–30, and "The Centrality of the Real in Haribhadra's Yoga Texts," in Olle Qvarnström and N. K. Wagle (eds) *Approaches to Jaina Studies: Philosophy, Logic, Rituals and Symbols*, Toronto, University of Toronto Centre for South Asian Studies, 1999, pp. 91–100.

19 *Yogaviṃśikā* 1.

20 *Yogadṛṣṭisamuccaya* I.11: *atas tv ayogo yogānāṃ yogaḥ para udāhītaḥ/mokṣa-yojanabhāvena sarvasaṃnyāsalakṣaṇaḥ//.*

21 *Yogadṛṣṭisamuccaya* passim.

22 O. Qvarnström, "Haribhadra and the Beginnings of Doxography in India," in Qvarnström and Wagle (eds) *Approaches to Jaina Studies*, pp. 169–210.

23 For an annotated English translation of the entire *Yogaśāstra* in the light of the autocommentary, the *Svopajñavṛtti*, see Qvarnström, *The Yogaśāstra of Hemacandra*). In Hemacandra's *Anyayogavyavachedika* (I.1) and *Triṣaṣṭiśalākāpuruṣacaritra* (Johnson, *Harmless Souls*, pp. 134, 259, 269, 285, 312, 319, 337), Vardhamāna (Mahāvīra) is portrayed as superior to all yogins (= mendicants). However, neither the Jina nor the mendicants are referred to as yogins in the *Abhidhānacintāmaṇi* (24–25). The Digambara author, Śubhacandra, ascribes the epithet *yogikalpatarum*, "the foremost yogin," and *yogīndra*, the king of yogins," to the Jina in his *Jñānārṇava* (I.2, 6), and the mendicants are frequently referred to as "yogins" (see, e.g. *Jñānārṇava* I.2, 6, 40; XXI. 6).

24 *Yogaśāstra* I.15: *caturvarge 'graṇīr mokṣo yogas tasya ca kāraṇam/ jñānaśraddhānacāritrarūpaṃ ratnatrayaṃ ca saḥ//.* "Liberation is the foremost among the four goals [of human objectives (*puruṣārtha*)] the means of which is yoga. This [yoga, which also is designated] the three jewels (*ratnatraya*), consists of [correct] knowledge (*jñāna*), faith (*śraddhāna*) and conduct (*cāritra*)." On yoga as a yogic dance, see *Yogaśāstra* I.8. The term *tāṇḍava* refers usually in Hindu classical mythology and poetry to the dance of death appropriate to Śiva in his destructive aspect, but it is also used in connection with yoga stressing their intimate connection. See Wendy Doniger, *Women, Androgynes, and Other Mythical Beasts*, Chicago, University of Chicago Press, 1980, pp. 130–133, 136.

25 See E. J. Thomas, *The History of Buddhist Thought*, London, Kegan Paul, Trench, Trübner & Co., 1933, pp. 231ff.

26 On Jaina tantrism, see (with references) P. Dundas, "Becoming Gautama. Mantra and History in Śvetāmbara Jainism," in John Cort (ed.) *Open Boundaries*, pp. 31–52; ibid., "The Jain Monk Jinapati Sūri Gets the Better of a Nāth Yogī," in David Gordon White (ed.) *Tantra in Practice*, Princeton, NJ, Princeton University Press, 2000, pp. 231–238; John Cort, "Tantra in Jainism: The Cult of Ghaṇṭākarṇ Mahāvīr, the Great Hero Bell-Ears," *Bulletin d'Études Indiennes*, 1997, vol. 15, pp. 115–133; O. Qvarnström "Jain Tantra: Divinatory and Meditative Practices in the 12th Century *Yogaśāstra* of Hemacandra," in David Gordon White (ed.) *Tantra in Practice*, pp. 595–604.

27 Cf. O. Qvarnström, "Stability and Adaptability: A Jain Strategy for Survival and Growth," *Indo-Iranian Journal*, 1998, vol. 41, pp. 33–55.

28 *Svopajñavṛtti* ad *Yogaśāstra* VIII. 78. For the available sources on the life of Hemacandra, see G. Bühler, *The Life of Hemacandrācārya*, trans. Manilal Patel, Śāntiniketan, Singhī Jaina Jñānapīṭha, 1936, pp. ix–xi, 1–5; John Cort, *Crossing Boundaries*, p. 108, n. 16; and R. C. C. Fynes's translation of Hemacandra's *The Lives of the Jain Elders*, Oxford, Oxford University Press, 1998, pp. ix–xii.

29 See *Yogaśāstra* XII.39, 40 and 41 (*amanaska*), 43 (*vimanska*), 25 (*unmanībhāva*); *Svopajñavṛtti* ad *Yogaśāstra* XII.21, 54 (*unmanībhāva*), 52 (*amanaskatā*).

30 On the five major fluctuations (*vṛtti*) of the mind, see Vyāsa ad *Yoga Sūtra* I.6–10.

31 See Gavin Flood, *An Introduction to Hinduism*, Cambridge, Cambridge.

32 *Svopajñavṛtti* ad *Yogaśāstra* V.1.

33 *Triṣaṣṭiśalākāpuruṣacaritra* II.264.

34 See e.g. Śubhacandra's *Jñānārṇava*, chapter 22.

35 See W. N. Brown, "Theories of Creation in the Rig Veda," *Journal of the American Oriental Society*, 1965, vol. 85, pp. 27–28, 33–34.

36 *Bṛhadāraṇyaka Upaniṣad* III.8.8; 4.1.6; Muṇḍaka Upaniṣad II.1.2.

37 See e.g. *Brahma Upaniṣad* 2 (*amanaska*); *Brahmabindu* 4 (*unmanībhāva*).

38 *Gauḍapādīyakārikā* III.31–32 (*amanastā, amanībhāva*). See Richard King, *Early Advaita Vedānta and Buddhism: The Mahāyāna Context of the Gauḍapādīya-Kārikā*, Albany, NY, State University of New York Press, 1995, pp. 149–150.

39 *Upadeśasāhasrī* 1.3.4; 1.13.12; 1.13.13; 1.14.38; 2.1.7 (*amanas*); 1.13.15; 1.14.34; 1.14.38 (*amanaska*); 1.13.1; 1.13.15 (*amanastva*).

40 *Dīghanikāya* I.223; I.184.

41 See Qvarnström, "Stability and Adaptability," (with references).

42 *Tantrāloka* XXIX.274c (*unmanasī sthitiḥ*), 275a (*unmanogatyā*). For this information, I am indebted to Dr Harunaga Isaksson (Universität Hamburg).

43 See Qvarnström, "Stability and Adaptability."

44 See A. K. Majumdar, *Chaulukyas of Gujarat: A Survey of the History and Culture of Gujarat from the Middle of the Tenth to the End of the Thirteenth Century*, Bombay, Bharatiya Vidya Bhavan, 1956, p. 294; Bühler, *The Life of Hemacandrācārya*, p. 26; K. K. Handiqui, *Yaśastilaka and Indian Culture; or, Somadeva's Yaśastilaka and Aspects of Jainism and Indian Thought and Culture in the Tenth Century*, Sholapur, Jaina Saṃskrti Saṃrakshaka Sangha, 1949, p. 240; *Svopajñavṛtti* ad *Yogaśāstra* IV.102.

45 David White, *The Alchemical Body: Siddha Traditions in Medieval India*, Chicago, IL, University of Chicago Press, 1996, p. 99. The following references to the Nāth tradition are based on White's excellent book on Siddha traditions in medieval India.

46 *Yogaśāstra* I.14cd; cf. White, *The Alchemical Body*, pp. 9, 321.

47 White, *The Alchemical Body*, pp. 9–10, 117–119.

48 Bühler, *The Life of Hemacandrācārya*, pp. 20–21, 46, 56.

49 White, *The Alchemical Body*, pp. 114ff.

50 White, *The Alchemical Body*, p. 119.

51 G. W. Briggs, *Gorakhnāth and the Kānphata Yogīs*, Delhi, Motilal Banarsidass, 1973. Calcutta, p. 72, n. 1.

52 See Paul Dundas, "The Jain Monk Jinapati Sūri Gets the Better of a Nāth Yogī," in White, *Tantra in Practice*, pp. 231–238.

53 See Jambūvijaya 1986: 1179–1184, n. 1. On the date and authorship of the *Amanaskayoga*, see Jan Gonda, *Medieval Religious Literature in Sanskrit*, Wiesbaden, Harrassowitz, 1977, pp. 221–222.

54 See e.g. *Haṭhayogapradīpikā* IV.3–4 (*unmanī* = *manonmanī* = *amanaska*), 20, 63 (*manonmaṇi*), 46, 60, 79, 103, 105 (*unmanī*).

55 Cort, *Open Boundaries*; Qvarnström, *The Yogaśāstra of Hemacandra* (Introduction with references).

56 TAS II.1.

8

YOGA IN EARLY HINDU TANTRA

David Gordon White

In his masterful book, *Kāpālikas and Kālāmukhas*, David Lorenzen makes the following cogent point concerning the goals of yogic practice.[1]

> In spite of abundant textual references to various *siddhis* [supernatural powers] in classical yoga texts, many modern Indian scholars, and like-minded western ones as well, have seized on a single *sūtra* of Patañjali (3.37) to prove that magical powers were regarded as subsidiary, and even hindrances, to final liberation and consequently not worthy of concentrated pursuits. This attitude may have been operative in Vedāntic and Buddhist circles and is now popular among practitioners imbued with the spirit of the Hindu reformist movements, but it was not the view of Patañjali and certainly not the view of mediaeval exponents of *haṭhayoga*.

It suffices to cast a glance at the *Yoga Sūtra*[2] to see that the acquisition of *siddhis* was at the forefront of yogic theory and practice in the first centuries of the common era: nearly all of the fifty-five *sūtras* of book three of this work are devoted to the *siddhis*, and the "disclaimer" in verse 37 of this book – that "these powers are impediments to *samādhi*, but are acquisitions in a normal fluctuating state of mind" – seems only to apply, in fact, to the *siddhis* enumerated in the two preceding verses. This is a view shared by P. V. Kane.[3] One finds very little of yogic practice, in the sense of techniques involving fixed postures (*āsanas*) and breath control (*prāṇāyāma*), in the *Yoga Sūtra*. They are, of course, the third and fourth limbs of Patañjali's eight-limbed yoga (2.29); however, in the seven *sūtras* (2.46–52) he devotes to them, Patañjali gives absolutely no detail on these matters, save perhaps a veiled reference to diaphragmatic retention, which he terms *stambha-vṛtti* (2.50). References to the subtle body, the channels (*nāḍīs*) and energy centers (*cakras*), are entirely absent from this work; they are also absent from Vyāsa's fifth-century commentary (although Vyāsa does give an account of a limited number of *āsanas*). It would appear in fact that the *c.* sixth century BCE *Chāndogya Upaniṣad* (8.6.6) has already gone far beyond Patañjali and his commentators when it states that "There are a hundred and one channels of the heart. One of these passes up to the crown of the head. Going up by it, one goes to immortality. The others are for departing in various directions."

In this essay, I will trace the development of a number of elements specific to *haṭha yoga* such as emerged in a number of Hindu and Buddhist sources between the eighth and twelfth centuries CE. These sources are the eighth-century Buddhist *Hevajra Tantra* and the following Hindu sources: the eighth- to tenth-century *Bhāgavata Purāṇa* and *Tantrasadbhāva Tantra*; the ninth- to tenth-century *Kaulajñānanirṇaya*; the *c.* tenth-century *Kubjikāmata* and *Jayadrathayāmala*; the eleventh-century *Tantrāloka* of Abhinavagupta; the eleventh- to twelfth-century *Rudrayāmala Tantra*; and the twelfth-century *Śrīmattotara Tantra*. In my historical analysis, I will discuss (1) the emergence of the subtle body system of the *cakras*; (2) the projection of powerful feminine figures from the external world of Tantric ritual onto the grid of the subtle body; and (3) the role of these now internalized feminine energies, including that known as the *kuṇḍalinī*, in the male practitioner's attainment of *siddhis*.

One need not go back very far to find the principal source of the seemingly timeless system of the six plus one *cakras*: it is Arthur Avalon's edition and translation of a late text, the *Ṣaṭcakranirūpaṇa*, as an appendix to his seminal work, *The Serpent Power*.[4] Perhaps due to the power of the illustrations of this configuration in Avalon's work, many scholars have taken it to be an immutable, eternal system, as old as yoga itself, and grounded, perhaps, in the yogin's actual experience of the subtle body. A case in point is a recent work by Rahul Peter Das which, while it offers an encyclopedic account of subtle body systems in Bengal, is constantly plagued by the author's frustration in the face of the inconsistencies and contradictions between those systems.[5] In fact, there is no "standard" system of the *cakras*. Every school, sometimes every teacher within each school, has had their own *cakra* system. These have developed over time, and an "archaeology" of the various configurations is in order.

Cakras

The six plus one *cakra* system of Hindu *haṭha yoga* is one that we are so familiar with as to assume that it emerged, fully formed, like Athena out of the Zeus's forehead. This of course was not the case. The earliest discussions of the *cakras*, "circles" or "wheels" of subtle energy located within the human body, are to be found in such early Buddhist Tantric works as the *c.* eighth century CE *Caryāgīti* and the *Hevajra Tantra*,[6] which locate four *cakras* within the human body, at the levels of the navel, heart, throat and head. These *cakras* are identified with four geographical sites (*pīṭhas*), which appear to correspond to points of contact between the Indian subcontinent and inner Asia: these are Kāmākhyā (Gauhati, Assam); Uḍḍiyāna (Swat Valley); Pūrṇagiri (location unknown), and Jālandhara (Kashmir/Punjab). This tradition is known to Gorakṣanātha, who identifies the same set of four *pīṭhas* with sites aligned along the spinal column within the subtle body.[7] The *Hevajra Tantra*[8] also identifies these four centers with a rich array of scholastic tetradic categories, including Buddha bodies, seed-mantras, goddesses, truths, realities, schools etc.[9] Their locations in the subtle body appear to correspond as well to the mystic locations of the mind in its four states as described in the Hindu *Brahma Upaniṣad*, one of the Saṃnyāsa *Upaniṣads*, which states that while one is (1) in a waking state, the mind dwells in the navel; (2) during dreamless sleep, it dwells in the heart; (3) during dream sleep, it dwells in the throat; (4) when it is in the "fourth state" only attainable by the yogin, it resides in the head.[10] This so-called Upaniṣad, and the collection to which it belongs, as well as another collection known as the yoga *Upaniṣads* are, however, substantially later than this and other early Buddhist sources containing data on the four *pīṭhas* or *cakras*. Later sources locate ten, and still later fifty-one *pīṭhas* (identified with the Sanskrit phonemes) within the subtle body.[11]

The vertical configuration of *cakras* that we identify with the Hindu mapping of the subtle body emerges slowly, in the course of the latter half of the first millennium CE. One such early Hindu source is the eighth to tenth century CE *Bhāgavata Purāṇa*,[12] which states that:

> the sage should, having pressed his heel into the anus, indefatigably raise the breath into the six sites (*ṣaṭsu . . . sthāneṣu*). Drawing [the breath situated] in the (1) navel (*nābhī*) upward into the (2) heart (*hṛd*), he should then raise it along the path of the up-breath into the (3) breast (*uras*). Then, the wise one, conjoining [breath] with knowledge, brings it slowly to (4) the root of the palate (*svatālumūlam*). From there, he whose seven paths [i.e. the eyes, ears, nostrils and mouth] have been blocked [and] who is without distraction brings it to the (5) place between the eyebrows (*bhruvorantaram*). Remaining [in this state] for twenty-four minutes, he whose gaze is sharp, having pierced his (6) cranial vault (*mūrdhan*), will then surge upward into the beyond (*param*).

What is the source of this enumeration in the *Bhāgavata Purāṇa*? A glance at the early medical literature indicates that these sites correspond quite exactly to anatomical notions of the vital points ([*mahā-*] *marman*, pl. *marmāṇi*) or the supports of the vital breaths (*prāṇāyatana*). These are listed in the *c.* 100 CE *Caraka Saṃhitā* as follows: head (*mūrdhan*), throat (*kaṇṭha*), heart (*hṛdaya*), navel (*nābhī*), bladder (*basti*) and rectum (*guda*).[13] Certain later sources add the *fraenum*,[14] the membrane that attaches the tongue to the lower jaw, to this list: this would correspond to the root of the palate (*svatālumūlam*) listed in the *Bhāgavata Purāṇa*.

Śaiva Siddhānta sources, which are slightly earlier than the *Bhāgavata Purāṇa*, give a slightly different account of the centers. These most commonly list five centers, which they call either sites (*sthānas*), knots (*granthis*), supports (*ādhāras*) or lotuses – but almost never *cakras*. These are the heart (*hṛt*); throat (*kaṇṭha*); palate (*tālu*); the place between the eyebrows (*bhrūmadhya*), and the fontanelle (*brahmarandhra*). Quite often, the *dvādaśānta* (the "End of the Twelve," the site twelve finger-breadths above the fontanelle) will also be mentioned in these sources, but not as a member of this set. So, too, these sources will sometimes evoke the root support (*mūlādhāra*), often in tandem with the *brahmarandhra*, but to the exclusion of the intervening centers.[15] Another early source with a five-*cakra* system is the *Kubjikāmata*. This work, whose system comprises groups of *devīs*, *dūtīs*, *mātṛs*, *yoginīs* and *khecarī* deities aligned along the vertical axis of the yogic body, nearly never refers to these groupings as *cakras*. According to Dorothea Heilijger-Seelens, the meaning of the term *cakra* at the time of the *Kubjikāmata* (ninth to tenth century) was restricted to the groups of deities located in a mandala, which was their base or support.[16]

The first Hindu source to both list the locations found in the *Bhāgavata Purāṇa* and apply the term *cakra* to them, is the ninth- to tenth-century *Kaulajñānanirṇaya* of Matsyendranātha:

> The various spokes [of the wheels] of divine maidens (*divyakanyāra*) are worshipped by the assembled gods, in (1) the secret place (genitals), (2) navel, (3) heart, (4) throat, (5) mouth, (6) forehead, and (7) crown of the head. [These maidens] are arrayed along the spine (*pṛṣṭamadhye*) [up] to the trident (*tridaṇḍakam*) [located in] the fontanelle (*muṇḍasandhi*). These *cakras* are of eleven sorts and possessed of thousands [?of maidens], O Goddess! [They are] five-spoked (*pañcāram*) and eight-leaved (*aṣṭa-pattram*), ten and twelve-leaved, sixteen and one hundred-leaved, as well as one hundred thousand-leaved.[17]

This passage continues with a discussion of these divine maidens, through whom various *siddhis* are attained, each of whom is identified by the color of her garb (red, yellow, smoky, white etc.). So it is that we find in this source a juxtaposition of (1) the locations of the *cakras*; (2) the use of the term *cakra*; (3) a description of the *cakras* as being composed of spokes *and* leaves (but not petals); and (4) a portrayal of divine maidens as dwelling in or on the spokes of these *cakras*. The problematic remark in this passage, that the *cakras* are in some way elevenfold, or of eleven sorts, appears to be explicated in the seventeenth chapter of the same source, which names eleven sites, of which six correspond to the six places or *cakras* of earlier traditions:

> The (1) rectum, (2) secret place, along with the (3) navel [and] (4) the downturned lotus (*padma*) in the heart, (5) the *cakra* of breath and utterances (*samīrastobhakam*) [i.e. the throat], (6) the cooling knot (*granthi*) of the uvula, (7) the root (or tip) of the nose, and the (8) End of the Twelve,[18] the (9) [site] located between the eyebrows; (10) the forehead, and the brilliant (11) cleft of brahman, located at the crown of the head: it is the stated doctrine that [this] elevenfold [system] is located in the midst of the body (*dehamadhyataḥ*).[19]

In addition to using the term *cakra*, this passage also refers to the downturned *lotus* (and not wheel) in the heart, as well as to a knot (*granthi*) located at the level of the uvula.[20] Its enumeration of eleven centers, an obvious expansion on the seven *cakras* listed in *Kaulajñānanirṇaya* 5.25–27, is directly appropriated by the eleventh-century Abhinavagupta, who acknowledges his great debt to and respect for Matsyendranātha in the seventh verse of the opening chapter of his massive *Tantrāloka*. The subtle body system of the Trika Kaula, as set forth by Abhinavagupta, is a system of *cakras* depicted as spoked wheels which, while they are five in number (*mūlādhāra*, *nābhicakra*, *hṛdayacakra*, *kaṇṭhacakra*, *bhrumadhyacakra*), are supplemented by a number of other subtle body locations (*lalāṭa*; *tālu*; *triveṇibrahmarandhra* or *dvādaśānta*) which, when taken together, tally with the eleven centers found in the *Kaulajñānanirṇaya*. Abhinavagupta's system also features a trident (*triśula*), located at the level of the fontanelle, and the thousand-spoked End of the Twelve.[21] This preponderance of evidence indicates that the subtle body system of the Trika Kaula was strongly influenced by that of Matsyendranātha, the author of the *Kaulajñānanirṇaya* revered as the founder of the entire Kaula system, and father of the Kaula orders. However, we must note that whereas the *Kaulajñānanirṇaya* discusses these centers as wheels possessed of spokes or leaves, or as lotuses, the *cakras* of the Trika Kaula subtle body are whirling spoked wheels which, in the body of the non-practitioner, become inextricable tangles of coils called knots (*granthis*) because they knot together spirit and matter.[22]

Returning to the *Kaulajñānanirṇaya*, a third discussion of subtle body mapping occurs in this source under the heading of sites (*sthānas*). Here, it describes eleven of these in terms of their spokes, leaves, and petals (*dalas*): in order, they are the four-leaved, eight-spoked, twelve-spoked, five-spoked, sixteen-spoked, sixty-four-petaled, one hundred-leaved, one thousand-petaled, ten million-leaved, five million-leaved and thirty million-leaved.[23] It then goes on to discuss a number of other subtle sites (*vyāpaka*, *vyāpinī*, *unmana* etc.) identified with the upper cranial vault, that one encounters in such coeval Kaula sources as the *Svacchandabhairava Tantra* and *Netra Tantra*.[24]

A final *Kaulajñānanirṇaya* discussion of the workings of the subtle body will serve to orient us toward another early Tantric work containing an extended discussion of yoga, the *c.* tenth-century *Kubjikāmata*. Under the heading of the yogic "seals" (*mudrās*), the *Kaulajñānanirṇaya* (14.92a) states that "one should pierce that door whose bolts are well-fitted" (*bhedayettatkapāṭañ cārgalāyā-susañcitā*). Similar language is found in the *Kubjikāmata*. Here, the statement "applications of the bolts on the openings of the body,"[25] occurs at the beginning of this work's discussion of "upward progress" (*utkrānti*),[26] which appears to be a type of hathayogic practice. The *Kubjikāmata* passage continues: "The rectum, penis, and navel, mouth, nose, ears and eyes: having fitted bolts in these places (i.e. the nine 'doors' or bodily orifices), one should impel the crooked one upward (*kuñcika-urdhvam niyojayet*)."[27] There next follows a discussion of a number of yogic practices – including the Cock Posture (*kukuṭṭāsana*) – which effect the piercing of the knot[s], confer numerous *siddhis*, and afford firmness of the self.[28]

Bhairava, the divine revealer of this text, next states that he will provide a description of what he calls the "bolt practices" of the knife etc. (*kṣurikād-yargalābhyāsa*), which effect upward progress (*utkrānti-kāraṇam*) in him who is qualified to use it, and great affliction in the unqualified. Having entered into a terrifying forest, one uses one's blood to trace a fearsome diagram (*maṇḍala*), at whose six corners one situates fearsome goddesses. One is to worship these with *mantras*, and then place them within one's own body (*ātmānaṃ madhyato nyaset*). They are then to be worshipped with pieces of (one's own) flesh, and compelled to return that offering through an offering of blood. Then, having pierced one's eight body parts (hands, breast, forehead, eyes, throat and middle of the back), and mixed this blood and flesh together with urine, feces and some liquor, one should place the mixture in the offering bowl. Having offered one's own bodily constituents, one then worships these goddesses with food offerings, incense etc.[29]

Next, having conjoined knowledge to bodily constituent, one offers one hundred *japas* to these goddesses, who are named in the following order: Kusumamālinī ("She Who is Garlanded with Flowers"[30]), Yakṣiṇī, Śaṅkhinī, Kākinī, Lākinī, Rākiṇī and Ḍākinī. A shorter, variant list of these Yoginīs is found in two places in the *Kaulajñānanirṇaya*; chapter 4 of the *Kaulajñānanirṇaya*, which is on the subject of Tantric sorcery, appears to be a source for the later Kubjikā traditions.[31]

What these Yoginīs are offered is of signal interest here: the first of these, Kusumamālinī is urged to take or swallow (*gṛhṇa*) the practitioner's "principal constituent," i.e. semen; the second, Yakṣiṇī, to crush his bone(s); the third, Śaṅkhinī, to take his marrow; the fourth, Kākinī, to take his fat; the fifth, Lākinī, to eat his flesh; the sixth, Rākiṇī, to take his blood; and the seventh, Ḍākinī, to take his skin.[32] These Yoginīs are named in nearly identical order in the eighteenth chapter of the *Śrīmattottara Tantra*, a later text of the same Kubjikā tradition. Here, the names are, in order, Ḍākinī, Rākiṇī, Lākinī, Kākinī, Śākinī, Hākinī, Yākinī and Kusumā.[33] They are listed in the same order in *Agni Purāṇa* 144.28b–29a (this passage belongs to that portion of the AP comprised by material inserted from Kubjikā sources in the eleventh century CE). Here, moreover, their names are listed in a description of the construction of the six-cornered Kubjikā *maṇḍala*, with the enumeration proceeding from the northwest corner.[34]

According to the *Kubjikāmata*, the person who has so sacrificed his body then exhorts these goddesses: "Take now that which is given by me . . . Afflicted am I, drained of blood am I, broken in pieces am I . . . O ye goddesses, quickly take this, my own body, that has been given by me . . ." The passage then concludes: "When he whose body has been so drained of blood [performs this] daily, then the resplendent yoginīs come on the seventh day." Pleased, these confer supernatural knowledge (*jñānasiddhi*) on the practitioner; or, if the rites are turned against others, their destruction and death.[35]

Clearly, the bodily constituents these goddesses are urged to consume constitute a hierarchy. These are, in fact, the standard series of the seven *dhātus*, the "bodily constituents" of the Hindu medical tradition (with the sole exception being that skin has here replaced *chyle* [*rasa*]), which are serially burned in the fires of digestion, until semen, the "principal bodily constituent," is produced. With each goddess invoked in this passage, the practitioner is offering the products of a series of refining processes.

Recall here that the description of this ritual of self-sacrifice is presented as a special form of a "bolt practice" that "impels the crooked one upward." To all appearances, this is a rudimentary form of *haṭha yoga*. What is missing, however, is an identification of the goddesses to whom one's hierarchized bodily constituents are offered with subtle body locations inside the practitioner. This connection is made, however, in another *Kubjikāmata* passage, which locates six Yoginīs, called the "regents of the six fortresses," as follows: Ḍāmarī is located in the *ādhāra*, Rāmaṇī in the *svādhiṣṭhāna*, Lambakarṇī in the *maṇipura*, Kākī in the *anāhata*, Sākinī in the *viśuddhi* and Yakṣiṇī in the *ājñā*.[36] In another chapter, the *Kubjikāmata* lists two sequences of six goddesses as *kulākula* and *kula* respectively. The first denotes the "northern course" of the six *cakras*, from the *ājñā* down to the *ādhāra*, and the latter the "southern course," in reverse order. The former group is creative, and the latter – comprised of Ḍakinī, Rākiṇī, Lākinī, Kākinī, Sākinī, and Hākinī – is destructive.[37]

A number of later sources,[38] beginning with the *c.* twelfth-century *Rudrayāmala Tantra*, identify these goddesses, whom it calls Yoginīs, with both the *cakras* and their corresponding *dhātus*. The *Rudrayāmala Tantra's* ordering identifies these Yoginīs with the following subtle body locations: Ḍākinī is in the *mūlādhāra*; Rākiṇī in the *svādhiṣṭhāna*; Lākinī in the *maṇipura*; Kākinī in the *anāhata*; Śākinī in the *viśuddhi*; and Hākinī in the *ājñā*.[39] Kusumamālā, who is missing from this listing, is located in the feet in the *Śrīmattotara Tantra*;[40] other works place a figure named Yākinī at the level of the *sahasrāra*.[41]

These are, of course, the standard names of the *cakras* of hathayogic tradition. They are, in fact, first so called by name in the *Kubjikāmata*, which correlates the six standard yogic body locations with its Yoginīs of the "northern course." Mark Dyczkowski has argued that it is in the milieu of the Kubjikā Kaula that the six-*cakra* configuration was first developed into a fixed coherent system.[42] The *Kubjikāmata*, the root Tantra of the Kubjikā Kaula, locates the *cakras* and assigns each of them a number of "divisions" (*bhedas*) or "portions" (*kalās*) which approximates the number of "petals" assigned to these "lotuses" in later sources.[43]

We also encounter in the *Kubjikāmata* the notion of a process of yogic refinement or extraction of fluid bodily constituents, which is superimposed upon the vertical grid of the subtle body, along the spinal column, leading from the rectum to the cranial vault. Nonetheless, it would be incorrect to state that there is a hathayogic dynamic to the *Kubjikāmata's* system of the *cakras*. What appear to be lacking are the explicit application of the term *cakra* to these centers, the explicit identification of these centers with the elements,[44] and the deification or hypostasization of the principle or dynamic of this refinement process: here I am referring to that commonplace of hathayogic theory, the female *kuṇḍalinī* or serpent power – who has perhaps been evoked, albeit not by name, in the statement made in this source that one should, through *utkrānti*, "impel the crooked one upward" (*Kubjikāmata* 23.114a).

Kuṇḍalinī and the channeling of feminine energies

The *Kubjikāmata* makes a number of other statements that appear to betray its familiarity with a notion of this serpentine feminine nexus of yogic energy.[45] In *Kubjikāmata* 5.84, we read that "feminine energy (*śakti*) having the form of a sleeping serpent [is located] at the End of the Twelve . . . Nevertheless, she is also to be found dwelling in the navel . . ."[46] This serpentine (*bhuja*[*ṅ*]*ga-ākārā*) Śakti is connected in this passage to mantras and subtle levels of speech, through which she is reunited with Śiva. A later passage (*Kubjikāmata* 12.60–67) describes the sexual "churning" (*mathanam*) of an inner phallus (*liṅgam*) and vulva (*yoni*) that occurs in the *maṇipura cakra*, i.e. at the level of the navel. Here, however, the language is not phonematic, but rather fluid: the churning of Śiva and Śakti produces a flood of nectar. This is not, however, the earliest mention of this indwelling female serpent to be found in Hindu literature. This distinction likely falls to the *c.* eighth-century *Tantrasadbhāva Tantra*,[47] which similarly evokes her in a discussion of the phonematic energy that also uses the image of churning:

> This energy is called supreme, subtle, transcending all norm or practice . . . Enclosing within herself the fluid drop (*bindu*) of the heart, her aspect is that of a snake lying in deep sleep . . . she is awakened by the supreme sound whose nature is knowledge, being churned by the *bindu* resting in her womb . . . Awakened by this [luminous throbbing], the subtle force (*kalā*), Kuṇḍalī is aroused. The sovereign *bindu* [Śiva], who is in the womb of Śakti, is possessed of a fourfold force (*kalā*). By the union of the Churner and of She that is being churned this [*kuṇḍali*] becomes straight. This [Śakti], when she abides between the two *bindus*, is called Jyeṣṭhā . . . In the heart, she is said to be of one atom. In the throat she is of two atoms. She is known as being of three atoms when permanently abiding on the tip of the tongue . . .

In this passage, we may be in the presence of the earliest mention of a coiled "serpent energy"; however, the term that is used here is *kuṇḍalī*, which simply means "she who is ring-shaped."[48] This is also the term that one encounters in the *Kaulajñānanirṇaya*, which evokes the following goddesses in succession as the Mothers (*mātṛkās*) who are identified with the "mass of sound" (*śabdarāśi*), located in "all of the knots" (*sarva-granthesu*) of the subtle body: Vāmā, Kuṇḍalī, Jyeṣṭhā, Manonmanī, Rudra-śakti, Kāmākhyā and Ugraṇī.[49] The same source describes the goddess named Vāmā as having a circular or serpentine form (*kuṇḍalākṛti*) and extending from the feet to the crown of the head: the raising of this goddess from the rectum culminates with her absorption at the End of the Twelve.[50] Once again, the imagery of the *kuṇḍalinī* serpent appears to be present in everything but exact name.

Perhaps the earliest occurrence of the term *kuṇḍalinī* (as opposed to *kuṇḍalī*) is found in the third hexad (*ṣaṭka*) of the *c.* tenth-century *Jayadrathayāmala* which, in a discussion of the origin of mantras, relates the *kuṇḍalinī* to phonemes as well as to the *kalās*:

> Māyā is the mother of the phonemes and is known as the fire-stick of the mantras. She is the *kuṇḍalinī* Śakti, and is to be

known as the supreme *kalā*. From that spring forth the mantras as well as the separate clans, and likewise the Tantras . . .[51]

Before continuing, I wish to dwell for a moment on the names of the Mother goddesses evoked in *Kaulajñānanirṇaya*. In Śaiva Siddhānta metaphysics, the Goddess Jyeṣṭhādevī, mentioned in the *Kaulajñānanirṇaya* and *Tantrasadbhāva* passages cited above, is described as assuming eight forms, by which she represents the eight *tattvas*: these are Vāmā (earth), Jyeṣṭhā herself (water), Raudrī (fire), Kālī (air), Kalavikaraṇī (ether), Balavikaraṇī (moon), Balapramathanī (sun) and Manonmanī (Śiva-hood). This group of eight are said to be the *śaktis* of the eight male Vidyeśvaras, of the Śaivasiddhānta system, the deifications of the eight categories of being that separate the "pure" worlds from the "impure."[52] With this enumeration, we can safely say that Matsyendranātha's source is an earlier Saiddhāntika work.[53] In addition, we see once more a hierarchization of internalized goddesses, identified here with the five elements (and a number of their subtler evolutes), a hierarchization identified with the ordering of phonemes (*śabdarāśi*) within the subtle body. That these are projected upon the grid of the subtle body is made clear by the fact that they are said to be located "in all the knots." Finally, this list of deities from the Saiddhāntika system is complemented by the Mother named Kuṇḍalī whom the *Kaulajñānanirṇaya* locates between Jyeṣṭha (earth) and Vāmā (water). It is a commonplace of later subtle body mapping to identify the five lower *cakras* with the five elements: Kuṇḍalī would thus be located, according to this schema, between the rectal *mūlādhāra* (earth) and the genital *svādhiṣṭhāna* (water). All of the foregoing discussion, of the correlations between goddesses, *cakras*, vital constituents, and subtle body locations, are presented in table 8.1, found on p. 156 at the end of this chapter.

Both the *Kaulajñānanirṇaya* account of the raising of the *kuṇḍalākṛti* Goddess Vāmā from the level of the rectum to the *dvādaśānta*, and the statement, in *Kubjikāmata* 5.84, to the effect that *śakti* dwells in the form of a sleeping serpent in both the cranial vault and the navel, are precursors of the dynamic role the *kuṇḍalinī* would play in later hathayogic sources. Abhinavagupta, who clearly took his inspiration from both of these sources, develops this principle in his discussion of the upper and lower *kuṇḍalinīs*, which are for him two phases of the same energy, in expansion and contraction, which effects both the descent of transcendent consciousness into the human microcosm, and the return of human consciousness toward its transcendent source. In spite of the highly evocative sexual language he employs, Abhinavagupta's model is nonetheless one of phonematic, rather than fluid expansion and contraction.[54] It is in the *Rudrayāmala Tantra* and the later hathayogic classics attributed to Gorakṣanātha that the *kuṇḍalinī* becomes the vehicle for fluid, rather than phonematic, transactions and transfers.

This role of the *kuṇḍalinī* in the dynamics of subtle body fluid transfer is brought to the fore in a portion of the Tantric practice of the five anti-sacraments, the *pañcamakāra* (literally, "M-words"), which Agehananda Bharati describes in the following manner:

> When the practitioner is poised to drink the liquor (*madya*, the third "M"), he says "I sacrifice"; and as he does so, he mentally draws the coiled energy of the Clan (*kula-kuṇḍalinī*) from her seat in the base *cakra*. This time, however, he does not draw her up into the thousand-petaled *sahasrāra* in the cranial vault, but instead he brings her to the tip of his tongue and seats her there. At this moment he drinks the beverage from its bowl, and as he drinks she impresses the thought on his mind that it is not he himself who is drinking, but the *kula-kuṇḍalinī* now seated on the tip of his tongue, to whom he is offering the liquid as a libation. In the same manner he now empties all the other bowls [containing food offerings, including sexual fluids] as he visualizes that he feeds their contents as oblations to the Goddess – for the *kula-kuṇḍalinī* is the microcosmic aspect of the universal Śakti.[55]

Here, the *kuṇḍalinī* at the tip of the practitioner's tongue is not spitting phonemes, as in the *Tantrasadbhāva Tantra* passage quoted above, but rather drinking ritual fluids, which are so many substitutes for, or actual instantiations of, vital bodily fluids.

I am at a loss to explain why it is that the feminine principle of yogic energy comes to be represented as a serpent, now coiled, and now straightened. Of course, there seems to be some sort of elective affinity between the *kuṇḍalinī's* function and form – however, the avian *haṃsa*, which doubles for the *kuṇḍalinī* in a number of sources, appears to fulfill the same function, of raising energy from the lower to the upper body. Lillian Silburn suggests that it is the serpent's coiling and straightening that would explain its projection onto the subtle body: a venomous serpent, when coiled, is dangerous; straightened, it is no longer dangerous. This would be of a piece with the characterization of the *kuṇḍalinī* as "poison" when she lies coiled in the lower body and "nectar" when she is extended upward into the cranial vault. Or, Silburn suggests, the image of the *kuṇḍalinī* is one that borrows from the Vedic serpents Ahir Budhnya and Aja Ekapād, or the Puranic Śeṣa/Ananta. I am more inclined to see the *kuṇḍalinī's* origins in the role of the serpent in Indian iconography. Temples and other buildings are symbolically supported by a serpent that coils around their foundations: a certain number of Hindu temples in Indonesia reproduce this image architecturally. Similarly, images of the Buddha and later of Kṛṣṇa are figured with a serpent support and canopy. Finally, the phallic emblem of Śiva, the *liṅgam*, is often figured with a coiled serpent around its base, whose spread hood serves as its canopy. This is a particularly evocative image when one recalls that the *kuṇḍalinī* is figured, in the classical hathayogic sources, as sleeping coiled three and a half times around an internal *liṅgam*, with her hood or mouth covering its top. When the yogin awakens her through his practice of postures and breath control, she pierces the lower door to the medial *suṣumṇā* channel, and "flies" upward to the place of Śiva in the cranial vault.

The Yoginīs in the subtle body

It is this image of the *kuṇḍalinī* as flying upward through the six *cakras*, to union with Śiva in the cranial vault, that points to what I believe to have been the origin of this staple of subtle body imagery. The *kuṇḍalinī*, a goddess into whose mouth one offers oblations of wine and vital fluids, who flies upward when satisfied by the same, has her prototype in the Yoginīs or Ḍākinīs of early Kaula tradition. Out of the multitude of descriptions of these powerful feminine figures, two salient features emerge: they love to eat human flesh and drink human vital fluids; and they fly through the air. The two are intimately connected, as a passage from the eighth-century *Mālatī-Mādhava* of Bhavabhūti makes abundantly clear:[56]

> Beholding by the power of resorption the eternal universal soul in the form of Siva – who, superimposed upon the circles (*cakras*) of my six body parts, manifests himself in the midst of the heart lotus – here I have now come without experiencing any fatigue from my flight by virtue of my extraction of the five nectars of people, [which I have effected] by the gradual filling of the channels.

Commenting on this verse, Jagaddhara states that this female figure's power of flight is acquired through her extraction (*ākāśagāmitva-utkarṣā-pratipādanāt*) of the five constituent elements of the human body (*śarirasya pañcabhūtātmakasya*). The female figure in question is Kapālakuṇḍalā ("She Who has Skulls for Earrings"), the consort, the Yoginī, of a Kāpālika named Aghoraghaṇṭa ("Hell's Bells"); and in this scene, she is flying to a cremation ground. Thus we are in the presence of a commonplace of medieval Indian literature, which locates Kaula practitioners and Yoginīs together in cremation grounds. In the case of the latter, they are always there to consume human flesh, a role that extends as far back as literature on multiple goddesses takes us.[57] These hosts of female figures live on, delight in, and are energized by the consumption of human flesh; and it is through their *extraction of the essence* of the bodies they eat that they are afforded the power of flight. Yoginīs or Ḍākinīs *need* human flesh in order to fly. To those who offer human flesh (their own or someone else's), they offer their form of grace, i.e. *siddhis*, of which the power of flight figures prominently.

For the unfortunate non-initiate, becoming "food for the Yoginīs" was the end: he was toast. The Yoginīs would descend upon him, and drain him of his blood, flesh, fat, bone, marrow, and seed, extracting his essence and leaving behind an empty husk. However, for the Kaula *yogin*, the male counterpart to the Yoginī (also called the Vīra, the virile consort of the Yoginī; or Siddha, the perfected partner of the Yoginī), one could have it both ways. That is, one could offer one's vital fluids, extracted from them by the Yoginī through sexual intercourse, and yet survive and, more than this, revel together with this consort in magical flight. This was effected through the numerous Kaula techniques for the intermingling (*melaka*) and shared enjoyment (*bhoga*) of sexual fluids. It could be effected through *vajrolī mudrā*, in which the male partner extracted his own essence back from the Yoginī through urethral suction; or through the drinking of the mingled sexual fluids of himself and the Yoginī. In both cases, the male partner gained what he was lacking (the "clan nectar," the fluid of gnosis naturally present in the Yoginī), while the female partner gained raw materials necessary for her refinement of the high performance fuel that powered her flight.

As the *Mālatī-Mādhava* passage and Jagaddhara's commentary make clear, the Yoginī's flight was fueled by her "extraction of the essence" of the five nectars (human semen, blood, urine, excrement and marrow)[58] or five elements (earth, water, air, fire, ether) of the human body. This is precisely the role played by the *kuṇḍalinī* in the subtle body of hathayogic practice. As she rises or flies upward along the medial channel, she implodes earth into water at the level of the *svādhiṣṭhāna* (genitals), water into fire at the *maṇipura* (navel), fire into air at the *anāhata* (heart), and air into the ether through which she flies at the *viśuddhi* (throat). The *cakras* that she pierces in this process of extraction or refinement are characterized as cremation grounds in a number of hathayogic sources; this is the locus of the Yoginīs' anthropophagy in the outside world.[59]

The body of evidence provided by this eighth-century source is a clear indication that the system of fluid transactions that formed the core of "tantric sex," of which *haṭha yoga* was an internalization, were originally grounded in the cremation ground-based anthropophagy of the Yoginīs or Ḍākinīs. It is this as well that is represented in the elaborate erotic sculptures found on the walls of Hindu temples from the Kaula period. Finally, it is this that accounts for the unique architectural plan of the Yoginī temples, which date from the same eighth- to tenth-century period and are found in the same Vindhya-mountain regions of central and eastern India as those in which the Kaula flourished. The Yoginī temples are circular and roofless, open to the sky. On the inner walls of these temples are figured voluptuous and terrible images of the (usually) sixty-four Yoginīs (often figured with severed human appendages in their hands or mouths), while an ithyphallic image of Bhairava stands at the center of the edifice.[60]

This configuration perfectly reproduces the schema of Yoginī *maṇḍalas*, in which the sixty-four Yoginīs, arrayed in eight clans, converge on their divine regent Bhairava, who is located at the heart of the diagram. It is also entirely functional *vis-à-vis* the purpose of the Kaula practice: initiation into the flow chart of the clan lineage, and mutual gratification and the *shared* power of flight enjoyed by Siddha and Yoginī alike. The circular Yoginī temples, open to sky, were landing fields and launching pads for Yoginīs and their male consorts. These circles of Yoginīs became internalized into the *cakras* of hathayogic practice, while their cultic practices – in which love and death become intimately intertwined through their extraction of the essence of their male lovers/victims – were internalized into the raising of the *kuṇḍalinī*.

Table 8.1 Six *cakras* in early Hindu sources (ninth to twelfth century CE)

Element	*Name of Jyeṣṭhā or Mother Goddess*	*Location*	*Dhātu*	*Yoginī associated with dhātu*	*Yoginī associated with cakra*	*"Standard" cakra*	*Number of petals*
Text	*KJñN*[61] *Śaivasiddhānta sources*[67]	*BhagP*[62] *KJñN*[68]	*KM*[63]	*KM*[64]	*RYT*[65]	*KM*[66]	
[ātman]	Manonmanī	cranial vault	semen	Kusumamālinī		[sahasrāra]	1,000
[sun]	[Balapramathanī]						
[moon]	[Balavikaraṇī]	eyebrows	marrow	Śaṅkhinī	Hākinī	ājñā	2
ether	[Kalavikaraṇī]	throat	bone	Yakṣinī	Śākinī	viśuddhi	16
air	Kālī	heart	fat	Kākinī	Kākinī	anāhata	12
fire	Raudrī	navel	flesh	Lākinī	Lākinī	maṇipura	8
water	Jyeṣṭhā Kuṇḍalī	genitals	blood	Rākiṇī	Rākiṇī	svādhiṣṭhāna Kuṇḍalī	6
earth	Vāmā	rectum	skin/*rasa*	Ḍākinī	Ḍākinī	mūlādhāra	4

Notes

1 David Lorenzen, *Kāpālikas and Kālāmukhas: Two Lost Śaivite Sects*, New Delhi, Thomson Press, 1972, pp. 93–94.

2 *Yoga Philosophy of Patañjali containing his Yoga aphorisms with commentary of Vyāsa* by Swami Hariharananda Aranya, rendered into English by P. N. Mukherji, Calcutta, University of Calcutta, 1981.

3 Lorenzen, *Kāpālikas*, citing Arthur Koestler, *The Lotus and the Robot*, London, Hutchinson, 1960, pp. 110–111. A similar situation may be found in early Buddhism, in which admonitions in the Vinaya Piṭaka against magical powers may be contrasted with statements to the effect that "a magical feat quickly converts an ordinary person": John S. Strong, *The Legend of King Aśoka: A Study and Translation of the Aśokavadāna*, Princeton, Princeton University Press, 1983, p. 75.

4 The *Ṣaṭcakranirūpaṇa* is included as an appendix to Sir John Woodroffe, *The Serpent Power*, Madras, Ganesh, 1973.

5 Rahul Peter Das, "Problematic Aspects of the Sexual Rituals of the Bauls of Bengal," *Journal of the American Oriental Society*, 1992, vol. 112, pp. 388–422.

6 *Hevajra Tantra* 2.4.51–55, in David L. Snellgrove, *The Hevajra Tantra, a Critical Study*, London, Oxford University Press, 1959, 2 vols, vol. 2, Sanskrit and Tibetan Texts, p. 68.

7 *Siddha Siddhānta Paddhati* 2.1c, 2b, 8b, 9c, in *Siddha Siddhānta Paddhati and Other Works of the Natha Yogis*, edited with an introduction by Kalyani Mallik, Poona, Oriental Book House, 1954. It is also known to Matsyendra, who in his *Kaulajñānanirṇaya* (8.20–22) substitutes Arbuda (Mount Abu) for Pūrṇagiri: *Kaulajñānanirṇaya and some Minor Texts of the School of Matysyendranātha*, ed. by Prabodh Chandra Bagchi, Calcutta Sanskrit Series, no. 3, Calcutta, Metropolitan, 1934.

8 *Hevajra Tantra* 1.7.12. A similar list is found in the coeval Buddhist *Sādhanamālā*, *Sādhanamālā*, ed. by Benoytosh Bhattacharya, Gaekwad's Oriental Series nos 26, 41, Baroda, Oriental Institute, 1925, 1928, 2 vols, vol. 2, pp. 453, 455, and the Hindu *Kālikā Purāṇa* (64.43–45): on these sources see D. C. Sircar, *The Śākta Pīṭhas*, Second revised edn, Delhi, Motilal Banarsidass, 1972, pp. 11–14.

9 *Hevajra Tantra* 1.1.22–30, discussed in David Snellgrove, *Indo-Tibetan Buddhism: Indian Buddhists and their Tibetan Successors*, Boston, Shambhala, 1987, vol. 1, p. 248. The *c.* tenth-century Hindu *Kubjikāmata* locates these four *pīṭhas* in the *viśuddhi cakra*: *Kubjikāmata* 11.50, 60 etc., in Teun Goudriaan and J. A. Schoterman, eds, *The Kubjikāmatatantra, Kulālikāmnāya Version, Critical Edition*, Leiden, Brill, 1988.

10 *Brahma Upaniṣad* 2. 82–83, in Patrick Olivelle, *Saṃnyāsa Upaniṣads: Hindu Scriptures on Asceticism and Renunciation*, New York, Oxford University Press, 1992, p. 149. So too, the *Malinīvijayottara Tantra* (11.35) describes four centers: *mūlādhāra* (anus), *kanda* (above the genitals), palate, and *dvādaśānta* ("End of the Twelve": see below, text to note 15) with their respective effects on the practitioner: André Padoux, "Transe, Possession ou Absorption Mystique?" in *La possession en Asie du Sud (Purusartha 21)*, ed. Jacky Assayag and Gilles Tarabout, Paris, Editions EHESS, 1999, p. 139.

11 For a discussion, see Sircar, *Śākta Pīṭhas*, pp. 17–18, and Pratapaditya Pal, *Hindu Religion and Iconology According to the Tantrasāra*, Los Angeles, Vichitra Press, 1981, pp. 24–29.

12 *Bhāgavata Purāṇa* 2.2.19b–21b, *Bhāgavata Purāṇa*, ed. and trans. by C. L. Goswami, Gorakhpur, Gita Press, 1971. It has been dated to the eighth century by Dennis Hudson, "The Śrīmad Bhāgavata Purāṇa in Stone: The Text as an Eighth-Century Temple and its Implications," *Journal of Vaisnava Studies*, 1995, vol. 3, pp. 137–138, 177.

13 *Caraka Saṃhitā* 4.7.9, cited in Arion Roșu, "Les *marman* et les arts martiaux indiens," *Journal Asiatique*, 1982, vol. 264, p. 418. Over time, the number of vital points or organs rises to 107: ibid., pp. 419–426.

14 *Rasanabandha*, listed in the *Aṣṭāṅgahṛdaya* and *Aṣṭāṅgasaṃgraha* of Vāgbhaṭa, *Viṣṇudharma*, and other sources: Roșu, "*Marman*," p. 418.
15 Helène Brunner, "The Place of Yoga in the Śaivāgamas," in Jean Filliozat, S. P. Narang, C. P. Bhatta, eds, *Pandit N. R. Bhatt Felicitation Volume*, Delhi, Motilal Banarsidass, 1994, pp. 436–438.
16 Dorothea Heilijger-Seelens, *The System of the Five Cakras in Kubjikāmatatantra 14–16*, Groningen, Egbert Forsten, 1994, pp. 34–35, 38.
17 *Kaulajñānanirṇaya* 5.25–27.
18 This mention of the *dvādaśānta* appears to be out of place, unless some other subtle center, within the contours of the body, is intended.
19 *Kaulajñānanirṇaya* 17.2b–4b.
20 In this, it mirrors Śaiva Siddhānta terminology to a certain extent: only the heart is termed a lotus, with the other centers generally termed *granthis*: Brunner, "Place of Yoga," p. 438.
21 Discussed in Lillian Silburn, *Kuṇḍalinī, Energy of the Depths*, trans. by Jacques Gontier, Albany, NY, SUNY Press, 1988, pp. 27–35.
22 Ibid., pp. 25–26.
23 *Kaulajñānanirṇaya* 3.6a–8a.
24 *Kaulajñānanirṇaya* 3.9–12. See André Padoux's discussion of *Svacchanda Tantra* 4 and *Netra Tantra* 22 in his *Vāc: The Concept of the Word in Selected Hindu Tantras*, trans. by Jacques Gontier, Albany, NY, SUNY Press, 1990, pp. 404–411. The *Svacchanda Tantra* has been published as *The Svacchanda Tantram with Commentary – "Udyota" by Kshema Raja*, ed. by Vraj Vallabh Dwivedi, Delhi, Parimal Publications, 1985, 2 vols.
25 *Kubjikāmata* 23.112b: *dvāreṣu argalasaṃyogam kuryāc codghāṭanaṃ*. An excellent discussion of many elements of subtle body system of the *Kubjikāmata*, together with a fine translation of chapters 14 through 16 of the text is Heilijgers-Seelens, *System of the Five Cakras*.
26 Teun Goudriaan, "Some Beliefs and Rituals Concerning Time and Death in the Kubjikāmata," *Selected Studies on Ritual in the Indian Religions. Essays to D. J. Hoens*, ed. by Ria Kloppenborg, Leiden, Brill, 1983, pp. 96–98, defines *utkrānti* as follows: "the method by which a *yogin* may choose to take leave of mundane existence."
27 *Kubjikāmata* 23.113b–114a.
28 *Kubjikāmata* 23.115–125.
29 *Kubjikāmata* 23.126–140.
30 Heilijger-Seelens, *System of Five Cakras*, p. 124, n. 14, opines that her name "seems to express the idea of the *ātman* being represented by a flower," citing the use of flowers in Balinese ritual. See also Gaya Charan Tripathi, "The Daily Puja Ceremony," in Anncharlott Eschmann *et al.*, eds, *The Cult of Jagannāth and the Regional Tradition of Orissa*, New Delhi, Manohar, 1978, pp. 297, 301, on Tantric uses of the same.
31 In the mantra following 4.15, the *Kaulajñānanirṇaya* names Kusumālinī, Ḍākinī, Rākṣasī, Lākinī and Yoginī; the mantra following *Kaulajñānanirṇaya* 9.5 lists Lākinī Ḍākinī, Śākinī, Kākinī and Yākinī.
32 *Kubjikāmata* 23.140. Their names correspond closely to those goddesses whose *bījas* were given at the beginning of this passage. The language with which these goddesses are invoked is quite similar to that addressed to disease-causing Mothers in *Agni Purāṇa* 299.50, quoted in Jean Filliozat, *Le Kumāratantra de Rāvaṇa et les textes parallèles indiens tibétains, chinois, cambodgien et arabe*, Cahiers de la Société Asiatique, 1è série, vol. 4, Paris, Imprimerie Nationale, 1937, p. 70.

33 *Śrīmattotara Tantra* 18.8–57, discussed in Heilijger-Seelens, *System of Five Cakras*, p. 147.
34 Marie-Thérèse de Mallmann, *Enseignements iconographiques de l'Agni-Purana*, Paris, Presses Universitaires de France, 1963, pp. 205–206.
35 *Kubjikāmata* 23.141–146.
36 *Kubjikāmata* 15.49b–54a, cited in Heilijger-Seelens, *System of Five Cakras*, pp. 137–138. These *cakras* are also described, independent of any identification with these Yoginīs, in earlier *Kubjikāmata* chapters. The *viśuddhi* is discussed in *Kubjikāmata* 11.44–99a; the *anāhata* in 11.99b–12.29; the *maṇipura* in 12.30–69; the *svādhiṣṭhāna* in 12.70 to 13.36; the *ādhāra* in 13.37–52; and the *ājñā* in 13.53–86.
37 *Kubjikāmata* 14.3–4, discussed in Heilijger-Seelens, *System of Five Cakras*, p. 146.
38 These include the *Vidyārṇava Tantra*, *Saundaryalaharī*, *Śrīmattotara Tantra* and *Lalitā Sahasranāma*: Vidya Dehejia, *Yoginī Cult and Temples: A Tantric Tradition*, New Delhi, National Museum, 1986, pp. 48–49.
39 *Rudrayamala Tantra* 27.54b–56b, *Rudrayāmalam*, ed. by Yogatantra Department, Benares, Sampurnanand Sanskrit Vishavavidyalaya, 1980. The identification is made by juxtaposition; in addition, six forms of Śiva are also listed.
40 *Śrīmattotara Tantra*, chapters 19 and 27, cited in Dehejia, *Yoginī Cult*, pp. 48–49.
41 Some of these works further identify these Yoginis with the *dhātus* they are offered in the *Kubjikāmata*; however, these same works alter their hierarchical arrangement along the vertical axis of the subtle body. The *Vidyārṇava Tantra*, *Saundaryalaharī*, and *Lalitā Sahasranāma* place Sākinī (bone) in the *mūlādhāra*; Kākinī (fat) in the *svādhiṣṭhāna*; Lākinī (flesh) in the *maṇipura*; Rākiṇī (blood) in the *anāhata*; Ḍākinī (skin) in the *viśuddhi*; Hākinī (marrow) in the *ājñā*; and Yākinī (semen) in the *sahasrāra*: Dehejia, *Yoginī Cult*, pp. 48–49.
42 Mark S. G. Dyczkowski, "Kubjikā the Erotic Goddess. Sexual Potency, Transformation and Reversal in the Heterodox Theophanies of the *Kubjikā Tantras*," *Indologica Taurinensia*, 1995–1996, vols 21–22, p. 139.
43 *Kubjikāmata* 11.34b–37b. This source calls the *mūlādhāra* "gudam." It assigns four "portions" ("petals" in later literature) to it; six to the *svādhiṣṭhāna*; twelve to the *maṇipura*; ten to the *anāhata*; sixteen to the *viśuddhi*; and two to the *ājñā*.
44 Heilijger-Seelens, *System of Five Cakras*, p. 38.
45 This source actually uses the term *kuṇḍalinī*, but in no case does it have the hathayogic sense of female serpent energy. It is rather employed to signify a *japa-mālā* thread (5.118); as a synonym for Śakti (6.4); and as a synonym for the *yoni* (6.108). It is used in a mantra (following 18.43); at the end of the description of the highest path of practice, the *śāmbhava-adhvan* (in 18.111); and in a discussion of visions leading to the power of prognostication (19.76).
46 *śakti prasupta-bhujaga-ākārā dvādaśānte varānane / nābhiṣṭhā tu tathāpy evaṃ draṣṭavyā parameśvari //.*
47 Dated by Alexis Sanderson, "Trika Śaivism," in *Encyclopedia of Religion*, ed. by Mircea Eliade, New York, Macmillan, 1986, vol. 13, p. 14. This passage is quoted by both Kṣemarāja in his *Śiva Sūtra Vimarṣinī* (2.3) and Jayaratha in his commentary on TĀ 3.67, vol. 2, p. 429. It is translated in Padoux, *Vāc*, pp. 128–130.
48 The same terminology is found in Śaiva Siddhānta sources: Brunner, "Place of Yoga," p. 438.
49 *Kaulajñānanirṇaya* 20.11a–12b. Jyeṣṭhā is named in the same context in the *Tantrasadbhāva Tantra* passage cited in the previous footnote.

50 *Kaulajñānanirṇaya* 17.23: *āpādatalamūrddhāntā vāmākhy[a] kuṇḍalākṛtim / gudasthamudayantasyā dvādaśānte layam punaḥ*. Here Kuṇḍalī is not a distinct goddess, but simply a quality of Vāmā.

51 *Jayadrathayāmala*, third hexad (NNA MSS no. 5.1975, Śaiva Tantra 429, Reel A 152/9, fol. 169b).

52 This group of eight is found in the Purāṇas, Tara Michael, *La Légende immémoriale du dieu Shiva, Le Shiva-purāṇa,* Paris, Gallimard, 1991, p. 157, note 3; Mallmann, *Enseignements*, pp. 55 and 57, citing *Agni Purāṇa* 74 and 308, and *Garuḍa Purāṇa* 23; as well as Śaivasiddhānta works (*Īśānagurudevapaddhati* 3.5.12–14 and *Tantrasamuccaya* 7.46). Cf. T. A. Gopinath Rao, *Elements of Hindu Iconography*, vol. 1, part 2, pp. 398–400, citing the *Siddhāntasārāvali* of Trilocana Śivācārya.

53 The same sequence figures in Śaivasiddhānta soteriology. "A wife ascends [the hierarchy of the ancestors] in step with her husband. She is a Rudrāṇī (wife of Rudra) until incorporation (*sapiṇḍikaraṇam*). Then she becomes first a Balavikaraṇī, then a Balapramathanī, and finally a Bhūtadamanī. These three are the highest of the eight goddesses that surround the goddess Manonmanī on the thirty-second cosmic level (*śuddhavidyātattvam*), the first of those which make up the pure (i.e. liberated) segment of the universe (*śudhādhvā*)": Alexis Sanderson, "Meaning in Tantric Ritual," p. 35, citing *Īśānaśivagurudevapaddhati* (*Siddhāntasāra*), Kriyapada 17.217c–19b; and *Svacchandatantra* 10.1142c–1146b. Cf. Brunner, "Place of Yoga," p. 453, on the subtle body as *puryaṣṭaka*.

54 Silburn, *Kuṇḍalinī*, pp. 15–83, passim.

55 Agehananda Bharati, *The Tantric Tradition*, New York, Samuel Weiser, 1975, p. 260.

56 *Mālatī-Mādhava* Act 5, verse 2, in M. R. Kale, ed. and trans., *Bhavabhūti's Mālatī-Mādhava with the Commentary of Jagaddhara*, reprint of third edn, Delhi, Motilal Banarsidass, 1983, pp. 95–96.

57 Among the hundreds of references to this found in the Kaula literature, the *Kaulajñānanirṇaya* (11.18) states: "By whatever means, one should always devour [the victim one is] attracting (*ākṛṣṭim*), one should honor the horde of *yoginīs* with food and [sexual] pleasure."

58 *Kaulajñānanirṇaya* 11.11. Certain Buddhist Tantras list brains and flesh in place of urine and feces.

59 *Haṭhayogapradīpika* 3.4. Nepali images of the "Eight *Śmaśānas*" (at which a Yoginī, a Bhairava, and a Siddha are located) situate these in the heart *cakra*: P. H. Pott, *Yoga and Yantra: Their Interrelation and their Significance for Indian Archaeology*, The Hague, Nijhoff, 1966, p. 84. This is in conformity with *Svacchanda Tantra* 2.175–180, with Kṣemarāja's commentary.

60 Dehejia, *Yoginī Cult*, p. 63.

61 *Kaulajñānanirṇaya* 20.11a–12b.

62 *Bhāgavata Purāṇa* 2.2.19b–21b.

63 In the unnumbered mantras following *Kubjikāmata* 23.140a. Alternate listings of these six (or seven) Yoginis are found elsewhere in the text: one of these (*Kubjikāmata* 10.138–40) is identical to that found in the *Rudrayāmala Tantra*: see below, note 65.

64 Ibid. However, the identification between the "standard" six cakras and Yoginīs uses an alternate list, found in *Kubjikāmata* 15.49b–54a. See above, notes 36 and 37.

65 *Rudrayāmala Tantra* 27.54b–56b. The same ordering is found in *Agni Purāṇa* 144.28b–29a, cited in Mallmann, *Enseignements*, pp. 205–206. In the Lālitā

Māhātmya of the *Brahmāṇḍa Purāṇa* (20.15–18), the order is: Yakṣinī, Śaṅkhinī, Lākinī, Hākinī, Śākinī, Dākinī and Hākinī a second time.

66 *Kubjikāmata* 11.44–13.86. This "standard listing" is also found in numerous later sources, including the *Rudrayāmala Tantra* (cited in Dehejia, *Yoginī*, p. 45).

67 Rao, *Elements of Hindu Iconography*, vol. 1, pp. 398–400; *Svacchandatantra* 2.68a–70b; 10.1145a–1146b; *Soma-śambhu-paddhati*, ed. Helène Brunner-Lachaux, Institut Français d'Indologie, no. 25, pts. 1–4 (Pondicherry: 1963, 1968, 1977, 1998), vol. 1, p. 170.

68 *Kaulajñānanirṇaya* 5.25–27.

9

METAPHORIC WORLDS AND YOGA IN THE VAIṢṆAVA SAHAJIYĀ TANTRIC TRADITIONS OF MEDIEVAL BENGAL

Glen Alexander Hayes

Introduction[1]

One of the most interesting areas of inquiry for the historian of South Asian religions concerns the many ways in which yoga – understood in both its classical and later forms of development – has been adopted and adapted by diverse Tantric traditions.[2] The issues of embodiment, freedom, and the nature of the material world are central to both traditions, although Tantrics have typically approached these issues in their own way, and have often used psychosexual ritual practices not found in classical yoga. But it seems clear that problems related to the "body" (physical, yogic, and other) and the material world are of primary importance to many (if not most) of the Yogic and Tantric traditions that we study. This short essay will deal not only with "the what" of my research into Tantric yoga (the description and presentation of Tantric texts, traditions, and personalities) but especially with "the so what?" (articulating the basic issues raised by our studies, connecting them to other areas of inquiry, and suggesting new methodologies for the study of yoga and tantra). I will suggest some new ways of analyzing and understanding the problems of embodiment and the material world in some branches of the Vaiṣṇava Sahajiyā Tantric traditions of medieval Bengal (which flourished during the sixteenth through nineteenth centuries). This methodology has helped me to understand some medieval interpretations of yoga, as well as the structures and processes underlying Vaiṣṇava Sahajiyā ideas of body, world, and transformation. I hope that it might also prove to be of some use to my colleagues in other areas of Yogic studies.

Basic issues and methodology

The subject of *dehatattva* (ideas and practices relating to cosmophysiology) is of major importance in most Tantric Yogic traditions (and certainly so among the medieval Vaiṣṇava Sahajiyās). This technical term refers to a number of yogic concerns, many of them relating to issues of embodiment, freedom, and transformations of the material world. If the basic goal for Tantra is some form of final liberation from the phenomenal world and realization of an underlying unity or state of cosmic consciousness, then the condition of embodiment in the material world may be said to present the basic religious "problem" for Tantrism. Since human beings begin the Tantric quest from this condition of embodiment and materiality, it is the intention of Tantric Yogic traditions first of all to analyze this condition, second to place it in a larger cosmic context or worldview, and finally to prescribe a system of psychophysical ritual practices (*sādhana*) which will resolve the apparent problem of embodiment and materiality.

For the historian of religions, the challenge to understanding *dehatattva* is one of discerning the essential structures and processes behind the cosmophysiology, connecting them to the ritual process, and placing them in the overall sociocultural context of the tradition. In this essay I will argue that a very useful and productive way of engaging this hermeneutical challenge is to examine the various metaphors and metaphorical entailments (the implications or subtleties of metaphors) used by Tantrics to express not only a cosmophysiology (the model *of* assumed reality), but which also serve to structure an appropriate ritual process (the model *for* dealing with that reality). People typically use metaphors for quite commonplace things (such as staying in "touch" with someone via email), often not realizing that they are indeed using metaphors. But beyond this everyday use of metaphors, amply illustrated by George Lakoff and Mark Johnson in *Metaphors We Live By*,[3] the historian of religions can make use of the fact that metaphors are far more than just linguistic devices. As Lakoff and Johnson note, "metaphor is pervasive in everyday life, not just in language but in thought and action. Our ordinary conceptual system, in terms of which we both think and act, is fundamentally metaphorical in nature."[4] What this leads to is the appreciation that metaphors provide people with powerful and tangible ways of expressing abstract notions in relatively concrete terms. By analyzing the use of metaphor in *dehatattva* and *sādhana*, the historian of religions can not only "unpack" (a container/luggage metaphor) the structure and processes of Yogic and Tantric worlds, but also find ways of connecting these esoteric systems to more everyday human problems, perceptions, and tendencies. If a major goal of our scholarship is to show meaningful patterns and functions of religion, illustrating the dynamics of text and context, then a methodology employing metaphorical analysis may help us to illuminate these issues, providing a "bridge" (conduit metaphor) to those of us outside of the hermeneutical "window" (another conduit metaphor).

In his later work on metaphors and embodiment, *The Body in the Mind: The Bodily Basis of Meaning, Imagination, and Reason*,[5] Mark Johnson discusses the centrality of what he terms the "imaginative structuring of experience" in human life, which consists of "forms of imagination that grow out of bodily experience, as it contributes to our understanding and guides our reasoning."[6] The two primary types of imaginative structures identified and treated by Johnson are what he terms "image schemata" and "metaphorical projections." Both concepts are useful to the study of *dehatattva* and *sādhana*. According to Johnson, an "image schema is a recurring, dynamic pattern of our perceptual interactions and motor programs that gives coherence and structure to our experience."[7] There are many important image schemata, such as the verticality schema (and the meanings of "up-down" phenomena) and the container schema (which can "mark off" a mental space or turn an idea into a "vessel"). Since all such schemata derive from a combination of bodily experience in the world and the ways we express those experiences, it is not surprising that these notions may help us to understand the intricacies of *dehatattva* and *sādhana* in tantra and yoga.

Many image schemata may well be more or less universal to humans, but others may be more specific to certain cultures and some may even be limited to certain groups and individuals. It seems likely, for example, that advanced practitioners of yoga and other psychophysical practices would develop rather distinctive image schemata appropriate to their experiences and *sādhana*, transmitted by specific *gurus* and teaching lineages. The medieval Vaiṣṇava Sahajiyās took a range of image schemata from the context of medieval Bengal and developed them into quite distinctive patterns appropriate for their own religious and mystical uses. Such an appropriation of basic image schemata by other Tantric traditions is likely to be found as well. For example, the basic verticality schema identified by Johnson "emerges from our tendency to employ an up-down orientation in picking out meaningful structures of our experience."[8] Thus, most cultures develop a scale of values pertaining to relative verticality, so that "up is more/better" (superiority) and "down is less/worse" (inferiority). Furthermore, a variety of metaphorical projections are then used to express these schemata in terms of language, art, and other cultural forms.

This use of schemata and projection is frequently behind common expressions (such as "I'm feeling up today," or "Those people work under me"). However, when modified by an esoteric tradition like the Vaiṣṇava Sahajiyās, a basic image schema and its related metaphorical projections can take on specific and significant implications. First of all, the cosmos of yoga and tantra frequently entails an entire "inner" (*antara*), "secret" (*marma, rahasya*), and "subtle" (*sukṣma*) world-system or microcosm where "verticality" can take on complex new meanings. In fact, for most yogic traditions, there is the belief that the secondary, spiritual, or yogic "body" is *both* "within" and "above" the physical body of flesh and blood. In other words, the standard notion of three dimensions – and the basic verticality schema – undergoes important transformations, and we are really dealing with a multidimensional cosmos. Thus, it not surprising that some quite elaborate and profound metaphorical and symbolic language is used to express this complex worldview. This complexity and subtlety is found in various mystical and esoteric traditions in the history of religions, and helps to explain why mystics have often employed metaphors to express both their model *of* reality (cosmology and cosmography) and model *for* reality (ethos and ritual systems).[9] For these and other reasons, we often find quite complex elaborations of basic image schemata. For Tantrics like the medieval Vaiṣṇava Sahajiyās, elaborations of basic image schemata and metaphorical projections may be found in concepts such as a "crooked river" (*bāṅkānadī*) which "flows upwards against the current" (*srotera-ujāna*) from the human genitals into the Yogic body and higher cosmic regions, including an ascending series of four "lotus-ponds" (*padma-sarovara*), and idyllic "villages" (*grāma*) such as "The Place of Eternal Bliss" (*sadānandapur*) and "The Place of the Hidden Moon" (*guptacandrapur*). These are just a few examples of the Sahajiyā use of different metaphors, including those of container, conduit, flower, fluid, and substance.

In Johnson's analysis, metaphor is a special type of "embodied imaginative structure" related to image schemata. He regards metaphor as:

> conceived as a pervasive mode of understanding by which we project patterns from one domain of experience in order to structure another domain of a different kind. So conceived, metaphor is not merely a linguistic mode of expression; rather, it is one of the chief cognitive structures by which we are able to have coherent, ordered experiences that we can reason about and make sense of. Through metaphor, we make use of patterns that obtain in our physical experience to organize our more abstract understanding.[10]

Of interest here is not only the argument that metaphors are far more than just linguistic modes of expression, but that they work together with bodily experience and image schemata to create coherent metaphoric worlds or what Johnson terms "mappings." It is precisely this process of "mapping" that we can find in Tantric Yogic notions of *dehatattva* and *sādhana*, for this "mapping" (itself a metaphor) allows for not just analysis and manipulation of the embodied condition, but for the gradual transformation of *both* the body and the material world, resulting in final liberation – at least as experienced by the practitioner.

The basic process of extending our understanding from the concrete to the abstract (and, subsequently, from the abstract back to the concrete) makes use of bodily experience in at least two ways. Johnson summarizes the process as follows:

> First, our bodily movements and interactions in various physical domains of experience are structured (as we saw with image schemata), and that structure can be projected by metaphor onto abstract domains. Second, metaphorical understanding is not merely a matter of arbitrary fanciful projection from anything to anything with no constraints. Concrete bodily experience not only constrains the "input" to the metaphorical projections but also the nature of the projections themselves, that is, the kinds of mappings that can occur across domains.[11]

Thus, our understanding moves from a bodily experience, conditioned by the image schemata we are used to, through metaphorical projections and on "out" to the world and people around us. Although this may at first seem somewhat mechanistic or simplistic, Johnson argues that the process is more of a gestalt; in a mathematical sense, we could say that it is not a simple linear process, but rather one of multiple interconnected dimensions. It would also seem that this process has long been understood by yogins, and that the various kinds of *sādhanas* rely on these connections between bodily experience, the senses, imagination, and reality.

The historian of religions would add to Johnson's analysis the importance of the dynamic between text and context. That is, the kind of "mappings" or worldviews that result from this complex process are not just "arbitrary fanciful projections from anything to anything with no constraints," but are definitely shaped and constrained by the surrounding geographical, social, cultural, linguistic, political, and religious contexts. This fundamental viewpoint of the historian of religions has been amply demonstrated, but needs to be cited as a major factor in the process of learning and conveying relevant image schemata from one generation to the next (or from *guru* to *chela*), and also as pivotal in the transmission of appropriate metaphorical projections from those images and associated bodily experiences. So, in the case of the Vaiṣṇava Sahajiyās, the kinds of bodily experiences, image schemata, and metaphorical projections have been influenced by, for example, medieval Bengali language, culture, religion, and even geography. The world of the Vaiṣṇava Sahajiyās was one of many rivers and streams, of ponds filled with lotuses, bordered by groves and gardens, adjacent to small villages, and often having stone landing-stairs (*ghāṭ*). It was also a world influenced by the great devotional and philosophical tradition of Gauḍīya Vaiṣṇavism, various Tantric and Yogic traditions, and also Sufi forms of Islam (to mention just a few influences). So, as we examine the expressions of bodily experience and metaphoric worlds in Vaiṣṇava Sahajiyā traditions, we should always keep in the mind the surrounding context.

Studying the Vaiṣṇava Sahajiyā traditions: problems and texts

Before examining some metaphors and entailments from the medieval Vaiṣṇava Sahajiyā traditions, I would like to provide some basic background information regarding the academic study of these traditions and problems relating to their texts and authors. Having done this, we will then look into metaphoric worlds and interpretations of yoga in medieval Vaiṣṇava Sahajiyā traditions. This is not the place to present the basic beliefs and practices of the Vaiṣṇava Sahajiyās, since this has in the main already been done by scholars such as Manindramohan Bose, Shashibhusan Dasgupta, Gopinath Kaviraja, Edward C. Dimock, Jr, and Paritos Dāsa, but some general observations may be helpful for those not familiar with Vaiṣṇava Sahajiyā traditions.[12] Essentially (and greatly oversimplifying a complex process), the Vaiṣṇava Sahajiyās combined tantric yoga with Gauḍīya Vaiṣṇava bhakti to form quite distinctive systems of belief, practice, and community. Although certain aspects of the Vaiṣṇava Sahajiyās have been studied, they are far from being as well understood as the Tibetan schools of Buddhist Tantra or the Hindu Śākta and Śaiva Tantric traditions. Those who have studied the Vaiṣṇava Sahajiyās have realized that they are one of the more "unsystematic" Tantric groups which, unlike the better-known Śākta, Śaiva, or Vajrayāna traditions, can scarcely be described in terms of a definitive textual corpus. In contrast to these other Tantric traditions, we have virtually no evidence of a written commentarial tradition – so vital to our understanding of Indian, Tibetan, Chinese, and Japanese Tantra. Without such a tradition of commentaries by learned and informed disciples, we are faced with many problems in hermeneutics – complicating an already difficult task. In part, this is due to the extremely esoteric nature of the teachings and practices themselves, as well as to the secrecy imposed upon generations of followers. Additionally, the esoteric vocabulary and semantics are very much a type of "coded system" in which an apparently ordinary reference, like *rasa* ("juice") or *bhiyāna* ("candy") may refer to any number of hidden meanings – whose gist was often handed down either orally or in special commentaries attached to the core texts and word lists. For modern scholars to move beyond basic vocabulary to the analysis of metaphors is thus even more difficult.

Although scholars have long known which texts are generally considered authoritative within the Śākta, Śaiva, Vajrayāna, and other Tantric schools, the student of the Vaiṣṇava Sahajiyās is faced with the dilemma of identifying exactly which texts are considered authoritative by the tradition itself. It is difficult, if not impossible, to precisely locate most extant Vaiṣṇava Sahajiyā texts within a distinctive textual tradition. Currently, there are several hundred Sahajiyā manuscripts known to scholars, but we lack sufficient information about the texts and their authors to attribute the material beyond the most rudimentary of levels. As mentioned earlier, there is apparently no surviving written commentarial tradition to help us as in other Tantric traditions, and there may have been pressure from Muslim and British authorities, as well as higher-caste and Westernized Hindus, to impose a veil of secrecy. We can roughly date the probable composition of some texts, but establishing the immediate teachers and students of the particular author is often impossible, for most of the small manuscripts (*puṅthi*) which have survived lack either the information or the beginning and closing folia upon which such information is usually inscribed.

Having reviewed and translated numerous Vaiṣṇava Sahajiyā texts and manuscripts over the past two decades, I would argue that there are at least four distinct general types or "genres" of Vaiṣṇava Sahajiyā literature.[13] The first, most representative of the popular or folk level, is the *pada* or short lyrical poem of ten to twenty couplets, based upon the earlier (fourteenth to fifteenth century) style of Vidyāpati, the later "Caṇḍīdāsas," and the Gauḍīya Vaiṣṇava poetry of the sixteenth and seventeenth centuries.[14] The second type or "genre" of Vaiṣṇava Sahajiyā literature is longer (approx. 300–700 couplets), usually blends popular and learned traditions and materials (including occasional Sanskrit quotations), and is represented by texts such as the *Amṛtaratnāvalī*, *Ānanda-bhairava*, *Amṛtarasāvalī*, and the *Āgamasāra*.[15] A third type is represented by texts like the *Ātmatattva*: short, carefully organized, non-lyrical philosophical treatises on cosmology and liberation.[16] The fourth type which I have found is represented by the *Vivarta-vilāsa* of Ākiñcana-dāsa (*c.* 1700 CE) a lengthy text of approximately 3,000 couplets which is essentially a Vaiṣṇava Sahajiyā commentary on the renowned *Caitanya-caritamṛta* of Kṛṣṇa-dāsa Kavirāja.[17] Much to the outrage of orthodox Gauḍīya Vaiṣṇavas, the *Vivarta-vilāsa* claims that leading Vaiṣṇava figures like Caitanya and Nityānanda were secretly Sahajiyās.[18] It also presents a fairly comprehensive survey of one later Sahajiyā lineage. Until we can make a more exhaustive, systematic study of the many unstudied and unknown manuscripts, we cannot make much more than the above admittedly impressionistic comments concerning textual styles.

Many Sahajiyā texts provide us with glimpses into their *dehatattva* and *sādhana*. One that I have studied and translated, the *Amṛtaratnavali* or

The Necklace of Immortality, attributed to one Mukunda-dāsa or Mukunda-deva (*c.* 1600–1650 CE), provides perhaps the best access to medieval Vaiṣṇava Sahajiyā metaphoric worlds and their entailments for three reasons.[19] First of all, as Manindramohan Bose has shown, it is as close to an "authoritative" text as we can find in the traditions. Bose cites a passage from a very popular later (late seventeenth to early eighteenth century) work by one Gaurī Dāsa, the *Nigūḍhārtha-prakāśāvalī*, wherein the *Necklace*, along with the *Ānanda-bhairava*, *Amṛtarasāvalī*, and the *Āgamasāra* are said to be the "primary" (*āge*) Vaiṣṇava Sahajiyā books.[20] Second, it is clearly intended to be a compact yet comprehensive treatment of the intricacies of Vaiṣṇava Sahajiyā *dehatattva* and *sādhana*; basically, a Yogic text dealing with cosmophysiology and liberation. Third, it is a text which is known to scholars, having been consulted by Dimock, Bose, Gopinath Kaviraja, and Paritos Dāsa. Finally, it exists in at least two manuscript editions at the University of Calcutta, which I was able to read and compare to the printed form found in Dāsa's *Caitanyottara prathama cāriṭi Sahajiyā puṁthi*.[21]

The most likely date for the composition of the *Necklace* is early in the seventeenth century, although the two manuscripts which have been consulted date from the late eighteenth and mid-nineteenth centuries.[22] Most of the approximately 330 verses in both manuscripts are composed in a four-footed couplet or *payāra* metre, although the *tripadī* metre – a six-footed couplet – has been used in several places. There are numerous points of agreement between the two manuscripts, but they frequently diverge dramatically (and from the printed version). Both manuscripts and the printed version close with: "Śri Mukunda-dāsa narrates (*kahe*) the *Amṛtaratnāvalī*."[23]

Yoga, embodiment, and transformation in *The Necklace of Immortality*: selected metaphors and entailments

There are many metaphors in *The Necklace of Immortality* that express yogic ideas about embodiment and liberation, but in this essay only a few will be analyzed to illustrate the potential uses of this methodology. To begin with, *sādhana* itself is referred to using the metaphor of a "journey" (NI:154):

> This path of *sādhana* is difficult to traverse, it is near-yet-far;
> from a distance it seems close, from close up it seems distant.

Central to the Vaiṣṇava Sahajiyās, as well as most other Tantric and Yogic traditions, is the basic metaphor of "*sādhana* is a journey," which here is given the additional paradoxical perceptual meanings of being "near-yet-far," an image often used by the Vaiṣṇava Sahajiyās. Since a journey covers a path, and thus a surface, the entailments of this metaphor are thus:

> since "a journey defines a path"
> and "a path defines a surface"
> then "*sādhana* defines a path"
> and "*sādhana* covers a surface."

Such a seemingly basic metaphor (and its additional meanings or entailments) helps to generate not only a complicated model *of* reality, but a model *for* reality as well. Based upon this need to travel down a "path" and cover "surface," it is Mukunda's task in the *Necklace* to outline just how one finds the path, where the path leads to, and which "surfaces" must be covered before final liberation *in* Sahaja (Sahaja itself being treated as a "container" metaphor here).[24]

Yet implied in the "journey" metaphor is the image of the journeyer, the traveler and explorer who undertakes the path and surfaces. And just as the traveler must move his or her body along the path and over the surfaces, so does Vaiṣṇava Sahajiyā *sādhana* require a body – but not just the ordinary body. It is here that we encounter some fascinating metaphoric expressions in the *Necklace*; in presenting just what kind and quality of body is needed for the journey to Sahaja, Mukunda draws upon the diverse influences of Gauḍīya Vaiṣṇavism and Tantric yoga. In contrast to many South Asian traditions which hold that final liberation is best achieved "without a body" (*videha*), Vaiṣṇava Sahajiyās accept the positions generally held by Tantric yoga and Gauḍīya Vaiṣṇavism, essentially that liberation may be achieved "with a body" (*saṃdeha*), taking advantage of the embodied state.[25] That is one reason why *dehatattva*, the "principles" or "truths" of the "body," is of major importance. Far from being an obstacle to liberation, the human body (or at least some kind of "body") provides a "vehicle" for liberation (again, the "container" metaphor is being used here). This imagery also recalls the classical yogic metaphor of the chariot, horses, and driver, found in the *Upaniṣads* and later texts, in which the body is likened to a chariot which moves along the road of the sense-objects.[26]

Immediately following the couplet stating that *sādhana* is "near-yet-far," Mukunda connects *sādhana* to body knowledge and warns of the consequences for those ignorant of this (NI:155):

> You must be able to know the principles of your own body (*dehatattva*).
> Whoever does not know the body [suffers] the consequences.

Since the body must take a journey through a variety of surfaces and paths to a destination, this implies not only the importance of some kind of topological or topographical domain, but a very special kind of inner world through which this journey proceeds. To reach this inner world, there must be a powerful transformation of the material world through *sādhana*, especially using the practice of ritual sexual intercourse (*rati-sādhana*) between the male and female Sahajiyā adepts. Not surprisingly, the *Necklace* presents (in a cryptic manner) such esoteric practices and seeks to outline the contours and qualities of that inner world, a mystical place which leads to the final bliss (*ānanda*) of Sahaja itself. However, in contrast to the worldly journeys which most of us are limited to, the Vaiṣṇava Sahajiyās see the path as going not "out" into the physical world, but rather "within the body" (*deha-antara*) and "upwards against the current" (*srotera-ujāna*) to the blissful celestial regions.

The embodied journeyer must proceed along a path of many "surfaces." This engagement with "surfaces" begins with the physical bodies of man and woman, moves along the "crooked river" (*bāṅkānadī*; a type of Yogic channel) that connects the genitals to four lotus "ponds" (*sarovara*) within the divine body, and culminates in the highest eternal regions (*nitya-dhāma*). However, one must first find an experienced guide and pathfinder; and thus it is essential to have a knowledgeable and experienced Sahajiyā *guru*. Mukunda is quite specific about the need for not just one, but two, *gurus* (NI:14–16; 25–27):

> The first step is to seek refuge at the place of the *mantra-guru*.
> Ordinary birth is from the womb, [but this only] leads to old age and to hell!
>
> When you find the *guru* you will be sheltered by [the power of] the *mantra*.
> Keep the instructions of the *guru* close to your heart!
>
> With great care, the *guru* who has initiated you with the *mantra* will guide your practices.
> As long as you practice, you must follow [those] instructions!
>
> At the time one receives the *mantra*, one also gains the lineage of the *guru*.
> You must [however] perform your *sādhana* according to the instructions of the śikṣāguru.[27]
>
> Through *sādhana*, the adept will acquire the finest obtainable body.
> Even aging men and women can learn about finding the mystical Mood (*bhāva*).

> The divine body (*deva-deha*) must be born within the [physical] body.
> Through what kinds of practices may men and women learn about it?

The first master, the *mantra-guru*, imparts the powerful seed-syllables and phrases that, in association with other ritual practices, will eventually help to transform the physical body of the journeyer into the subtle interior "divine body" (*deva-deha*). However, it is necessary to follow the acquisition of the *mantra* with initiation by the "teaching" or *śikṣā-guru*, who will guide the subsequent practices of *sādhana*. Here we see the shared entailments between the "journey" metaphor and two other important metaphors, that of the "container" (as "body") and the "birth" metaphor (as source of the new "body" or "container"). An interesting expression of this metaphorical complexity is given by Ākiñcana-dāsa, associated with Mukunda's lineage, in the *Vivarta-vilāsa* (pp. 114–115) in a quite "pregnant" image:[28]

> The grace of the *guru* and the practitioners comes after the grace of mother and father.
> This tells you that there are two separate and distinct kinds of birth.
>
> One can't be born [in either manner] without uterine blood, semen, vagina, and penis.
> How can that be? Let me elaborate a bit.
>
> One's first birth is due to the mating of mother and father.
> But consider how just a little grace from the *guru* can cause a rebirth.
>
> That also involves uterine blood, semen, vagina, and penis.
> Clear your mind and listen, for I speak the essence of this!
>
> The chants to Kṛṣṇa (*harināma*) are like the uterine blood, while the seed-syllable (*mantra-bīja*) is like the semen.
> The *guru*'s tongue is like the penis, and the disciple's ear is like the vagina.
>
> So, your births should come about from these things.
> Understand that your [second] birth is due to the grace of practitioners.

This passage is obviously quite "pregnant" with meanings, but here we will only consider the implications for the metaphors of "journey," "body/container," and "birth." Since another "body" or "container" is required to traverse the path that leads from the ordinary to sacred realms, it is necessary for the *mantra-guru* (as "father") and the secret community of Sahajiyā adepts (as "mother") to serve as metaphorical "parents" of that secondary yogic body or "container." So, just as one's biological parents (according to the Bengali Hindu model of conception) provide the vital male and female fluids which generate the physical body, it is the *sādhana* learned from the *guru* and the mystical community that generate the "divine body" (*deva-deha*) of higher practices.[29] Metaphorically, the *mantras* imparted by the tongue of the *guru* (as "semen") *do* help to fashion the Yogic body, as they merge with the sounds of the communal devotional songs for Kṛṣṇa (as "blood") heard by the disciple's ear.[30] The homologies of tongue/penis and ear/vagina provide for a wealth of metaphors and entailments, revealing that basic processes of perception and communication are given powerful sexual and cosmic meanings. Another interesting point may be made, as two sonic, vibrational, and auditory phenomena (*mantra* and *hari-nāma*) are here treated as metaphors related to vital sexual fluids. If the physical bodily container results from biological parents joining these essences through penis and vagina, the metaphorical projection suggests that the divine body results from the joining of the transformed essences via ritual sexual intercourse, through obtaining a *mantra*, and by participating in communal praises for Kṛṣṇa (regarded by Sahajiyās as the cosmic masculine principle, not as a deity). Thus, this image, when examined through an analysis of its metaphors and entailments, provides us with a rather concise model for transformations of not just the body, but also the material and sonic worlds. It also shows us how medieval Vaiṣṇava Sahajiyās reinterpreted the classical Yogic notion of "yoking" or "joining" different cosmic aspects in pursuit of liberation.

Once the process of transformation has begun, according to Mukunda, there are three basic phases of the journeyer's path (NI:18): Beginner (*pravarta*), Accomplished (*sādhaka*), and Perfected (*siddha*). Corresponding to these three phases are three "stages" (*aśraya*; also "refuge" or "shelter"): *bhāva*, *rasa*, and *prema*. These three technical terms are difficult to translate into English, but here *bhava* may be glossed as an emotional or mystical "mood" or "condition," *rasa* as "aesthetic enjoyment," and *prema* as "divine love."[31] Although we cannot possibly do justice here to these pairs of triadic progressions, suffice it to say that the path is an ascending one, in terms of ontological status, ritual purity, and consciousness. Furthermore, the sequence of *bhāva*, *rasa*, and *prema* represents what we might call a "structuring of emotions," derived from the *rasa*-theory of classical Sanskrit aesthetics, but here adapted as a yogic technique. The beginner, using the sixty-four types of "external" (*vaidhi*) devotions developed by Gauḍīya Vaiṣṇavas (NI:23), begins the gradual transformation of the physical body. Such practices include singing and dancing in honor of Kṛṣṇa, and progress gradually towards adopting the role of a female character in the mythological drama of the love-play (*līlā*) between Rādhā and Kṛṣṇa.[32] This serves to establish the proper mystical "mood" (*bhāva*) which provides a foundation for later, more advanced and interior, practices.

The second and third levels of Accomplished (*sādhaka*) and Perfected (*siddha*) represent those phases of *sādhana* when the adepts begin the practice of ritual sexual intercourse (*rati-sādhana*) and advanced visualization procedures. The Beginner (*pravarta*) phase is one of the practitioner becoming familiar with what Lakoff and Johnson would term "imaginative structuring of experience," "image schemata," and "metaphorical projections" (learned via basic ritual practices and interactions with the *guru* and the Sahajiyā community or *sādhu-saṃgha*). It is a time of being socialized into the model of reality, and the start of the difficult process of *internalizing* that model (as well as of the metaphors and entailments, although they were probably not necessarily recognized as such by the practitioners).

With the second phase, the adept begins to use the metaphors to the point of occasionally losing one's self in them, as implied by the complex term *rasa*. In Sanskrit aesthetics and dramaturgy, as well as in Gauḍīya Vaiṣṇava devotionalism, *rasa* is an elevated state of religio-aesthetic appreciation, and for Mukunda it involves the critical beginning of transformation of the physical body and detachment from the outer material world. Finally, at the third phase of *siddha*, the adepts are able to experience the pure interactive flow of divine selfless love (*prema*), which, in a sense, is a perfection of the use of the metaphors. Much like the higher levels of classical *aṣṭāṅga-yoga*, such as *pratyāhāra* ("sense withdrawal"), *dhyāna* ("meditation"), and *dhāraṇā* ("concentration") can lead to the uninterrupted bliss of *samādhi* ("absorption"), the first two phases of Beginner and Accomplished can lead to the eternal bliss (*sadānanda*) of Sahaja and realization of the ultimate state of the *sahaja-mānuṣa*, the "innate being."

Underlying this transformative process is another use of the basic container metaphor, and involves what many Sahajiyās called *āropa-sādhana*, the "practice of attribution" of cosmic essence (*svarūpa*; "true form") to human embodiment (*rūpa*; "form").[33] Basically, the process requires that each Sahajiyā man try to discover, deeply within himself, the underlying cosmic male essence or "true form," called Kṛṣṇa, and for the Sahajiyā woman to realize her inner cosmic feminine essence or "true form," called Rādhā. Such a distinction separates the Vaiṣṇava Sahajiyās from the Gauḍīya Vaiṣṇavas, for this use of Kṛṣṇa and Rādhā is decidedly humanistic, not theistic. The goal is not to transcend to a heaven in order to view the god Kṛṣṇa and his consort Rādhā as they engage in erotic endeavors, but rather for an embodied man and an embodied woman to use love-making in order to attain heavenly status. But it is precisely this embodied condition of *rūpa* that allows them to realize that heavenly status and the cosmic essence of *svarūpa*. As Dimock observes in *The Place of the Hidden Moon*: "*Āropa* is the necessary and delicate process by which the Sahajiyā is taught to raise both feet from the clay."[34]

Yet this powerful transformative Yogic process, begun with the "birth" of the potential divine body upon initiation, continues with the practice of ritual sexual intercourse, called *rati-sādhana* ("practice with a desirable woman") by Mukunda, and *rāga-sādhana* ("passionate practice") by other Sahajiyās. Such practices continue the metaphorical world-creation begun by initiation and the first stage of *sādhana*, as they help to fully generate the inner divine body and reveal the path to Sahaja. But they are also terribly dangerous, and can lead to great peril. One of the many short Sahajiyā lyrical poems (*pada*) warns that: "The practice of ritual sexual intercourse (*rāga-sādhana*) is as the road for the traveler," implying that such activities are *not* the destination, but just a means to an end (and further illustrates use of the journey metaphor).[35] For the Vaiṣṇava Sahajiyās, as with most Tantrics, the sexual rituals (whether actual or visualized) are potent ways of transforming dangerous cosmic powers. The *Necklace* (e.g. NI:105) likens these dangerous powers of passion to a biting snake (*sarpa daṃśana*), which, reflecting Bengali cultural notions of snakes, can be either deadly poisonous or powerfully sacred. Those who are attracted to tantra because of the physical sexuality will fall off the path, poisoned by the senses and lust (*kāma*); but for those who follow the directions of the *gurus*, changing lust into pure love (*prema*), the results can be salvific. Mukunda (NI:115) states that: "The best kind of *sādhana* is with a desirable woman [and involves] sexual intercourse (*sambhoga*) and eroticism (*śṛngāra*). If you are successful at *sādhana* with a desirable woman, you will escape from worldly change (*vikāra*)."

The divine body (*deva-deha*) provides another body or yogic "container" which the soul of the practitioner uses for the "journey" along the path to Sahaja. In contrast to the physical bodies of the adepts, formed initially from the vital fluids of the biological parents, the divine body for Mukunda is androgynous, fashioned not only from the *mantra*-semen of the *guru*, and the *nāma*-uterine blood of the community, but also from the yogically reversed sexual fluids of the ritual partners. This is a curious metaphorical projection of both ritual practices and bodily substances in the pursuit of ultimate transformation, and versions of this are known as *ultā-sādhana* or *ujāna-sādhana* in various Tantric, Nātha, and *haṭha-yogic* traditions.[36] For the Sahajiyās, this process involves the male sexual partner not ejaculating during ritual intercourse, supposedly using his command over the non-striated muscles in the genital system to "reverse" (*ulṭā*) his semen (*rasa*) as well as the uterine fluids (*rati*) into the penis and urethra and into the Yogic channel, the "crooked river" (*bāṅkānadī*).[37] The implications for body imagery and metaphor are quite rich here, for the androgynous divine body, while initiated (literally) by the *guru* and the *sādhu-saṃgha*, is in effect self-generated by the ritual couple. The *bāṅkānadī* is said to flow inwards and "upwards against the current" (NI:180; *sroter-ujāna*), from the joined penis and vagina "into" the eternal regions (*nitya-dhāma*).

The *mantra* of the *guru* and the *hari-nāma* (sung praises) shared with the community provide the vibrational energy, if you will, of the divine body, but it is the yogically reversed sexual fluids of the ritual partners that constitute the "substance" (*vastu*) of the divine body.[38] This is interesting, for it may be seen as a way of providing the divine body, whose "birth" is commenced through mantric and devotional sounds, with a type of flesh, solidity, and substance. In fact, the term *vastu*, which in other South Asian traditions frequently means "truth" or "thing," is an important technical term not only among the medieval Vaiṣṇava Sahajiyās, but among modern-day Bāuls.[39] Mukunda uses the term no less than fifty-five times in the *Necklace*, either alone or in compounds like *sahaja-vastu* ("original substance"). *Vastu* may be glossed as an essential cosmic "stuff" or "substance," and serves somewhat as a Sahajiyā parallel to the Sāṃkhya notion of *prakṛti*, the fundamental cosmic substance. However, *vastu* is also regarded as a very special kind of yogic substance that is produced by ritual sexual intercourse, especially when the male and female sexual fluids are made to flow "upwards against the current" (*sroter-ujāna*) along the *bāṅkānadī* towards the four inner lotus ponds (*sarovara*) and Sahajiyā heavens (*nitya-dhāma*).

That Mukunda and other medieval Vaiṣṇava Sahajiyās would use a substantive term like *vastu* in their *dehatattva* is significant, for it illustrates the use of several different kinds of ontological metaphors identified by Lakoff and Johnson: entity, substance, and container metaphors. Abstractions like the experience of a "divine body" and associated states of consciousness are expressed and made more accessible through the use of such images. As Lakoff and Johnson note:

> Our experience of physical objects and substances provides a further basis for understanding – one that goes beyond mere orientation. Understanding our experiences in terms of objects and substances allows us to pick out parts of our experience and treat them as discrete entities or substances of a uniform kind. Once we can identify our experiences as entities or substances, we can refer to them, categorize them, group them, and quantify them – and, by this means, reason about them.[40]

Because of the use of such metaphors to express mystical experiences, the metaphoric world of the *Necklace* has a particular character or quality that distinguishes it from the metaphoric worlds of other Yogic and Tantric traditions, which often use different kinds of metaphors. Whereas the metaphoric world of the *Necklace* is expressed primarily through metaphors of substances and fluids, other types of Tantric and Yogic worlds, for example, those expressed using the better-known systems of *cakras* and *kuṇḍalinī-śakti*, use metaphors of energy, sound, power, and light.[41] Although this is not the place to delve into the many fascinating issues arising from such differences, it should be clear that, once a basic metaphorical world is established, certain entailments and outcomes are possible (while others are not). In other words, a cosmophysiology based primarily (though not exclusively) upon fluids and substances will probably have some dynamics or "feel" (to use a modern sensory metaphor) that vary from one based primarily upon energy, sound, and light.

Mukunda is quite clear about the importance of substance and fluid, for early in the text (NI:7–12), immediately after offering homage to notable Gauḍīya Vaiṣṇava authorities like Caitanya, Nityānanda, and the Gosvāmins, he discusses the importance of *rasa*, understood on several levels – as a religio-aesthetic experience, as a sexual substance, and even as an alchemical term (as mercury).[42] However, since the basic meaning of *rasa* is "juice" or "essence" (as from a sugar cane), this allows Mukunda to develop entailments based upon the core image of a "sweet fluid" that causes delightful sensations when "tasted." Thus, *rasa* can be the rapturous aesthetic or devotional experience of "sweet" emotions, and it can also be the essence that derives, not just from a cane, but from the penis. Furthermore, those who experience *rasa* are called *rasikas* ("aesthetes" or "tasters"), and Mukunda compares their experiences to floating along in a river (NI:8–9):

> Those devotees who are *rasikas* seek the blessed Body (*śrīrūpa*).
> Their minds are constantly bobbing about in the *rasa*.
>
> With minds submerged in *rasa*, they float along.
> *Rasa* can only be produced by keeping the company of *rasikas*.

Both meanings of *rasa* – as aesthetic experience and sexual substance – share similar entailments, for both "experience" and "semen" can "flow" like a river. This riverine entailment of the basic substance/fluid metaphor also helps to explain why the *dehatattva* of the *Necklace* consists of a system of a river and ponds, and not the more familiar *suṣumṇā-nāḍī* and *cakras* of other traditions: fluids naturally run through rivers and streams and into ponds. Recalling the earlier metaphor of *sādhana* as a journey, which defines a path and surfaces, if mystical experience is being expressed in terms of fluidic metaphors, then the later stages of the process of liberation may be expressed as passage along a river, being contained by the two banks of the river, flowing into a pond, and leaving the waters through landing-stairs (*ghāṭ*) to enter neighboring celestial villages (*grāma*). Of course, much of this also reflects the natural topology and climate of deltaic Bengal, with its innumerable streams, rivers, and bodies of water. In other words, the experiences of substances, fluids, rivers and bodies of water may have been adopted as metaphors and then projected in order to refer to, categorize, group, and quantify profound mystical and sexual experiences. (It is also possible to find parallels with Patañjali's classical notion of yoga as the suppression (*nirodha*) of the "mind waves" (*citta-vṛtti*), which may also be seen as a type of fluid metaphor.)

Concluding remarks

Although much more remains to be said about Vaiṣṇava Sahajiyā uses of metaphors and entailments to express ideas of embodiment, liberation, and transformations of the material world, I hope that this essay has demonstrated some useful new ways of approaching these important areas of inquiry. Because Mukunda makes such rich use of symbol and metaphor in the *Necklace*, I have found that such a method has helped me to better understand the extremely esoteric structures and processes presented by the text. It might prove useful for understanding *dehatattva* and *sādhana* in other Yogic and Tantric traditions as well.

Although I have long appreciated the role of symbolism in Yogic and Tantric *dehatattva*, it was not until I realized that those same familiar symbols (such as "pond" or "lotus") formed part of a larger metaphoric world that I began to appreciate the inherent dynamics and subtleties of yogic *dehatattva*. This is, of course, a highly phenomenological approach, as it seeks to describe the contours and processes of the Sahajiyā cosmos; but it is also one that emphasizes the functional aspects of the symbols that, taken together, constitute the metaphoric world of *dehatattva*. To repeat Lakoff and Johnson's observation from the beginning of this essay, "metaphor is pervasive in everyday life, not just in language but in thought and action. Our ordinary conceptual system, in terms of which we both think and act, is fundamentally metaphorical in nature."[43] I would extend this argument and say that metaphor is also fundamental to the religious imagination. Metaphors, and those all-important entailments, provide vital and dynamic ways of expressing and dealing with the abstract and mysterious dimensions of a sacred cosmos, rendering them accessible and meaningful. Metaphors, such as those of substance, fluid, entity, container, and conduit can help to structure and figuratively "flesh out" the boundaries, parameters, and dynamics of that otherwise-ineffable yogic cosmos. Seen this way, worldview and myth are thus structured by, and expressed through, symbols, metaphors, and entailments. Rituals and *sādhana* become, then, enactments of those very symbolic and metaphoric structures through the medium of the human body.

It seems to me that much of yoga and tantra involves (at least in some way) what Johnson has called the "imaginative structuring of experience." The Tantric Yogic quest for mastery over sexuality, the physical body, and the material world is certainly based upon the process of *sādhana* as an "imaginative structuring of experience" guided by the *guru*. Since two of the basic types of such "structuring" are "image schemata" (which shape and guide our perceptions and motor activities) and "metaphorical projections" (which extend bodily experiences out into the world), it is only natural that *dehatattva* and *sādhana* should make creative use of metaphor. For scholars of yoga and tantrism, this allows us to approach the problems of embodiment, liberation, and transformation of the material world in a systematic manner. With an esoteric Vaiṣṇava Sahajiyā text like the *Necklace*, I have tried to analyze not just the basic symbolism, but how the symbolism is used to create a dynamic cosmos and ritual system. "Fluids" don't just sit there; they flow – and thus need to be directed or suppressed. "Containers" don't just contain; they have contents, openings, and may serve as "conduits" to another "container." "Lotuses" are not just static floral symbols; they float on fluids, draw fluids up through their roots, send scents out into the air, attract buzzing bees, have vertical dimensions (facing "up" to heaven, but rooted "down" into the mud) as well as horizontal dimensions (with rows of colored petals, and a center). Only by taking all of these images as metaphors, and exploring their subtle entailments and implications, can the scholar of the Vaiṣṇava Sahajiyās hope to do justice to the vivid sensory worlds painted by these texts. As the interface between "body" and "cosmos," between microcosm and macrocosm, Vaiṣṇava Sahajiyā *dehatattva* represents what we might call a "sensuous cosmology." Only by *sensing* the material world, in terms of both "making sense of" and "perceiving" that world with the body, can the transformation of both be realized, and liberation attained.

For Mukunda, the path of *sādhana* is indeed quite sinuous as well as sensuous, with many shapes and surfaces to be encountered, mastered, and left behind. Although we have not had time to consider them here, he makes use of many interesting sensory and emotional metaphors as he unfolds his "sensuous cosmology." The divine body comes fully equipped, as it were (a cybernetic metaphor?), with a complete array of senses and capacities for that transformative journey along the path to Sahaja. Thanks to the *mantra-guru*, the *sādhu-saṃgha*, and the *śikṣā-guru*, the Sahajiyā adepts have a very special body that they can use for realizing the "original" cosmic state of Sahaja. And just as sensible people in the ordinary world like to dress appropriately for any given occasion, Mukunda has thoughtfully provided that divine body with its own *Necklace of Immortality*.

Notes

1 Earlier versions of this essay were presented at the Tantric Studies Seminar during the 1996 Annual Meeting of the American Academy of Religion in New Orleans and at An International Seminar on the yoga Traditions held at Loyola Marymount University in 1997. Portions of this current essay will also appear in my forthcoming essay, "The Guru's Tongue: Metaphor, Ambivalence, and Appropriation in Vaiṣṇava Sahajiyā Traditions," in *In the Flesh: Eros, Secrecy, and Power in the Tantric Traditions of India and Nepal*, ed. by Hugh B. Urban, Glen A. Hayes and Paul Ortega-Muller, Albany, NY, SUNY Press.

2 This is not the place to address the thorny issue of terminology, for scholars do not agree on just what "tantra" as a tradition includes. For a concise recent overview of this issue, see Andre Padoux, "Concerning Tantric Traditions," in Gerhard Oberhammer (ed.) *Studies in Hinduism II: Miscellanea to the Phenomenon of Tantras*, Vienna, Osterreichische Akademie der Wissenschaften, 1998, pp. 9–20. See also Douglas Renfrew Brooks, *The Secret of the Three Cities: An Introduction to Hindu Śākta Tantrism*, Chicago, University of Chicago Press, 1990, esp. pp. 46–72. Another useful overall perspective is given in the introduction to David Gordon White (ed.) *Tantra in Practice*, Princeton, Princeton University Press, 2000, pp. 3–38.

3 George Lakoff and Mark Johnson, *Metaphors We Live By*, Chicago, University of Chicago Press, 1980. See also the later work by Mark Johnson, *The Body in the Mind: The Bodily Basis of Meaning, Imagination, and Reason*, Chicago, University of Chicago Press, 1987. Other useful studies of metaphor include: George Lakoff, *Women, Fire, and Dangerous Things: What Categories Reveal about the Mind*, Chicago, University of Chicago Press, 1987; George Lakoff and Mark Turner, *More than Cool Reasoning: A Field Guide to Poetic Metaphor*, Chicago, University of Chicago Press, 1989; George Lakoff and Mark Johnson, *Philosophy in the Flesh: The Embodied Mind and its Challenge to Western Thought*, New York, Basic Books, 1999; *On Metaphor*, ed. by Sheldon Sacks, Chicago, University of Chicago Press, 1979; Paul Ricoeur, *The Rule of Metaphor: Multidisciplinary Studies of the Creation of Meaning in Language*, Toronto, University of Toronto Press, 1977. The literature of contemporary metaphor theory is quite vast, but the above should provide the reader with adequate introductions to the field.

4 Lakoff and Johnson, *Metaphors We Live By*, p. 3.

5 Johnson, op. cit.

6 Johnson, p. xiv.

7 Ibid., p. xiv.

8 Ibid., p. xiv.

9 I am using Clifford Geertz's ideas of model of and model for reality. See Clifford Geertz, *The Interpretation of Cultures*, New York, Basic Books, 1973, esp. chapter 4, "Religion as a Cultural System," and chapter 5, "Ethos, World View, and the Analysis of Sacred Symbols."

10 Johnson, *The Body in the Mind*, pp. xiv–xv.

11 Ibid., p. xv.

12 Standard scholarly works on the Vaiṣṇava Sahajiyās in English are Shashibhusan Dasgupta, *Obscure Religious Cults*, third edn, Calcutta, Firma K. L. Mukhopadhyay, 1969, esp. pp. 113–156; Manindramohan Bose, *The Post-Caitanya Sahajiā* [*sic*] *Cult of Bengal*, Calcutta, University of Calcutta, 1930, reprint edn Delhi, Gian Publishing House, 1986; and Edward C. Dimock, Jr,

The Place of the Hidden Moon: Erotic Mysticism in the Vaiṣṇava-Sahajiyā Cult of Bengal, Chicago, University of Chicago Press, 1966; reprint edn Phoenix Books, 1989. My own works include: "Shapes for the Soul: A Study of Body Symbolism in the Vaiṣṇava-Sahajiyā Tradition of Medieval Bengal," PhD dissertation, University of Chicago, 1985; "On the Concept of Vastu in the Vaiṣṇava-Sahajiyā Tradition of Medieval Bengal," in Purusottama Bilimoria and Peter Fenner (eds) *Religions and Comparative Thought: Essays in Honour of the Late Dr. Ian Kesarcodi-Watson*, Delhi, Sri Satguru Publications/Indian Books Centre, 1988, pp. 141–149; "Boating Upon the Crooked River: Cosmophysiological Soteriologies in the Vaiṣṇava Sahajiyā Tradition of Medieval Bengal," in Tony K. Stewart (ed.) *Shaping Bengali Worlds, Public and Private*, South Asia Series Occasional Paper No. 37, East Lansing, Asian Studies Center/Michigan State University, 1989, pp. 29–35; "The Vaiṣṇava Sahajiyā Traditions of Medieval Bengal," in Donald S. Lopez, Jr (ed.) *Religions of India in Practice*, Princeton, Princeton University Press, 1995, pp. 333–351; "Cosmic Substance in the Vaiṣṇava Sahajiyā Traditions of Medieval Bengal," *Journal of Vaiṣṇava Studies*, 1996–1997, vol. 5, pp. 183–196; "The Churning of Controversy: Vaiṣṇava Sahajiyā Appropriations of Gauḍīya Vaiṣṇavism," *Journal of Vaiṣṇava Studies*, 1999, vol. 8, pp. 77–90, and "*The Necklace of Immortality*: A Seventeenth-Century Vaiṣṇava Sahajiyā Text," in White, *Tantra in Practice*, pp. 308–325. Scholarly works in Bengali include: Manindra Mohan Basu (Bose), *Sahajiyā sāhitya*, Calcutta, University of Calcutta, 1932; Paritos Dāsa, *Caitanyottara prathama cāriṭi Sahajiyā puṅthi*, Calcutta, Bharati Book Stall, 1972; *Sahajiyā o Gauḍīya Vaiṣṇava dharma*, Calcutta, Firma K. L. M. Private Ltd, 1978; and Gopinath Kaviraja, *Tantrik sādhana o siddhānta*, 2 vols, Burdhwan, Bardhaman Visvavidyalaya, 1969–1975, which covers the Vaiṣṇava Sahajiyās in various places. Excellent introductions to Hindu Tantrism, as well as useful studies of specific traditions, may be found in Douglas Renfrew Brooks, *The Secret of the Three Cities: An Introduction to Hindu Śākta Tantrism*, Chicago, University of Chicago Press, 1990 and Paul Eduardo Muller-Ortega, *The Triadic Heart of Śiva: Kaula Tantricism of Abhinavagupta in the Non-Dual Shaivism of Kashmir*, Albany, State University of New York Press, 1989.

13 I would like to acknowledge my own teacher, the late Edward C. Dimock, Jr of the University of Chicago, for helping over these many years as I have studied the Vaiṣṇava Sahajiyās. I would also like to thank my colleague Tony K. Stewart of North Carolina State University for his assistance in translations and interpretations.

14 An interesting selection of *padas* can be found in Basu, *Sahajiyā sāhitya*. Several examples can be found in my contribution to Lopez, *Religions of India in Practice*, pp. 339–344

15 The Bengali versions of each of these texts may be found in Dāsa, *Caitanyottara prathama*. The *Amṛtaratnāvalī*, *Ānanda-bhairava*, and *Āgama-sāra* may also be found in Basu, *Sahajiyā sāhitya*. A selection from the *Amṛtarasāvalī* may be found in my contribution to Lopez, *Religions of India in Practice*, pp. 344–347. A selection from the *Amṛtaratnāvalī* may be found in my contribution to White, *Tantra in Practice*, pp. 308–325.

16 The Bengali text may be found in Satyendranath Basu (ed.) *Vaiṣṇava-granthāvalī*, Calcutta, Basumati Sahitya Mandir, 1342 BS [1936], pp. 151–152.

17 The *Vivarta-vilāsa* has been repeatedly issued in inexpensive paper editions. I have used the fourth edition, published in 1948 in Calcutta by Taracand Das. The best study and translation of the *Caitanya Caritāmṛta* is Edward C.

Dimock, Jr, *Caitanya Caritāmṛta of Kṛṣadāsa Kavirāja*, ed. by Tony K. Stewart, Cambridge, Dept. of Sanskrit and Indian Studies, Harvard University, 1999.

18 On the controversy between Sahajiyās and Gauḍīya Vaiṣṇavas, see my article, "The Churning of Controversy: Vaiṣṇava Sahajiyā Appropriations of Gauḍīya Vaisnavism," *Journal of Vaiṣṇava Studies*, 1999, vol. 8, pp. 77–90.

19 Selections from this text may be found in my contribution to White, *Tantra in Practice*, pp. 308–325.

20 Manindra Mohan Bose, *The Post-Chaitanya Sahajiā* [*sic*] *Cult of Bengal*, Calcutta, University of Calcutta, 1930, p. 180. The Bengali word *āge* can also mean "earliest," but the context suggests that it does in fact mean "primary."

21 Dāsa, *Sahajiyā puṁthi*, pp. 131–157.

22 The two manuscripts belong to the collection of the University of Calcutta Department of Bengali. The first one consulted, #595, is dated 1206 BS, corresponding to 1799 CE. It is written upon "country-made" paper 11.5 by 5.5 inches in size, containing folia 2–13 with twelve lines per side. The second manuscript, #6451, dates from BS 1261, approximately 1850 CE. Fortunately, it is complete in twelve folia, and is physically similar to #595. Although this version does not have couplet numbers, I have assigned them myself. Unless otherwise noted, all references to the text (using the abbreviation NI) will be from #6451, with couplet numbers added by me. It should be noted that even the late eighteenth century is comparatively old for a Bengali *puṁthi*, most having been either lost or subjected to environmental degradation like mold, ants, water, and such.

23 *amṛtaratnāvalī kahe śrīmukundadāsa*; NI:330; Dāsa, *Sahajiyā puṁthi*, p. 157.

24 On the container metaphor, see Lakoff and Johnson, *Metaphors*, pp. 29–32. The Sanskrit and Bengali word *sahaja* is derived from the prefix *saha-* ("together with") and the verb *ja-* ("to be born"). Although a popular colloquial meaning is "easy," it may also be rendered as "original, innate," "spontaneous," and even as "together-born." The basic meaning for Vaiṣṇava Sahajiyās is as a final cosmic state wherein all dualities are collapsed and a state of unity and bliss is achieved. For the term as used by earlier Buddhist Tantrics, see Per Kvaerne, "On the Concept of Sahaja in Indian Buddhist Tantric Literature," *Temenos*, 1975, vol. 11, pp. 88–135.

25 For discussions of *videha* versus *samdeha*, especially the state of "living liberation" (*jīvanmukta*), see Andrew O. Fort and Patricia Y. Mumme (eds) *Living Liberation in Hindu Thought*, Albany, SUNY Press, 1996.

26 See, for example, *Katha Upanisad* 3.3ff.

27 There are two types of gurus for Sahajiyās: the first dispenses the mantra, while the second, the *śikṣāguru*, imparts the esoteric teachings. Elsewhere, it is suggested that the best *śikṣāguru* for a male adept is a woman, from whom he may gradually learn the sexual *sādhana*. One assumes that a female adept will take a man as her respective *śikṣā-guru*. On the role of *gurus* in Sahajiyā traditions, see Dimock, *Place of the Hidden Moon*, pp. 192–200. For the Gauḍīya Vaiṣṇava notions of the types of *gurus*, see David L. Haberman, *Acting as a Way of Salvation: A Study of Rāgānugā Bhakti Sādhana*, New York, Oxford University Press, 1988, pp. 117–123. On the importance of the lineage of the *guru* in tantrism, see Paul Muller-Ortega, *The Triadic Heart of Śiva*, pp. 55–63.

28 This is a slightly modified translation from that presented in my contribution to Lopez, *Religions of India in Practice*, p. 350.

29 On the Bengali Hindu ideas regarding conception and birth, see Ronald B. Inden and Ralph W. Nicholas, *Kinship in Bengali Culture*, Chicago, University of Chicago Press, 1977, esp. pp. 35–66.

30 Use of such standard Gauḍīya Vaiṣṇava practices is regarded by Sahajiyās as an important part of beginning levels of *sādhana*, and is called "external practice" (*bāhya-sādhana*) by other Sahajiyā texts. This contrasts to later and more advanced "inner practices" (*antara-sādhana*).

31 The first two terms, *bhāva* and *rasa*, figure prominently in the traditions of Sanskrit aesthetics and dramaturgy that were modified by Gauḍīya Vaiṣṇavas and adapted by Vaiṣṇava Sahajiyās, while *prema* is the condition of pure, selfless love experienced by Rādhā for Kṛṣṇa, and regarded by Sahajiyās as, among other things, an advanced state of emotional interaction between the male and female ritual partners. A very important "code reading" of *rasa* for Mukunda is "male semen." See my doctoral dissertation, "Shapes for the Soul," pp. 50–141, for more on this issue.

32 For details regarding Gauḍīya Vaiṣṇava devotional practices, see Haberman, *Acting as a Way of Salvation*; Sushil Kumar De, *Early History of the Vaiṣṇava Faith and Movement in Bengal*, 2nd edn, Calcutta, Firma K. L. Mukhopadhyay, 1961; Dimock, *Place of the Hidden Moon*, and Dimock, *Caitanya Caritāmṛta*.

33 Curiously, the term *āropa* is not found in the *Necklace*, although the principles are quite evident. On this term, see Dimock, *Place of the Hidden Moon*, p. 164. Found elsewhere in Indian philosophy, it appears in numerous Sahajiyā texts.

34 Dimock, *Place of the Hidden Moon*, p. 164.

35 Cited ibid., p. 163.

36 See, for example, Eliade, *Yoga: Immortality and Freedom*, Princeton, Princeton University Books, 1958, pp. 270, 318. This is also treated in David Gordon White, *The Alchemical Body: Siddha Traditions in Medieval India* Chicago, University of Chicago Press, 1996.

37 Retention of the sexual fluids as a way of gaining power is well documented in South Asian religious traditions. See, for example, Dimock, *Place of the Hidden Moon*, pp. 157, 179; G. Morris Carstairs, *The Twice-Born, A Study of a Community of High-caste Hindus*, London, Hogarth Press, 1957, pp. 83–84. See also Mircea Eliade, "Spirit, Light, and Seed," and White, *Alchemical Body*.

38 See my dissertation, pp. 50–141, for a longer discussion of the comparison of Sahajiyā *vastu* with Sāṃkhya *prakṛti* as well as my "On the Concept of Vastu" and "Cosmic Substance in the Vaiṣṇava Sahajiyā Traditions of Medieval Bengal," noted above.

39 The term *vastu*, like *rasa*, is a complicated term and illustrates the problems associated with studying Sahajiyā terminology. Derived from the Sanskrit root *vas* ("to dwell, live, stop [at a place], stay . . .; to remain, abide with or in"; see Sir M. Monier-Williams, *Sanskrit-English Dictionary*, reprint edn, Oxford, Oxford University Press, 1976, p. 932, col. 2. It is often translated as "any really existing or abiding substance or essence, thing, object, article" as well as "the pith or substance of anything" (see ibid., col. 3).

40 Lakoff and Johnson, *Metaphors*, p. 25.

41 This is not to say that Mukunda does not make some use these other metaphors, especially sound and color/light, or that other traditions eschew metaphors of fluid and substance. However, Mukunda clearly emphasizes the primacy of the substance/fluid metaphors over these others. I will explore these issues further in my forthcoming book.

42 See Monier-Williams, p. 869, cols 2–3. On the Gauḍīya Vaiṣṇava and Vaiṣṇava Sahajiyā interpretations, see Dimock, *Place of the Hidden Moon*, pp. 20–24. An extensive treatment of alchemy made be found in White, *Alchemical Body*.
43 Lakoff and Johnson, *Metaphors*, p. 3.

BIBLIOGRAPHY

Primary sources

Abhidhānacintāmaṇi of Hemacandra. Edited by O. Boehtlingk and C. Rieu. Osnabrück, Biblio Verlag, 1972. Originally published, St Petersburg, 1847.

Amanaskayoga. Edited and translated by B. Singh. Delhi, Svami Kesavananda Yoga-Samsthana-Prakasana, 1987.

Amṛtaratnāvalī of Mukunda-dāsa. Edited and trans. by Paritos Dāsa, in *Caitanyottara Prathama Cāriṭi Sahajiyā Puṅthi*. Calcutta, Bharati Book Stall, 1972, 131–157.

Anyayogavyavacchedikā with the Commentary of Malliṣeṇa. *The Syādvādamañjarī. The Flowerspray of the Quodammodo Doctrine*. Translated by Frederick William Thomas. Berlin, Akademie-Verlag, 1960.

Bhagavadgītā. Edited and trans. by Franklin Edgerton. 2 vols. Cambridge, MA., Harvard University Press, 1944.

Bhagavadgītā. Translated by Sarvepalli Radhakrishnan. London, George Allen & Unwin, 1948.

Bhagavadgītā with the Commentary of Saṅkara. *Śrimad Bhagavadgītā Bhāṣya of Śrī Śaṅkarācārya*. Edited and trans. by A. G. Krishna Warrier. Madras, Ramakrishna Math, 1983.

Bhāgavata Purāṇa. Bhāgavata Purāṇa. Edited and trans. by C. L. Goswami. Gorakhpur, Gita Press, 1971.

Brahma Bindu Upaniṣad. See *Upaniṣads*, 1990, 687–690.

Brahma Upaniṣad. See *Upaniṣads*, 1990, 725–732.

Brahmasūtra Bhāṣya of Saṅkara. *Complete works of Śrī Śaṅkarācārya in the original Sanskrit, vol. 7*. Madras, Samata Books, 1981.

Bṛhadāraṇyaka Upaniṣad with the Commentaries of Śaṅkara and Ānandagiri. *Bṛhadāraṇyakopaniṣat: Ānandagirikṛtaṭīkāsaṃvalita Śāṅkarabhāṣyasametā*. Edited by Kasinatha Sastri Agashe. Poona, Ānandāśrama Press, 1982.

Bṛhadāraṇyaka Upaniṣad with the Commentaries of Sureśvara and Ānandagiri. *Bṛhadāraṇyakopaniṣadbhāṣyavārtikam Ānandagiriṭīkāsaṃvalitam*. Edited by S. Subrahmanya Śāstri. Mt Abu, Mahesanusandhana Samsthanam, 1982.

Bṛhadāraṇyaka Upaniṣad. See *Upaniṣads*, 1996, 3–94.

Caitanya Caritāmṛta. Caitanya Caritāmṛta of Kṛṣadāsa Kavirāja. Translated by Edward C. Dimock, Jr, ed. by Tony K. Stewart, Cambridge, Dept of Sanskrit and Indian Studies, Harvard University, 1999.

Chāndogya Upaniṣad with the Commentaries of Śaṅkara and Ānandagiri. *Chāndogyopaniṣat: Ānandagirikṛtaṭīkāsaṃvalita Śāṅkarabhāṣyasametā.* Edited by Kasinatha Sastri Agashe. Poona, Ānandāśrama Press, 1983.

Dīghanikāya. Edited by T. W. Rhys Davids and J. E. Carpenter. London, Pali Text Society, 1890–1911.

Dīghanikāya. Dialogues of the Buddha. Translated by T. W. Rhys Davids. London, Pali Text Society, 1899.

Gauḍapādīyakārikā of Gauḍapāda. *The Āgamaśāstra of Gauḍapāda.* Edited and trans. by Vidhushekhara Bhattacharya. Calcutta, University of Calcutta, 1943. Reprint, Delhi, Motilal Banarsidass Publishers, 1989.

Haṭhayogapradīpikā. Edited and trans. by S. Iyengar. Bombay, 1893. Revised edn *The Adyar Library Bulletin* 36, 1972.

Jaina Āgama. Gaina Sūtras. Translated by Hermann Jacobi. 2 vols. Oxford, The Clarendon Press, 1884–1895.

Jñānārṇava of Śubhacandra. Edited by H. L. Jain, K. Ch. Siddhantacharya and A. N. Upadhye. Sholapur, 1977.

Kaulajñānanirṇayaḥ with the Commentary of Prabodh Chandra. Bagchi. *Kaulajñānanirṇayaḥ and some Minor Texts of the School of Matsyendranātha.* Edited by Prabodh Chandra. Bagchi. Calcutta, Metropolitan Printing & Pub. House, 1934.

Kubjikāmatatantra. Edited and trans. by Teun Goudriaan and J. A. Schoterman, Leiden, E. J. Brill, 1988.

Maitrī Upaniṣad. See *Upaniṣads*, 1897.

Mālatī-Mādhava of Bhavabhuti. *Bhavabhuti's Mālatī-Mādhava* [with the Commentary of Jagaddhara.] Edited and trans. by M. R. Kale. Dehli, Motilal Barnarsidass, 1983.

Muṇḍaka Upaniṣad. See *Upaniṣads*, 1996, 266–277.

Naiṣkarmya Siddhi of Sureśvarācārya. *The realization of the absolute: the Naiṣkarmya Siddhi of Srī Sureśvara.* Edited and trans. by A. J. Alston. London, Shanti Sadan, 1971.

Nyāyadarśana with the Commentaries of Vātsyāyana, Uddyotakara, Vācaspatimiśra and Viśvanātha. *Nyāyadarśanam with Vātsyāyana's Bhāṣya, Uddyotakara's Vārttika, Vācaspati Miśra's Tātparyaṭīkā & Viśvanātha's Vṛtti.* Edited by Taranatha Nyaya-Tarkatirtha and Amarendramohan Tarkatirtha. New Delhi, Munshiram Manoharlal Publishers, 1985.

Pātañjala-yogasūtra-bhāṣya vivaraṇam of Śaṅkarācārya. *Pātañjala-yogasūtra-bhāṣya vivaraṇam of Śaṅkara-Bhagavatpāda.* Edited by Polakam Sri Rama Sastri and S. R. Krishnamurthi Sastri. Madras, Government Oriental Manuscript Library, 1952.

Ṛg Veda Saṃhitā. Translated by K. F. Geldner. 3 vols. Cambridge, Harvard University Press, 1951.

Rudrayāmala Tantra. Rudrayāmalam. Edited by Yogatantra Department. Benares, Sampurnanand Sanskrit Svavidyalaya, 1980.

Sādhanamālā. Edited by Benoytnosh Bhattacharyya. 2 vols. Baroda, Central Library, 1925.

Sahajiyā O Gauḍīya Vaiṣṇava Dharma, Calcutta, Firma K. L. Mukhopadhyay, 1978.

Saṃnyāsa Upaniṣads. Saṃnyāsa Upaniṣads: Hindu Scriptures on Asceticism and Renunciation. Translated by Patrick Olivelle. New York, Oxford University Press, 1992.

Sarvadarśanasaṃgraha of Sāyana Mādhava. *The Sarvadarśanasaṃgraha, or, Review of the Different Systems of Hindu Philosophy.* Translated by E. B. Cowell and A. E. Gough. London, Kegan Paul, Trench, Trübner & Co., 1904.

Sarvadarśanasaṃgraha of Sāyaṇa Mādhava. Edited by Mahamahopadhyaya Vasudev Shastri Abhyankar. Poona, Bhandarkar Oriental Research Institute, 1924. Reprint, 1978.

Sarvajñasiddhi of Haribhadrasūri. Sanskrit text along with the Hiṃsāṣṭaka, its *Svopajña Avacūri* and *Aṃdrastuti.* Edited by R. K. Saṃshtā, Rutlam, 1924.

Śatapathabrāhmaṇa. The Śatapatha-Brāhmaṇa, According to the Text of the Mādhyandina School. Translated by Julius Eggeling, Delhi, Motilal Banarsidass, 1963.

Siddhasiddhāntapaddhati. Siddha-siddhānta-paddhati and other works of the Natha yogis. Edited by Kalyani Mallik. Poona, Oriental Book House, 1954.

Śiva Purāṇa. La légende immémoriale du Dieu Shiva: Le Shiva-purāna. Translated by Tara Michaël. Paris, Gallimard, 1991.

Ślokavārttika of Kumārila Bhaṭṭa. Translated by G. Jhā. Calcutta, Asiatic Society of Bengal, 1900–1908.

Ṣoḍaśakaprakaraṇa of Haribhadrasūri. Sanskrit text together with Yaśobhadra's *vivaraṇa* and Yaśovijaya's *vyākhyā*, the *Yogadīpikā*. D.L.J.P. Fund Series, 1911.

Somasambhupaddhati. Edited by Hélène Brunner-Lachaux. Pondicherry, Institut Français d'Indologie, 1963–1998.

Śri Śāṅkaragranthāvaliḥ. Complete works of Śrī Śaṅkārācārya in the original Sanskrit. Madras, Samata Books, 1981.

Śrutisārasamuddharaṇa of Toṭakācārya. *Extracting the essence of the Śruti: The Śrutisārasamuddharaṇa of Toṭakācārya.* Edited and trans. by Michael Comans. Delhi, Motilal Banarsidass, 1996.

Svacchanda Tantra. The Svacchanda Tantram [with Commentary "Udyota" by Kshema Raja]. Edited by Kṣema Rāja. Delhi, Parimal Publications, 1985.

Taittirīya Upaniṣad with the Commentaries of Śaṅkara and Ānandagiri. *Taittirīyopaniṣat: Ānandagirikṛtaṭīkāsaṃvalita Śāṅkarabhāṣyopetā.* Poona, Ānandāśrama Press, 1977.

Tantrāloka of Abhinavagupta. *Luce delle sacre scritture.* Translated by Raniero Gnoli. Torino, Unione tipografico-editrice torinese, 1972.

Tantrāloka of Abhinavagupta with the Commentary of Jayaratha. Edited by R. C. Dwivedi and Navjivan Rastogi. 8 vols. Delhi, Motilal Banarsidass, 1987.

Tantras. Tantracūḍāmaṇi. Pīṭhanirnaya. The Śākta pīṭhas. Edited by Dineshchandra Sircar. Delhi, Motilal Banarsidass, 1973.

Tattvārtha Sūtra of Umāsvāti with the Commentaries of Pūjyapāda and Siddhasenagaṇi. *That which is = Tattvārtha Sūtra.* Translated by Nathmal Tatia. San Francisco, HarperCollins Publishers, 1994.

Tattvārthasūtra of Umāsvāti. Edited by J. L. Jain. Arah, 1920.

Tattvārthasūtra of Umāsvāti. *Eine Jaina-Dogmatik. Umāsvāti's Tattvārthādhigama Sūtra.* Edited and trans. by H. Jacobi. Leipzig, 1906.

Triṣaṣṭiśalākāpuruṣacaritra of Hemacandra. *The Lives of Sixty-three Illustrious Persons.* Translated by Helen Moore Johnson. Vol. 2. Baroda, Oriental Institute, 1931. Reprint, 1962.

Upadeśasāhasrī of Śaṅkarācārya. *Śaṅkara's Upadeśasāhasrī*. Edited and trans. by Sengaku Mayeda. Tokyo, Hokuseido Press, 1973.

Upaniṣads. Translated by Patrick Olivelle. Oxford, Oxford University Press, 1996.

Upaniṣads. *Sixty Upaniṣads of the Veda*. Translated by Paul Deussen, V. M. Bedekar and Gajanan Balkrishna Palsule. 2 vols. Delhi, Motilal Banarsidass, 1990. Originally published, Leipzig, *Sechzig Upanishads des Vedas, aus dem Sanskrit übersetzt und mit Einleitungen und Anmerkungen versehen*, 1897.

Uttarādhyayanasūtra. *The Uttarādhyayanasūtra, being the first mūlasūtra of the Śvetāmbara Jains*. Edited by Jarl Charpentier. Uppsala, Appelbergs Boktr, 1922.

Vivarta-vilāsa of Ākiñcana-dasa. Edited by Kṛṣṇa Bhaṭṭācārya. 4th edn. Calcutta, Taracand Dasa, 1948.

Yogabindu of Haribhadrasūri. *The Yogabindu of Ācārya Haribhadrasūri*. Edited and trans. by K. K. Dixit. Ahmedabad, Lalbhai Dalpatbhai Bharatiya Sanskrit Vidyamandira, 1968.

Yogadṛṣṭisamuccaya of Haribhadrasūri. *Yogadṛṣṭisamuccaya and the Yogaviṃśika of Haribhadrasūri*. Edited and trans. by K. K. Dixit. Ahmedabad, Lalbhai Dalpatbhai Bharatiya Sanskrit Vidyamandira, 1970.

Yogasārasaṃgraha of Vijñānabhikṣu. *An English Translation with Sanskrit Text of the Yogasāra-Saṃgraha of Vijñānabhikṣu*. Bombay, Tattva-Vivechaka Press, 1894.

Yogaśāstra of Hemacandra. *Yogaśāstraṃ Svopajñavṛttivibhūṣitam*. Edited by Jambūvijaya. 3 vols. Bombay, Jaina Sahitya Vikasa Maṇḍala, 1977, 1981, 1986. Translated into English by Olle Qvarnström, Cambridge, MA, Harvard University Press, 2002.

Yogaśataka of Haribhadrasūri. Edited by Puṇyavijaya. Ahmedabad, 1965.

Yogasūtra of Patañjali. *Pātañjalayogadarśana, with the Vyāsa-Bhāṣya of Vyāsa, the Tattva-Vaiśāradī of Vācaspati Miśra and the Rāja-Mārtaṇḍa of Bhoja Rāja*. Edited by Kāśīnātha Śāstrī Āgāśe. Poona, Ānandāśrama Sanskrit Series, 1904.

——. *Yogasūtra of Patañjali with the Yogasūtrabhāṣya of Vyāsa and the Tattvavaiśāradī of Vācaspatimiśra*. Poona, Ānandāśrama Sanskrit Series, 1932.

——. *Yogasūtra* of Patañjali with the Commentary of Bhojarāja. Edited by Dhuṇḍhirājaśāstri Sastri. Varanasi, Chaukhambhā Saṃskṛita Saṃsthāna, 1982.

——. *The Yoga-Sūtras of Patañjali with the Commentary of Vyāsa and the Gloss of Vācaspati Miśra*. Translated by Rāma Prasāda. Allahabad, The Panini Office, 1912. Reprint, New Delhi, Oriental Books Reprint Corporation, 1978.

——. *The Yoga-Sūtras of Patañjali*. Edited and trans. by Manilal N. Dvivedī. Madras, Theosophical Publishing House, 1930.

——. *Aphorisms of yoga, by Bhagwān Shree Patanjali; done into English from the original in Samskrit with a commentary by Shree Purohit Swāmi, and an introduction by W. B. Yeats*. London, Faber & Faber, 1938.

——. *Yoga Philosophy of Patañjali: Containing his Yoga Aphorisms with Vyasa's Commentary in Sanskrit and a Translation with Annotations Including Many Suggestions for the Practice of Yoga* by Swami Hariharananda Aranya. Rendered into English by P. N. Mukerji. Reprint. Albany, New York, State University of New York Press, 1983.

——. *The Yoga-Sūtra of Patañjali: A New Translation and Commentary*. Translated by Georg Feuerstein. Folkestone, UK, Wm. Dawson and Sons, Ltd, 1979.
——. *Yoga-Sūtras of Patañjali with the Exposition of Vyāsa: A Translation and Commentary*. Translated by Usharbudha Arya. Honesdale, PA, Himalayan International Institute, 1986.
——. *The Yogasūtras of Patañjali on Concentration of Mind*. Translated by Fernando Tola, Carmen Dragonetti and K. Dad Prithipaul. Delhi, Motilal Banarsidass, 1987.
——. *The Yoga Sūtras of Patañjali: An Analysis of the Sanskrit with Accompanying English Translation* by Christopher Chapple and Yogi Ananda Viraj (Eugene P. Kelly, Jr.) Delhi, Śri Satguru Publications, 1990.
Yogasūtravivaraṇa of Śaṅkarācārya. *The Complete Commentary by Śaṅkara on the Yoga Sūtras: a Full Translation of the Newly Discovered Text*. Translated by Trevor Leggett. London, Kegan Paul International, 1990.
Yogavārttika of Vijñānabhikṣu. *Yogavārttika of Vijñānabhikṣu: text, with English translation and critical notes, along with the text and English translation of the Pātañjala Yogasūtras and Vyāsabhāṣya*. Translated by T. S. Rukmani, 4 vols. New Delhi, Munshiram Manoharlal, 1981–1989.

Secondary sources

Asaṅga, *Mahāyāna-Sūtralamkāra, Exposé de la Doctrine du Grand Véhicule selon le Système Yogācāra*, trans. Sylvain Lévi, Paris, H. Champion, 1907.
Assayag, J. and G. Tarabout (eds) *La Possession en Asie Du Sud*, Paris, Ecole des Hautes Études en Sciences Sociales, 1999.
Bakker, Hans and Peter Bisschop, "Mokṣadharma 187 and 239–241 reconsidered," in *Asiatische Studien/Études Asiatiques*, 1999, vol. 53, pp. 459–472.
Basu (Bose), M. M., *Sahajiyā Sāhitya*, Calcutta, University of Calcutta, 1932.
Basu, S. (ed.) *Vaiṣṇava-Granthavali*, Calcutta, Basumati Sahitya Mandir, 1936.
Bedekar, V. M., "The Place of Japa in the Mokṣadharmaparvan (Mb. XII 189–193) and the Yoga-Sūtras: A Comparative Study," *Annals of the Bhandarkar Oriental Research Institute*, 1963, vol. 44, pp. 63–74.
——, "Yoga in the Mokṣadharmaparvan of the *Mahābhārata*," *Wiener Zeitschrift für die Kunde Südasiens und Archiv für indische Philosophie*, 1968–1969, vol. 12–13, pp. 43–52.
Bharati, A., *The Tantric Tradition*, New York, Samuel Weiser, 1975.
Biardeau, M., "Quelques Réflections sur L'apophatisme de Śaṅkara," *Indo-Iranian Journal*, 1959, vol. 3, pp. 81–101.
Bose, M. M., *The Post-Caitanya Sahajiā Cult of Bengal*, Calcutta, The University of Calcutta, 1930; see also Basu (Bose), M. M.
Briggs, G. W., *Gorakhnāth and the Kānphata Yogīs*, Delhi, Motilal Banarsidass, 1973. Calcutta, 1938.
Brockington, J. L., "Mysticism in the Epics," in Peter Connolly (ed.) *Perspectives on Indian Religion: Papers in Honour of Karel Werner*, Delhi, Sri Satguru, 1986, pp. 9–20.
——, "The Bhagavadgītā: Text and Context," in J. Lipner (ed.) *The Fruits of Our Desiring: An Enquiry into the Ethics of the Bhagavadgītā for Our Times*, Calgary, Bayeux, 1997, pp. 28–47.

——, *The Sanskrit Epics*, Leiden, Brill, 1998.
——, "Epic Sāṃkhya: Texts, Teachers, Terminology," *Asiatische Studien/Études Asiatiques*, 1999, vol. 53, pp. 473–490.
Bronkhorst, J., "On the Chronology of the Tattvārtha Sūtra and Some Early Commentaries," *Wiener Zeitschrift für die Kunde Südasiens und Archiv für Indische Philosophie*, 1985, vol. 29, pp. 155–184.
——, *The Two Traditions of Meditation in Ancient India*, Stuttgart, Franz Steiner Verlag Wiesbaden, 1986.
Brooks, D. R., *The Secret of the Three Cities: An Introduction to Hindu Śākta Tantrism*, Chicago, University of Chicago Press, 1990.
Brown, C. M., "Modes of Perfected Living in the *Mahābhārata* and the Purāṇas: The Different Faces of Śuka the Renouncer," in Andrew O. Fort and Patricia Y. Mumme (eds) *Living Liberation in Hindu Thought*, Albany, NY, State University of New York Press, 1996, pp. 157–183.
Brown, W. N., "Theories of Creation in the Rig Veda," *Journal of the American Oriental Society*, 1965, vol. 85, pp. 23–34.
Brunner, H., "The Place of Yoga in the Śaivāgamas," in N. R. Bhatt, Pierre-Sylvain Filliozat, Satya Pal Narang and C. P. Bhatta (eds) *Pandit N.R. Bhatt, Felicitation Volume*, Delhi, Motilal Banarsidass, 1994, pp. 436–438.
Bühler, G., *The Life of Hemacandrācārya*, trans. by Manilal Patel, Śāntiniketan, Singhī Jaina Jñānapīṭha, 1936. Originally published as *Über das Leben des Jaina-Mönches Hemacandra. Des Schülers des Devachandra aus der Vajraśākhā.* Wien, 1889.
Carpenter, D., "Language, Ritual and Society: Reflections on the Authority of the Veda in India," *Journal of the American Academy of Religion*, 1992, vol. 60, pp. 57–77.
——, "Revelation in Comparative Perspective. Lessons for Interreligious Dialogue: Bhartrhari and Bonaventure," *Journal of Ecumenical Studies*, 1992, vol. 29, pp. 175–188.
——, *Revelation, History, and the Dialogue of Religions: A Study of Bhartṛhari and Bonaventure*, Maryknoll, NY, Orbis, 1995.
Carstairs, G. M., *The Twice-Born, a Study of a Community of High-Caste Hindus*, London, Hogarth Press, 1957.
Chapple, C. K., "*Citta-Vṛtti* and Reality in the *Yoga Sūtra*," in *Sāṃkhya-Yoga: Proceedings of the IASWR Conference, 1981*, Stony Brook, NY, Institute for Advanced Studies in World Religions, 1983, pp. 103–119.
——, "Reading Patañjali without Vyāsa: A Critique of Four *Yoga Sūtra* Passages," *Journal of the American Academy of Religion*, 1994, vol. 62, pp. 85–105.
——, "Living Liberation in Sāṃkhya and Yoga," in Andrew O. Fort and Patricia Y. Mumme (eds) *Living Liberation in Hindu Thought*, Albany, NY, State University of New York Press, 1996, pp. 115–134.
——, "Haribhadra's Analysis of Pātañjala and Kula Yoga in the Yogadṛṣṭisamuccaya," in John Cort (ed.) *Open Boundaries: Jain Communities and Cultures in Indian History*, Albany, NY, State University of New York Press, 1998, pp. 15–30.
——, "The Centrality of the Real in Haribhadra's Yoga Texts," in Olle Qvarnström and N. K. Wagle (eds) *Approaches to Jaina Studies: Philosophy, Logic, Rituals and Symbols*, Toronto, University of Toronto Centre for South Asian Studies, 1999, pp. 91–100.

—— and Eugene P. Kelly, *The Yoga Sūtras of Patañjali: An Analysis of the Sanskrit with Accompanying English Translation*, Delhi, Sri Satguru Publications, 1990.

—— and M. E. Tucker (eds) *Hinduism and Ecology: The Intersection of Earth, Sky, and Water*, Cambridge, MA, distributed by Harvard University Press for the Center for the Study of World Religions, Harvard Divinity School, 2000.

Comans, M., "The Question of the Importance of Samādhi in Modern and Classical Advaita Vedānta," *Philosophy East & West*, 1993, vol. 43, pp. 19–38.

——, "Śaṅkara and the Prasaṅkhyānavāda," *Journal of Indian Philosophy*, 1996, vol. 24, pp. 49–71.

Cort, J., "Liberation and Well Being: A Study of the Śvetāmbar Mūrtipūjak Jains of North Gujarat," PhD dissertation, Harvard University, 1989.

——, "Tantra in Jainism: The Cult of Ghaṇṭākarṇ Mahāvīr, the Great Hero Bell-Ears," *Bulletin d'Études Indiennes*, 1997, vol. 15, pp. 115–133.

——, "Who is a King? Jain Narratives of Kingship in Medieval Western India," in John Cort (ed.) *Open Boundaries: Jain Communities and Cultures in Indian History*, Albany, NY, State University of New York Press, 1998, pp. 85–110.

—— (ed.) *Open Boundaries: Jain Communities and Cultures in Indian History*, Albany, NY, State University of New York Press, 1998.

Das, R. P., "Problematic Aspects of the Sexual Rituals of the Bāuls of Bengal," *Journal of the American Oriental Society*, 1992, vol. 112, pp. 388–422.

Dasa, P., *Caitanyottara Prathama Cāriṭi Sahajiyā Puṅthi*, Calcutta, Bharati Book Stall, 1972.

Dasgupta, S. B., *Obscure Religious Cults*, Calcutta, Firma K. L. Mukhopadhyay, 1969.

Dayal, H., *The Bodhisattva Doctrine in Buddhist Sanskrit Literature*, London, K. Paul Trench Trübner, 1932.

De, S. K., *Early History of the Vaisnava Faith and Movement in Bengal, from Sanskrit and Bengali Sources*, Calcutta, Firma K. L. Mukhopadhya, 1961.

Dehejia, V., *Yogini, Cult and Temples a Tantric Tradition*, New Delhi, National Museum, 1986.

Deussen, P., *Sixty Upaniṣads of the Veda*. See *Upaniṣads*.

Dimock, E. C., *The Place of the Hidden Moon; Erotic Mysticism in the Vaiṣṇavasahajiyā Cult of Bengal*, Chicago, University of Chicago Press, 1966.

Doniger, W., *Women, Androgynes, and Other Mythical Beasts*, Chicago, University of Chicago Press, 1980.

Dundas, P., *The Jains*, London, Routledge, 1992.

——, "Becoming Gautama. Mantra and History in Śvetāmbara Jainism," in John Cort (ed.) *Open Boundaries: Jain Communities and Cultures in Indian History*, Albany, NY, State University of New York Press, 1998, pp. 31–52.

——, "The Jain Monk Jinapati Sūri Gets the Better of a Nāth Yogī," in David Gordon White (ed.) *Tantra in Practice*, Princeton, NJ, Princeton University Press, 2000, pp. 231–238.

Dyczkowski, M. S. G., "Kubjikā the Erotic Goddess: Sexual Potency, Transformation and Reversal in the Heterodox Theophanies of the Kubjikā Tantras," *Indologica Taurinensia*, 1995–1996, vols 21–22, pp. 123–140.

Edgerton, F., "The Meaning of Sāṃkhya and Yoga," *American Journal of Philology*, 1924, vol. 45, pp. 1–46.

——, *The Beginnings of Indian Philosophy; Selections from the Rig Veda, Atharva Veda, Upanisads, and Mahābhārata*, London, G. Allen & Unwin, 1965.
Eliade, M., *Yoga: Immortality and Freedom*, trans. W. R. Trask, Princeton, N.J., Princeton University Press, 1969.
——, "Spirit, Light and Seed," *History of Religions*, 1971, vol. 11, pp. 1–30.
——, *Patañjali and Yoga*, trans. Charles Lam Markmann, New York, Schocken Books, 1975.
Feuerstein, G., *The Yoga-Sūtra of Patañjali: An Exercise in the Methodology of Textual Analysis*, New Delhi, Arnold-Heinemann, 1979.
——, *The Yogasūtra of Patañjali: A New Translation and Commentary*, Folkestone, Kent, Wm. Dawson and Sons Ltd, 1979.
——, *The Philosophy of Classical Yoga*, New York, St Martin's Press, 1980.
Filliozat, J., *Étude de Démonologie Indienne: Le Kumaratantra de Ravana et Les Textes Parallèles Indiens, Tibétains, Chinois, Cambodgien et Arabe*, Paris, Imprimerie Nationale, 1937.
Flood, G. D., *An Introduction to Hinduism*, Cambridge; New York, Cambridge University Press, 1996.
Forman, R. K. C., *The Innate Capacity: Mysticism, Psychology, and Philosophy*, New York, Oxford University Press, 1998.
Fort, A. O., *Jīvanmukti in Transformation: Embodied Liberation in Advaita and Neo-Vedanta*, Albany, NY, State University of New York Press, 1998.
——, "On Destroying the Mind: The Yogasūtras in Vidyāraṇya's Jīvanmukti-viveka," *Journal of Indian Philosophy*, 1999, vol. 27, pp. 377–395.
—— and P. Y. Mumme (eds) *Living Liberation in Hindu Thought*, Albany, NY, State University of New York Press, 1996.
Frauwallner, E., "Untersuchungen zum Mokṣadharma," (3 parts), *Journal of the American Oriental Society*, 1925, vol. 45, pp. 51–67; *Wiener Zeitschrift für die Kunde des Morganlandes*, 1925, vol. 32, pp. 179–296, and 1926, vol. 33, pp. 57–68.
——, *Geschichte der Indischen Philosophie*, Salzburg, O. Müller, 1953.
Fuller, C. J., *The Camphor Flame: Popular Hinduism and Society in India*, Princeton, NJ, Princeton University Press, 1992.
Fynes, R. C. C., *Hemacandra. The Lives of the Jain Elders*, Oxford; New York, Oxford University Press, 1998.
Geertz, C., *The Interpretation of Cultures: Selected Essays*, New York, Basic Books, 1973.
Gombrich, R. F., *How Buddhism Began: The Conditioned Genesis of the Early Teachings*, London; Atlantic Highlands, NJ, Athlone Press, 1996.
Gonda, J., *Medieval Religious Literature in Sanskrit*, Wiesbaden, Harrassowitz, 1977.
Gopinatha Rao, T. A., *Elements of Hindu Iconography*, New York, Paragon Book Reprint Corp., 1968. Originally published Madras, 1914.
Goudriaan, T., "Some Beliefs and Rituals Concerning Time and Death in the Kubjikāmata," in Ria Kloppenborg (ed.) *Selected Studies on Ritual in the Indian Religions*, Leiden, E. J. Brill, 1983, pp. 96–98.
Griffiths, P. J., *On Being Mindless: Buddhist Meditation and the Mind–Body Problem*, La Salle, IL, Open Court, 1986.
Grimes, R. L., *Beginnings in Ritual Studies*, Columbia, SC, University of South Carolina Press, 1995.

Haberman, D. L., *Acting as a Way of Salvation: A Study of Rāgānugā Bhakti Sādhana*, New York, Oxford University Press, 1988.
Halbfass, W., *Studies in Kumārila and Śaṅkara*, Reinbek, Inge Wezler, 1983.
——, *Tradition and Reflection: Explorations in Indian Thought*, Albany, NY, State University of New York Press, 1991.
——, *On Being and What There Is: Classical Vaiśeṣika and the History of Indian Ontology*, Albany, State University of New York Press, 1992.
—— (ed.) *Philology and Confrontation: Paul Hacker on Traditional and Modern Vedanta*, Albany, NY, State University of New York Press, 1995.
Handiqui, K. K., *Yaśastilaka and Indian Culture; or, Somadeva's Yaśastilaka and Aspects of Jainism and Indian Thought and Culture in the Tenth Century*, Sholapur, Jaina Saṃskrti Saṃrakshaka Sangha, 1949.
Hara, M., *Koten Indo No Kugyo* [*Tapas in the Mahabharata*], Tokyo, Shunjusha, 1979.
Hauer, J. W., *Die Anfänge der Yogapraxis Im Alten Indien: Eine Untersuchung über die Wurzeln der Indischen Mystik nach Ṛg Veda und Atharvaveda*, Berlin; Stuttgart, W. Kohlhammer, 1922.
——, *Der Yoga, Ein Indischer Weg zum Selbst; Kritisch-Positive Darstellung nach den Indischen Quellen*, Stuttgart, W. Kohlhammer, 1958.
Hayes, G. A., "Shapes for the Soul: A Study of Body Symbolism in the Vaiṣṇava-Sahajiyā Tradition of Medieval Bengal," PhD dissertation, University of Chicago, 1985.
——, "On the Concept of Vastu in the Vaiṣṇava-Sahajiyā Tradition of Medieval Bengal," in Ian Kesarcodi-Watson, Puruṣottama Bilimoria and Peter G. Fenner (eds) *Religions and Comparative Thought: Essays in Honour of the Late Dr. Ian Kesarcodi-Watson*, Delhi, India, Sri Satguru Publications, 1988, pp. 141–149.
——, "Boating Upon the Crooked River: Cosmophysiological Soteriologies in the Vaiṣṇava Sahajiyā Tradition of Medieval Bengal," in Tony Stewart (ed.) *Shaping Bengali Worlds, Public and Private*, East Lansing, MI, Asian Studies Center, Michigan State University, 1989, pp. 29–35.
——, "The Vaiṣṇava Sahajiyā Traditions of Medieval Bengal," in Donald S. Lopez (ed.) *Religions of India in Practice*, Princeton, NJ, Princeton University Press, 1995, pp. 333–351.
——, "Cosmic Substance in the Vaiṣṇava Sahajiyā Traditions of Medieval Bengal," *Journal of Vaiṣṇava Studies*, 1996–1997, vol. 5, pp. 183–196.
——, "The Churning of Controversy: Vaiṣṇava Sahajiyā Appropriations of Gauḍīya Vaiṣṇavism," *Journal of Vaiṣṇava Studies*, 1999, vol. 8, pp. 77–90.
——, "*The Necklace of Immortality*: A Seventeenth-Century Vaiṣṇava Sahajiyā Text," in David Gordon White (ed.) *Tantra in Practice*, Princeton, NJ, Princeton University Press, 2000, pp. 308–325.
——, "The Guru's Tongue: Metaphor, Ambivalence, and Appropriation in Vaiṣṇava Sahajiyā Traditions," in *In the Flesh: Eros, Secrecy, and Power in the Tantric Traditions of India and Nepal*, ed. by Hugh B. Urban, Glen A. Hayes and Paul Ortega-Muller, Albany, NY, SUNY Press, forthcoming.
Heilijgers-Seelen, D. M., *The System of Five Cakras in Kubjikamatatantra 14–16*, Groningen, the Netherlands, E. Forsten, 1994.
Hiltebeitel, A., *Rethinking the Mahābhārata: A Reader's Guide to the Education of the Dharma King*, Chicago, University of Chicago Press, 2001.

Hopkins, E. W., "Yoga-Technique in the Great Epic," *Journal of the American Oriental Society*, 1901, vol. 22, pp. 333–379.
Hudson, D., "The Śrīmad Bhāgavata Purāṇa in Stone: The Text as an Eighth-Century Temple and Its Implications," *Journal of Vaiṣṇava Studies*, 1995, vol. 3, pp. 137–182.
Inden, R. B. and R. W. Nicholas, *Kinship in Bengali Culture*, Chicago, University of Chicago Press, 1977.
Ingalls, D. H. H., "Śaṅkara's Arguments against the Buddhists," *Philosophy East & West*, 1954, vol. 3, pp. 291–306.
Jacob, G. A., *A Concordance to the Principal Upaniṣads and Bhagavadgītā*, Delhi, Motilal Banarsidass, 1971.
Jaini, P. S., *The Jaina Path of Purification*, Berkeley, University of California Press, 1979.
Jambūvijaya, *Yogaśāstram*. See *Yogaśāstra.*
Ježic, M., "The First Yoga Layer in the Bhagavadgītā," in J. P. Sinha (ed.) *Ludwik Sternbach Felicitation Volume*, Lucknow, Akhila Bharatiya Sanskrit Parishad, 1979, pp. 545–557.
——, "Textual Layers of the Bhagavadgītā as Traces of Indian Cultural History," in Wolfgang Morgenroth (ed.) *Sanskrit and World Culture: Proceedings of the Fourth World Sanskrit Conference*, Berlin, Akademie Verlag, 1986, pp. 628–638.
Johnson, M., *The Body in the Mind: The Bodily Basis of Meaning, Imagination, and Reason*, Chicago, University of Chicago Press, 1987.
Johnson, W. J., *Harmless Souls, Karmic Bondage and Religious Change in Early Jainism with Special Reference to Umāsvāti and Kundakunda*, Delhi, Motilal Banarsidass, 1995.
Kaelber, W. O., *Tapta Mārga: Asceticism and Initiation in Vedic India*, Albany, NY, State University of New York Press, 1989.
Kapani, L., *La Notion de Saṃskāra dans L'Inde Brahmanique et Bouddhique*, Paris, Collège de France: Dépositaire exclusif De Boccard, 1992.
Kaviraja, G., *Tantrik Sadhana O Siddhānta*, Burdhwan, Bardhaman Visvavidyalaya, 1969–1975.
Kesarcodi-Watson, I., P. S. Bilimoria and P. G. Fenner, *Religions and Comparative Thought: Essays in Honour of the Late Dr. Ian Kesarcodi-Watson*, Delhi, India, Sri Satguru Publications, 1988.
King, R., *Early Advaita Vedānta and Buddhism. The Mahāyāna Context of the Gauḍapādīya-kārikā*, Albany, NY, State University of New York Press, 1995.
Klostermaier, K. K., "Spirituality and Nature," in Krishna Sivaraman (ed.) *Hindu Spirituality: Vedas through Vedanta*, New York, Crossroad Publishing Company, 1989, pp. 319–337.
Koelman, G. M., *Pātañjala Yoga, from Related Ego to Absolute Self*, Poona, Papal Athenaeum, 1970.
Koestler, A., *The Lotus and the Robot*, New York, Macmillan, 1960.
Kvaerne, P., "On the Concept of Sahaja in Indian Buddhist Tantric Literature," *Temenos*, 1975, vol. 11, pp. 88–135.
Lakoff, G. and M. Johnson, *Metaphors We Live By*, Chicago, University of Chicago Press, 1980.
——, *Women, Fire, and Dangerous Things: What Categories Reveal about the Mind*, Chicago, University of Chicago Press, 1987.

——, *Philosophy in the Flesh: The Embodied Mind and its Challenge to Western Thought*, New York, Basic Books, 1999.
Lakoff, G. and Mark Turner, *More than Cool Reasoning: A Field Guide to Poetic Metaphor*, Chicago, University of Chicago Press, 1989.
Larson, G. J., *Classical Sāṃkhya: An Interpretation of Its History and Meaning*, Delhi, Motilal Banarsidass, 1979.
——, "An Old Problem Revisited: The Relation between Sāṃkhya, Yoga and Buddhism," *Studien zur Indologie und Iranistik*, 1989, vol. 15, pp. 129–146.
——, "Classical Yoga Philosophy and Some Issues in the Philosophy of Mind," *Religious Studies and Theology*, 1995, vols 13–14, pp. 36–51.
—— "Classical Yoga as Neo-Sāṃkhya: A Chapter in the History of Indian Philosophy," *Asiatische Studien/Études Asiatiques*, 1999, vol. 53, pp. 723–732.
—— and R. S. Bhattacharya (eds) *Sāṃkhya: A Dualist Tradition in Indian Philosophy*, Princeton, NJ, Princeton University Press, 1987.
Lopez, D. S. (ed.) *Religions of India in Practice*, Princeton, NJ, Princeton University Press, 1995.
Lorenzen, D. N., *The Kapalikas and Kalamukhas, Two Lost Saivite Sects*, New Delhi, Thomson Press, 1972.
Lubin, T., "Consecration and Ascetical Regimen: A History of Hindu Vrata, Dikṣa, Upanayana and Brahmacarya," PhD dissertation, Columbia University, 1994.
Majumdar, A. K., *Chaulukyas of Gujarat: A Survey of the History and Culture of Gujarat from the Middle of the Tenth to the End of the Thirteenth Century*, Bombay, Bharatiya Vidya Bhavan, 1956.
Malamoud, C., *Le Svādhyāya: Récitation Personnelle du Veda: Taittirīya-Āraṇyaka, Livre II*, Paris, Institut de Civilisation Indienne: Diffusion É. de Boccard, 1977.
Mallmann, M. T. d., *Les Enseignements Iconographiques de l'Agni-Purana*, Paris, Presses Universitaires de France, 1963.
Mayeda, S., *A Thousand Teachings: The Upadeśasāhasrī of Śaṅkara*, Albany, NY, State University of New York Press, 1992.
Monier-Williams, M., E. Leumann and C. Cappeller, *A Sanskrit-English Dictionary Etymologically and Philologically Arranged with Special Reference to Cognate Indo-European Languages*, Oxford, The Clarendon Press, 1899.
Müller, F. M., *The Six Systems of Indian Philosophy*, London, Longmans Green and Co., 1899.
Muller-Ortega, P. E., *The Triadic Heart of Śiva: Kaula Tantricism of Abhinavagupta in the Non-Dual Shaivism of Kashmir*, Albany, NY, State University of New York Press, 1989.
Oberhammer, G., *Strukturen Yogischer Meditation: Untersuchungen zur Spiritualität des Yoga*, Vienna, Verlag der Österreichischen Akademie der Wissenschaften, 1977.
——, *Studies in Hinduism II: Miscellanea to the Phenomenon of Tantras*, Vienna, Verlag der Osterreichischen Akademie der Wissenschaften, 1998.
O'Flaherty, W. D., *Asceticism and Eroticism in the Mythology of Śiva*, London, New York, Oxford University Press, 1973.
Olivelle, P., *Dharmasūtras: The Law Codes of Āpastamba, Gautama, Baudhāyana, and Vasiṣṭha*, Oxford; New York, Oxford University Press, 1999.

Padoux, A., "Contributions à l'Étude de Mantraśāstra. II: Le Japa," *Bulletin de l'École Française d'Extrême-Orient*, 1987, vol. 76, pp. 117–164.

——, *Vāc, the Concept of the Word in Selected Hindu Tantras*, Albany, NY, State University of New York Press, 1990.

——, "Concerning Tantric Traditions," in Gerhard Oberhammer (ed.) *Studies in Hinduism II: Miscellanea to the Phenomenon of Tantras*, Vienna, Verlag der Osterreichischen Akademie der Wissenschaften, 1998, pp. 9–20.

——, "Transe, Possession ou Absorption Mystique?" in Jackie Assayag and Gilles Tarabout (eds) *La Possession en Asie du Sud*, Paris, École des Hautes Études en Sciences Sociales, 1999, pp. 133–147.

Pal, P., *Hindu Religion and Iconology According to the Tantrasāra*, Los Angeles, Vichitra Press, 1981.

Pathak, K. B., "Kumārila's Verses Attacking the Jaina and Buddhist Notions of an Omniscient Being," *Annals of the Bhandarkar Oriental Research Institute*, 1930–1931, vol. 12, pp. 123–131.

Pensa, C., "On the Purification Concept in Indian Tradition, with Special Regard to Yoga," *East and West*, 1969, vol. 19, pp. 194–228.

Pflueger, L., "God, Consciousness, and Meditation: The Concept of Īśvara in the Yogasūtra," PhD dissertation, University of California, Santa Barbara, 1990.

——, "Discriminating the Innate Capacity: Salvation Mysticism of Classical Sāṃkhya-Yoga," in Robert K. C. Forman (ed.) *The Innate Capacity: Mysticism, Psychology, and Philosophy*, New York, Oxford University Press, 1998, pp. 45–81.

Pott, P. H., *Yoga and Yantra, Their Interrelation and Their Significance for Indian Archaeology*, The Hague, M. Nijhoff, 1966.

Potter, K. (ed.) *Advaita Vedānta up to Śaṅkara and His Pupils*, Delhi, Motilal Banarsidass, 1981.

Poussin, L., "Le Bouddhisme et le Yoga de Patañjail," *Mélanges Chinois et Bouddhiques*, 1936–1937, vol. 5, pp. 223–242.

Qvarnström, O., "Stability and Adaptability: A Jain Strategy for Survival and Growth," *Indo-Iranian Journal*, 1998, vol. 41, pp. 33–55.

——, "Haribhadra and the Beginnings of Doxography in India," in Olle Qvarnström and N. K. Wagle (eds) *Approaches to Jaina Studies: Philosophy, Logic, Rituals and Symbols*, Toronto, University of Toronto Centre for South Asian Studies, 1999, pp. 169–210.

——, "Jain Tantra: Divinatory and Meditative Practices in the 12th Century Yogaśāstra of Hemacandra," in David Gordon White (ed.) *Tantra in Practice*, Princeton, NJ, Princeton University Press, 2000, pp. 595–604.

——, *The Yogaśāstra of Hemacandra. A Twelfth Century Handbook on Śvetāmbara Jainism*, Cambridge, MA, Harvard University Press, 2002.

—— and N. K. Wagle (eds) *Approaches to Jaina Studies: Philosophy, Logic, Rituals and Symbols*, Toronto, University of Toronto Centre for South Asian Studies, 1999.

Radhakrishnan, S., *The Principal Upaniṣads*, Oxford, Oxford University Press, 1974.

Renou, L., *Vocabulaire du Rituel Védique*, Paris, C. Klincksieck, 1954.

Ricoeur, P., *The Rule of Metaphor: Multidisciplinary Studies of the Creation of Meaning in Language*, Toronto, University of Toronto Press, 1977.

Roşu, A., "Les *Marman* et les Arts Martiaux Indiens," *Journal Asiatique*, 1981, vol. 269, pp. 417–451.

Rukmani, T. S., "Tension between Vyutthāna and Nirodha in the Yoga-Sūtras," *Journal of Indian Philosophy*, 1997, vol. 25, pp. 613–628.

——, "Sāṃkhya and Yoga: Where They Do Not Speak in One Voice," *Études Asiatiques*, 1999, vol. 53, pp. 733–753.

Sacks, S. (ed.) *On Metaphor*, Chicago, University of Chicago Press, 1979.

Sanderson, A., "Meaning in Tantric Ritual," in Ann-Marie Blondeau (ed.) *Essais sur le Rituel II*, Louvain; Paris, Peeters, 1996, pp. 15–95.

Scharfstein, B.-A., *Mystical Experience*, Baltimore, Penguin Books, 1974.

Schreiner, P., "Yoga – Lebenshilfe oder Sterbetechnik?" *Umwelt & Gesundheit*, 1988, vols 3/4, pp. 12–18.

——, "What Comes First (in the *Mahābhārata*): Sāṃkhya or Yoga?" *Asiatische Studien/Études Asiatiques*, 1999, vol. 53, pp. 755–777.

Shee, M., *Tapas und Tapasvin in den Erzählenden Partien des Mahabharata*, Reinbek, Dr I. Wezler Verlag, 1986.

Shulman, D. D., *The Hungry God: Hindu Tales of Filicide and Devotion*, Chicago, University of Chicago Press, 1993.

Silburn, L., *Kuṇḍalini, Energy of the Depths*, Albany, NY, State University of New York Press, 1988.

Smith, F. M., "Nirodha and the Nirodhalakṣaṇa of Vallabhācārya," *Journal of Indian Philosophy*, 1998, vol. 26, pp. 489–551.

Snellgrove, D. L., *The Hevajra Tantra, a Critical Study*, 2 vols, London, Oxford University Press, 1959.

——, *Indo-Tibetan Buddhism*, 2 vols, Boston, Shambhala, 1987.

Stewart, T. K. (ed.) *Shaping Bengali Worlds, Public and Private*, East Lansing, MI, Asian Studies Center Michigan State University, 1989.

Strong, J., *The Legend of King Aśoka*, Princeton, NJ, Princeton University Press, 1983.

Sundaresan, V., "On Prasaṃkhyāna and Parisaṃkhyāna: Meditation in Advaita Vedānta, Yoga, and Pre-Śaṅkaran Vedānta," *The Adyar Library Bulletin*, 1998, vol. 62, pp. 51–89.

——, "What Determines Śaṅkara's Authorship? The Case of the Pañcīkaraṇa," *Philosophy East & West*, 2002, vol. 52, pp. 1–35.

Taber, J. A., *Transformative Philosophy: A Study of Śaṅkara, Fichte, and Heidegger*, Honolulu, University of Hawaii Press, 1983.

Taimni, I. K., *The Science of Yoga: a Commentary on the Yoga-Sūtras of Patañjali in the Light of Modern Thought*, Wheaton, IL, Theosophical Pub. House, 1967.

Tatia, N., *Studies in Jaina Philosophy*, Varanasi, Jain Cultural Research Society, 1951.

Thomas, E. J., *The History of Buddhist Thought*, London, Routledge and Kegan Paul, 1933.

Thrasher, A. W., *The Advaita Vedānta of Brahma-Siddhi*, Delhi, Motilal Banarsidass Publishers, 1993.

Tripathi, G. C., "The Daily Puja Ceremony," in Anncharlott Eschmann, Hermann Kulke and Gaya Charan Tripathi (eds) *The Cult of Jagannath and the Regional Tradition of Orissa*, New Delhi, Manohar, 1978, pp. 285–307.

Umesh, R. M., *Yoga, Enlightenment, and Perfection of Abhinava Vidyatheerth Mahaswamigal*, Chennai, Sri Vidyatheerth Foundation, 1999.
Varenne, J., *Yoga and the Hindu Tradition*, Chicago, University of Chicago Press, 1976.
Vetter, T., *Studien zur Lehre und Entwicklung Śaṅkaras*, Vienna, The De Nobili Research Library, 1976.
Vivekānanda, *The Complete Works of Swami Vivekānanda*, 8 vols, Calcutta, Advaita Ashrama, 1970.
Whicher, I., "Cessation and Integration in Classical Yoga," *Asian Philosophy*, 1995, vol. 5, pp. 47–58.
——, "The Final Stages of Purification in Classical Yoga," *The Adyar Library Bulletin*, 1997, vol. 61, pp. 1–44.
——, "Nirodha, Yoga Praxis and the Transformation of the Mind," *Journal of Indian Philosophy*, 1997, vol. 25, pp. 1–67.
——, "The Mind (Citta): Its Nature, Structure and Functioning in Classical Yoga," *Saṃbhāṣā*, 1997–1998, vols 18–19, pp. 35–62, 1–50.
——, *The Integrity of the Yoga Darśana: A Reconsideration of Classical Yoga*, Albany, NY, State University of New York Press, 1998.
——, "Yoga and Freedom: A Reconsideration of Patanjali's Classical Yoga," *Philosophy East & West*, 1998, vol. 48, pp. 272–322.
——, "Classical Sāṃkhya, Yoga and the Issue of Final Purification," *Études Asiatiques*, 1999, vol. 53, pp. 779–798.
White, D. G., *The Alchemical Body: Siddha Traditions in Medieval India*, Chicago, University of Chicago Press, 1996.
—— (ed.) *Tantra in Practice*, Princeton, NJ, Princeton University Press, 2000.
Wiley, K. L., "Āghatiyā Karmas: Agents of Embodiment in Jainism," PhD dissertation, University of California at Berkeley, 2000.
——, "Karmic Bondage and Kaṣāyas: A Re-Examination of 'Umāsvāti's Jainism,'" in V. P. Jain (ed.) *Proceedings of the International Seminar on Umāsvāti and His Works*, Delhi, Bhogilal Leherchand Institute of Indology, forthcoming,
Williams, R., *Jaina Yoga. A Survey of the Mediaeval Śrāvakācāras*, London, Oxford University Press, 1963.
Woodroffe, J. G., *The Serpent Power: Being the Sat-Cakra-Nirupana and Paduka-Pañcaka*, Madras India, Ganesh & Co., 1973.
Woods, J. H. (trans.), *The Yoga-System of Patañjali*, Cambridge, MA, Harvard University Press, 1914.
Zaehner, R. C., *Our Savage God*, London, Collins, 1974.

INDEX

Terms used in both roman and italic in the text are listed here in italic. Variant capitalizations/hypenations are listed under the majority usage. Terms used in both singular and plural forms are indicated here by *(s)*.

mind (*citta*) 26, 27, 34, 35, 38, 39, 42, 50 n. 109, 53, 55, 56, 64 n. 7, 74, 81 n. 9, 85, 91, 115, 130, 132, 134–6; *see also nirodha*; *vṛtti(s)*
misidentification 54–5, 57, 59
Miśra, Maṇḍana 120
models *of* and *for* reality 163, 165, 170, 174
mokṣa see liberation
Mokṣadharma 2, 13–15, 32, 33, 38
Mokṣadharmaparvan 2, 19, 22–3, 32
mokṣamārga (path to liberation) 7, 131
moral conduct 19–20
moral virtues 60
Mt Abu, Rajasthan 137
Mukunda-dāsa/deva 9, 169–70, 174–9

Nārāyaṇīya 17, 18
Nāth Sampradāya 8, 137–8
Nāth Siddhas (or Kānphaṭas) 8; relationship with Jainas 137–8
The Necklace of Immortality 9–10, 169–78
neo-Vedāntins 99–100
nine causes (*nava kāraṇāni*) 57–8
nirbīja-samādhi see samādhi, seedless
nirodha (cessation) 3–4, 5, 7, 8, 20, 26, 37, 39, 42, 52–6, 60–2, 71, 83, 85–6, 178; *cittanirodha* 7, 131, 132; *cittavṛttinirodha*, Śaṅkara on 103–9, 117, 119–21
nirvāṇa (release from karmic bondage) 37, 73, 130–1
nivṛtti (withdrawal from the world) 63, 74, 109, 118
niyama (observances) 88, 111, 116
niyama vidhi see vidhi(s)
non-activity (*ayoga(tā)*) 130–1, 133
non-acquisitive attitude (*akusīda*) 58
non-mind, state of 134, 136

Oṃ: meditation on 31–2, 33, 34–5, 40; *see also auṃ*
opposites, cultivation of 41

pañcamakāra (M-words) 153
parisaṃkhyā(na) meditation 105, 110, 119
Patañjala yoga 3, 6, 7, 38, 42, 44, 45, 51–2, 57, 58, 99; and Sāṃkhya-Yoga 4–5; role of practice in 25–45; *see also* Patañjali
Patañjali 3, 5, 6, 7, 21, 25–7, 41, 44, 51–5, 57, 61, 63, 70–2, 79, 84–9, 91–2, 132, 143–4, 178; on *abhyāsa* and *vairāgya* 35–40; on *avidyā* 55; on *dharma* 92; on *Īśvarapraṇidhāna* 34; on *kaivalya* 55; on *kriyāyoga* 45; on *saṃskāras* 40–1, 43; on *svādhyāya* 29–34; on *tapas* 28–9; *see also* Patañjala yoga; *Yoga Sūtra*
pedagogical context 57
penance *see tapas*
personal recitation *see svādhyāya*
phonemes *see* subtle body systems
pīṭhas (geographical sites) 145
plurality 75–6
postures 134–5; seated 115
power of higher awareness (*citi-śakti*) 6, 55, 93, 120
powers (*siddhis*) 8, 17 18, 21, 143, 144, 146, 155
Prajāpati 30, 31
prajñā (wisdom) 41–2, 58, 89, 111, 117
prakṛti(s) 3, 4–5, 15, 16, 36, 37, 42, 51, 53–4, 62, 89–91, 107, 118, 176; of the Lord Īśvara 112; role in *kaivalya* 56, 84; v. *puruṣa* 57, 60, 71, 73–8, 80, 82 n. 23, 62
prāṇa(s) 100, 114, 122 n. 10
praṇava see auṃ
prāṇāyāma (breath control) 20, 28–9, 31, 33, 39, 88, 93, 114–15, 116
prasarga see creation
prasava see pratiprasava
Praśna 113
Pratardana 18
pratiprasava (return to the source/ inverse evolution) 52–5, 77, 84, 91
pratyāhāra (sense withdrawal) 20–1, 33, 114–16, 174
pravṛtti (action in the world) 63, 109
prayojakam (the initiator) 91
prema (divine love) 173–4, 183 n. 31
psychology 42–4
purification 28, 34, 36, 44, 59, 62; *abhyāsa* as 39; role of *japa* 33; role of *kaivalya* 56; role of *tapas* 28–9
purificatory texts (*pāvanāni*) 32, 33
purity (*śauca*) 88, 90, 91, 111

CPSIA information can be obtained at www.ICGtesting.com
Printed in the USA
BVOW011513160512

290348BV00002B/79/P